AEROBATIC TEAMS
OF THE WORLD

Aerobatic Teams of the World

Adrian M. Balch

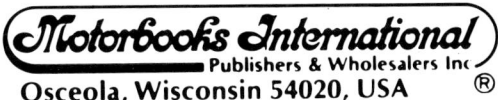
Publishers & Wholesalers Inc
Osceola, Wisconsin 54020, USA

Dedicated to all aerobatic team pilots whose skill and courage has given enjoyment to spectators the world over.

Published 1986 by Motorbooks International
Publishers & Wholesalers Inc.,
PO Box 2, 729 Prospect Avenue, Osceola, WI 54020 USA.

Copyright © Adrian M. Balch, 1986.

First published in England 1986
by Airlife Publishing Ltd.

All rights reserved. With the exception of quoting brief passages for the purposes of review no part of this publication may be reproduced without prior written permission from the publisher.

Motorbooks International is a certified trademark, registered with the United States Patent Office.

ISBN 0-87938-224-4

Printed and bound in the United Kingdom
by Livesey Ltd., Shrewsbury.

Contents

	Page		*Page*
AUSTRALIA	9	NORWAY	92
AUSTRIA	11	PAKISTAN	93
BELGIUM	13	PHILIPPINES	94
BRAZIL	16	PORTUGAL	96
CANADA	19	SOUTH AFRICA	97
CHINA — Republic of	26	SWEDEN	99
FINLAND	27	SWITZERLAND	102
FRANCE	28	UNITED STATES OF AMERICA	103
GERMANY	33	LESSER-KNOWN AEROBATIC TEAMS	135
GREAT BRITAIN	34		
GREECE	71	ARGENTINA BOLIVIA CHILE CHINA — People's Republic of CZECHOSLOVAKIA KOREA — Republic of SOVIET UNION SPAIN TURKEY	
INDIA	74		
IRAN	75		
ISRAEL	77		
ITALY	79		
JAPAN	84	APPENDIX I	137
NETHERLANDS	86	APPENDIX II	139
NEW ZEALAND	89	INDEX	145

Acknowledgements

The main source of photographs and information has kindly been supplied by the air arms themselves, *via* their London Air/Defence Attachés or direct from their Public Relations Offices. My thanks go to all that have contributed to this book, in particular the Air Attachés of the London embassies from Austria, Belgium, Brazil, Greece, Japan and Pakistan. For the RAF coverage, my thanks go to Denis Bateman of the MoD Air Historical Branch, Andrew Wilson of the Inspectorate of RAF Recruiting and Ken Hunter of the RAF Museum. My appreciation is expressed to the PR staff at British Aerospace's Warton and Kingston Divisions and to Rolls-Royce of Bristol for excellent photographs. Special thanks go to Len Lovell of the Fleet Air Arm Museum at Yeovilton, for research and photographs in the Royal Navy section. Also to Derek Morter, leader of Airwork's *Blue Herons* and Lieutenant Commander J. T. Lockwood of *The Sharks*. For information and photographs in the Canadian section, I would like to thank Colonel J. G. Boulet, CAF, Ian Geddes of Canadair Ltd., Fred Guthrie and Terry Waddington. For the Indian Section, I would like to thank Pushpindar S. Chopra.

I am indebted to famed warbird restorer, Robert Lamplough for obtaining some of the superb photographs in the Italian section. He just happened to be in the Italian MoD in Rome when my letter arrived, so translated it and brought back a huge selection of photographs and transparencies in conjunction with Captain Manca, Italian Air Force. I just wish I could have used them all.

Thanks are also due to Lieutenant-Colonel J. F. Bodére of the French Air Force Public Relations Office in Paris and Ensign A. E. F. Waling of the Royal Netherlands Air Force. I would like to express my gratitude to Paul A. Harrison in New Zealand for photographs and research and to Squadron Leader C. D. Cole of the RNZAF Public Relations Office. The Public Affairs Officers of the following teams have also been very generous with publicity material: USAF *Thunderbirds*, U.S. Navy *Blue Angels*, RAF *Red Arrows*, *Wings of Portugal*, Philippine Air Force *Blue Diamonds*, *Patrouille Suisse*, South African Air Force *Silver Falcons*.

For the Swedish section, I am extremely grateful to Gösta Norrbohm, Colonel (Retired) Royal Swedish Air Force for his research and enough photographs to make a book on Swedish aerobatic teams! I would also like to thank Lieutenant-Colonel Eric Solander, of the USAF Public Affairs Office for supplying all the photographs I asked for. Also, my thanks go to Theron Rinehart of Fairchild-Republic, Lois Lovisolo of the Grumman History Center, Robert A. Toliver and to Walter E. Williams, ex-leader of the Colorado ANG *Minute Men* for the kind loan of his precious publicity material. My appreciation is also expressed to Robert A. Carlisle of the U.S. Naval Public Affairs Office and to Harry Gann of McDonnell-Douglas, William T. Larkins and George Pennick, all of whom supplied valuable photographs. For additional research, information and useful addresses, I have to thank D. Y. Louie, Paul Coggan, Richard Hamblin and Gordon Swanborough.

Thanks go to my long-standing friend, Stephen Wolf for the use of his excellent colour slides and to my friend in Switzerland, Werner Gysin-Aegerter for the loan of negatives and transparencies. Peter R. March supplied photographs of aircraft from nearly all the teams seen in Europe since the early 1960s. They are much appreciated and if this book was twice the size, I could have used them all!

I would like to thank well-known aviation artist, Richard Ward, for many of the photographs in his archives. Finally, I am extremely grateful to David W. Menard for most generously supplying photographs and transparencies and for the loan of his precious negatives.

My interest in aerobatic teams was encouraged by Squadron Leader Ray Hanna and members of the 1966, '67 and '68 RAF *Red Arrows*, who allowed me to make frequent visits to their base at Kemble during those years and presented me with photographs on each visit. Thanks to you all.

Unfortunately, this is not the definitive work on this subject. If money was no object, I would like to have included many more photographs to show every colour scheme of every aircraft type in every team, together with colour profile drawings, but these can be found in other enthusiast publications. Although the object of an aerobatic team is to publicly demonstrate the efforts of a particular air arm, publicity material on some of the lesser-known teams was not forthcoming, in spite of much letter writing. As good quality photographs of some teams could not be obtained, pictures of other team's aircraft from the same air arm fill the pages to provide a visually-attractive book.

Foreword

by Air Commodore A. B. Blackley, CBE, AFC, BSc, RAF, Commandant, Central Flying School

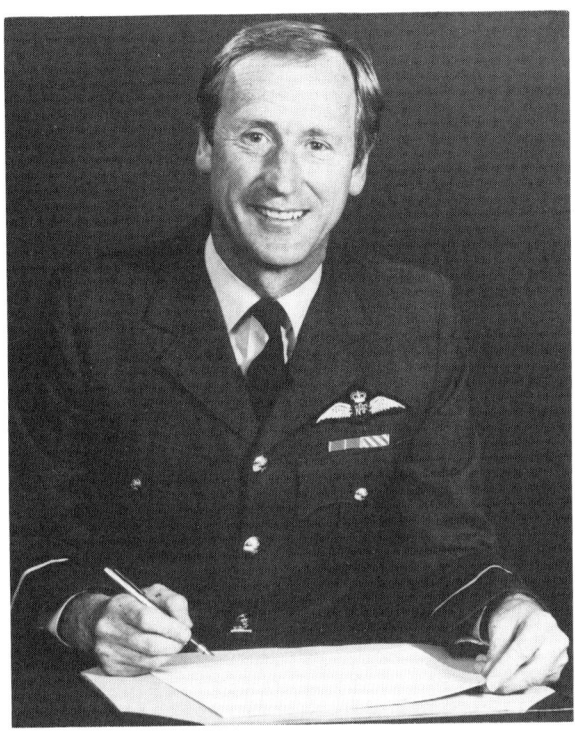

As Commandant of the Central Flying School I am responsible for the Royal Air Force Aerobatic Team, the *Red Arrows* and I am honoured to have the opportunity to say something of the airmanship required to produce the spectacle and artistry displayed by aerobatic teams today. The challenge of flying an aircraft to its limits not only accurately, but in formation with other aircraft, is a skill to be applauded and to combine this with the ability to fly sequences which are exhilarating and a delight to the eye is impressive indeed.

This book, which outlines the history of every known military aerobatic team, is an acknowledgement to those aviators who have demonstrated the quality of pilot training which has given them the ability to operate reliably to exacting standards and, most importantly, to work as a team. These skills are fundamental to effective military operations and so it should be remembered that they are the reason why we can enjoy the spectacle of military aerobatic teams today. I do hope that you enjoy the book.

RAF Scampton
September 1985

Introduction

Aerobatic teams have held a fascination for me, ever since seeing the RAF's *Black Arrows* Hunters perform at the 1958 Farnborough Air Show. An aerobatic team is usually the highlight of an air show and is good publicity for the air arm concerned. It can be fairly safe to assume that most of you have seen an aerobatic team perform and have been impressed or even thrilled by the display. Keeping the spectators interested in the display, perfect station-keeping and spectacular manoeuvres are top of the list, when judging a performance. One of the main features of the *Red Arrows* display, for example, is that they always try to have the whole or part of the team in front of the spectators at all times. Other teams often disappear for long periods while they reform, or display too high or too far away to do them justice. Smoke plays a very important part in highlighting any team's display and those without smoke soon lose the public's interest.

Colour schemes also play an important rôle in the presentation of a team. Most teams have very elaborate schemes, incorporating their country's national colours. The RAF made several experiments on the most visual colours, before red was decided as the most appealing and most visual colour for the RAF's aerobatic team, the *Red Arrows*. Several part-time teams, unfortunately, do not sport special schemes on their aircraft, as these machines cannot be spared for the team alone. Usually, they wear the standard training or fighting colours of their operational role, but may have a badge added where the same aircraft are used in the team.

With the larger air forces, aerobatic teams began making their appearance in the 1920s, after the air arms had recovered from the First World War. In general, it wasn't until after the Second World War that several countries formed a particular team to represent their air force at home and abroad, to 'show the flag'. This enabled the enthusiasts and public to compare manoeuvres and led to a competitive spirit and friendly rivalry between the teams.

Although the speed, with which manoeuvres are performed, has changed since the biplane days of the 1930s, the precision and basic display routine has remained the same. Formation is achieved by aligning one's aircraft with that of the leader. The formating pilot concentrates his reactions and energies into following the smallest movements, making his aircraft an extension of the leader's. To the basic pair, additional aircraft are added, on the wing and in line astern; and so the formation is gradually built up, each succeeding outside position requiring more concentration to accept the enlarged movements up and down the line. The leader begins a manoeuvre and flies the whole team as one. It is rather like flying a very large cumbersome aircraft through fighter-type manoeuvres. There has to be great trust and much hard work, both mentally and physically, as the formating pilots hang on.

No civilian aerobatic teams have been included in this book, for several reasons. There have been too many, varying in status, and to include them all would double the size and cost of this book. The majority of enthusiasts think generally of an aerobatic team comprising powerful military jets with garish colour schemes and trailing smoke across the sky. Due to the cost involved, most civil teams have only been equipped with light piston-engined types. As it is thought these generate less interest than the military teams, they have been omitted.

There have been several semi-official teams formed by squadrons for the odd display. These have not been included, as no special markings were carried and they are not widely publicised. It has been very difficult to decide which semi-official teams to include and which to omit, but generally if a team has performed at several public displays and represented an air arm, then it is included, if only as a brief mention in some cases.

Whether you are a photographer, spotter, historian or just have a passing interest in aerobatic teams, it is hoped you will enjoy this book which covers one of the most colourful aspects of military aviation.

Adrian M. Balch,
January 1986

AUSTRALIA
Royal Australian Air Force

One of the first opportunities for the Australian public to see the RAAF perform aerobatics was in 1934. On 10th November of that year, an impressive flying display was held at Laverton as a climax to the Melbourne Centenary celebrations, when C. W. A. Scott and T. Campbell-Black won the Mildenhall to Melbourne Air Race in the D.H. 88 Comet. At the air pageant were teams of Bulldogs and Moths. These teams performed at various displays during the 1930s, but it was not until well after the Second World War that named teams began emerging, when the RAAF became equipped with jet fighters.

In 1958, No. 77 Squadron flew a team of Meteor F.8s called *The Meteorites*. Apart from their overall natural metal finish, the team's Meteors wore medium-blue fins and wingtips. The team's name appeared on the nose on a shooting star, or rather 'meteorite', insignia. Team aircraft included A77-870, '871 and '874 of which the latter two are preserved at Wagga Wagga, N.S.W.

Sabre Teams

The RAAF had several teams flying the Commonwealth-built CA-27 Sabre, the first of which was *The Black Diamonds* formed by No.75 Squadron. This team was formed on the 40th Anniversary of the RAAF in 1961 and their Sabres were equipped to make smoke. On a basically natural metal airframe, the aircraft wore a black diamond insignia on the fuselage and black nose trim. When first formed, the tail marking comprised a 'hat and cane' insignia in a black and white diamond pattern, but was later appropriately changed to a large black diamond. *The Black Diamonds* disbanded at the end of the 1964 season, some of their aircraft being: A94-353, '352, '363, '369, '365 and '359.

Below: CA-27 Sabre Mk.31 A94-915, of RAAF aerobatic team, the *Marksmen,* from 2 OCU in 1968. Trim is black and yellow. Note the smoke-making pipe down the fuselage. (RAAF)

The second Sabre aerobatic team was formed by No. 76 Squadron at Williamtown, N.S.W. This was *The Black Panthers*, which were operational during 1962 and whose aircraft wore a large leaping black Panther insignia on the fuselage sides. Their Sabres included A94-352 and A94-359. *The Black Panthers* disbanded at the end of 1962 and No. 76 Squadron formed another Sabre team in 1963, called *The Red Diamonds*. The same aircraft were used, but the black Panther insignia was replaced by a large red diamond with lightning flash. Sabres wearing these markings included A94-942 and '947.

The RAAF were represented in the Far East by No. 3 Squadron's team of Sabres at Butterworth. Malaysia during 1966, but it wasn't until 1968 that the RAAF formed another aerobatic team in Australia. This team was called *The Marksmen* and was operated by No. 2 OCU at Williamtown, N.S.W. These Sabres had black and yellow striped fins and nose trim and like all the other Sabre teams, were equipped to make smoke. *Marksmen* Sabres included A94-365, '369 and '915, the team disbanding at the end of 1968.

Below: A7-002, one of the licence-built Aermacchi MB-326Hs of the RAAF *Telstars* aerobatic team, at Avalon, 1968. (Author's collection)

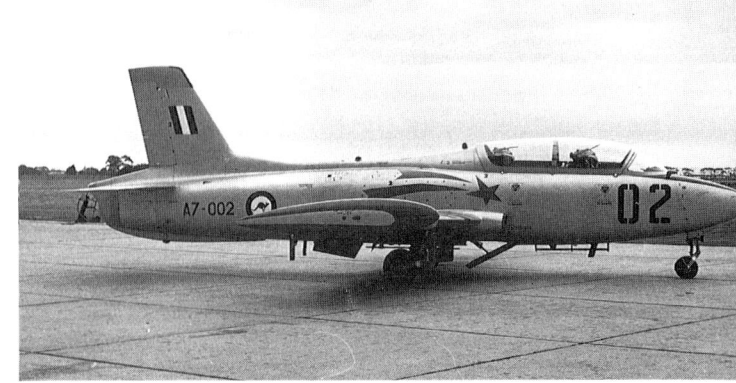

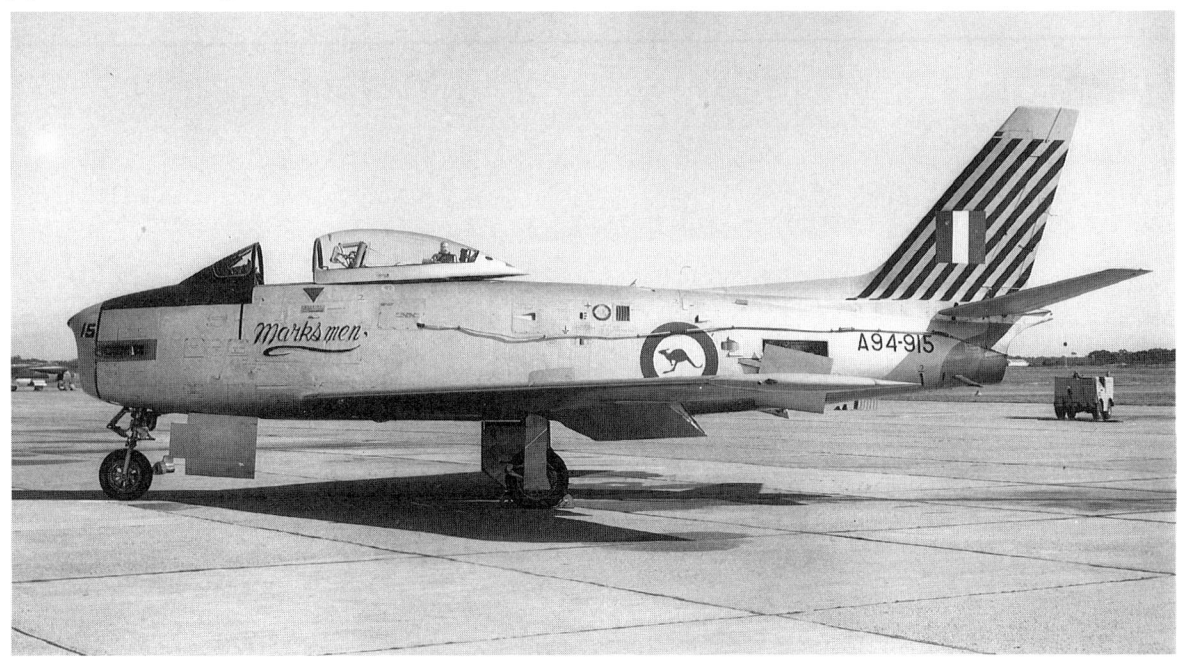

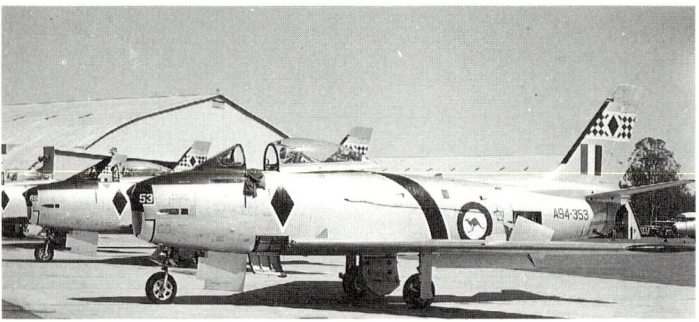

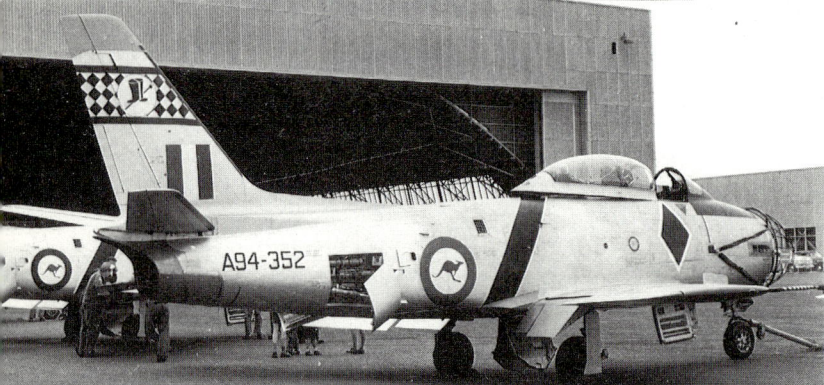

Two views of CA-27 Sabre Mk.31s from the RAAF's No. 75 Squadron *Black Diamonds* team during 1961. Note variations in tail markings. (d'E. C. Darby via R. Ward)

The Central Flying School started forming named teams in the early 1960s, one of the first being *The Telstars,* which formed at Edinburgh, N.S.W., in 1966 with Vampire T.33s. The Vampires retained their silver and dayglo training colours with the addition of a dark blue shooting star insignia on the nose. *The Telstars* re-equipped with Commonwealth-built Macchi MB-326 trainers in 1969 at East Sale, Victoria. On a silver-overall airframe, a large orange shooting star appeared down the fuselage and the wingtip tanks were orange and silver. The team's Vampires included A79-626 and '654, while two of their MB-326Hs were A7-002 and '008. *The Telstars* disbanded at the end of 1970, making way for the current RAAF aerobatic team, *The Roulettes,* which formed the following year. Flying Aermacchi MB-326Hs in the current RAAF training colours of orange and white, *The Roulettes* are now in their fifteenth year of operation as the official RAAF aerobatic team.

Apart from their standard training colours, a large red 'R' appears on the fin of each aircraft. 1981 was the Diamond Jubilee of the RAAF and the red 'R' was painted on the large pale blue diamond on the fin. MB-326Hs of *The Roulettes* team include A7-014, '026, '027, '057 and '090.

Below: A7-090 heads the line-up of Aermacchi MB-326Hs of the RAAF, CFS *Roulettes* team, at Williamtown, February 1981. (Author's collection)

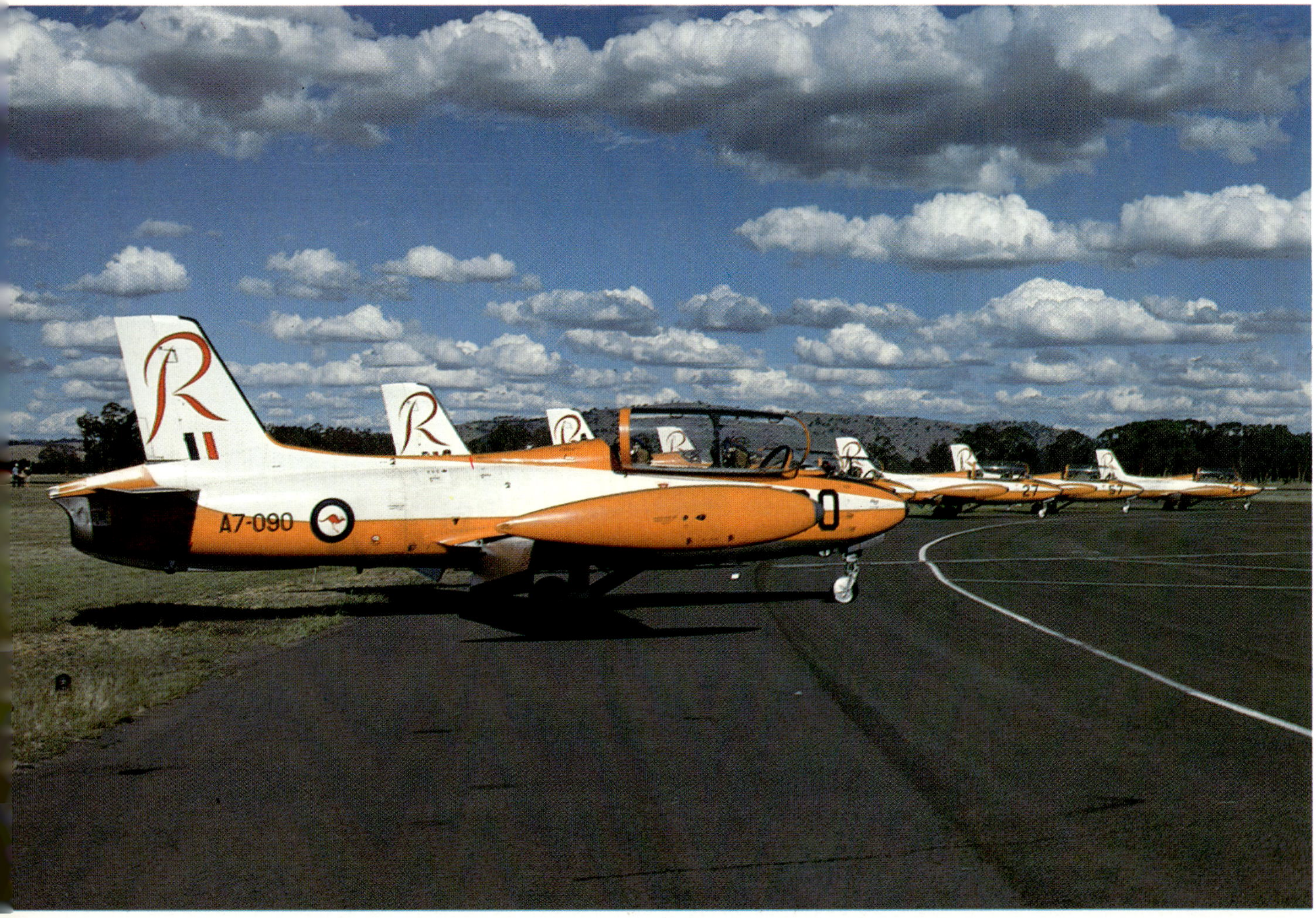

AUSTRIA
Austrian Air Force

1966-68 and 1975-76: "The Silver Birds", Graz/Thalerhof, then Zeltweg

The Silver Birds were the first named Austrian Air Force aerobatic team, formed in 1966 at Graz/Thalerhof with four Fouga CM-170 Magisters. The team was un-named until 1967 and has been led by OStv Dietmar Schönherr throughout its career. The team's Fouga Magisters were silver with dayglo orange extremities, one of their machines having the code, '4D-YK'. *The Silver Birds* performed mainly in Austria and disbanded at the end of 1968.

Below: The orange/black/yellow nose flash identifies these Austrian Air Force SAAB 105s as being the *Silver Birds* team in 1976. (Austrian Air Force)

In 1972, the SAAB 105 ÖE began to replace the Fouga Magister in Austrian Air Force service and in 1975, Dietmar Schönherr reformed *The Silver Birds* at Zeltweg with 4 SAAB 105 ÖEs. This team was most notable for its displays during the International Air Tattoo at Greenham Common, England in July 1976. The team flew their last display in September 1976, then disbanded once again, leaving *KARO AS* to represent the Austrian Air Force at displays throughout Europe. The SAAB 105 ÖE aircraft of *The Silver Birds* were natural metal overall, with dayglo red extremities and blue letter codes on their fins. Special team markings were applied in the form of red, yellow and black zig-zag nose markings. Neither the Fouga Magisters nor the SAAB 105s, in these teams, were equipped to make smoke.

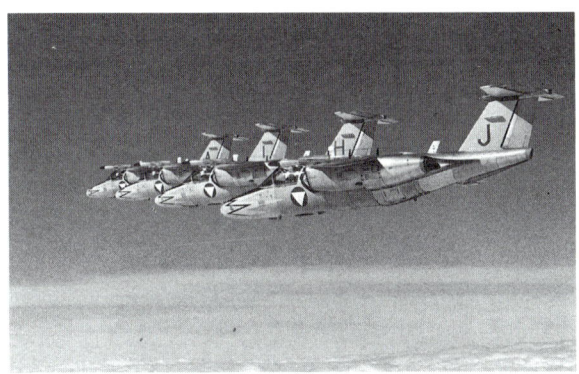

Below: SAAB 105 ÖEs of the Austrian Air Force aerobatic team *Karo AS*. (Austrian Air Force)

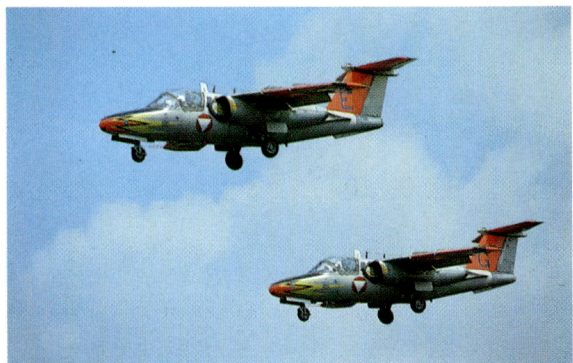

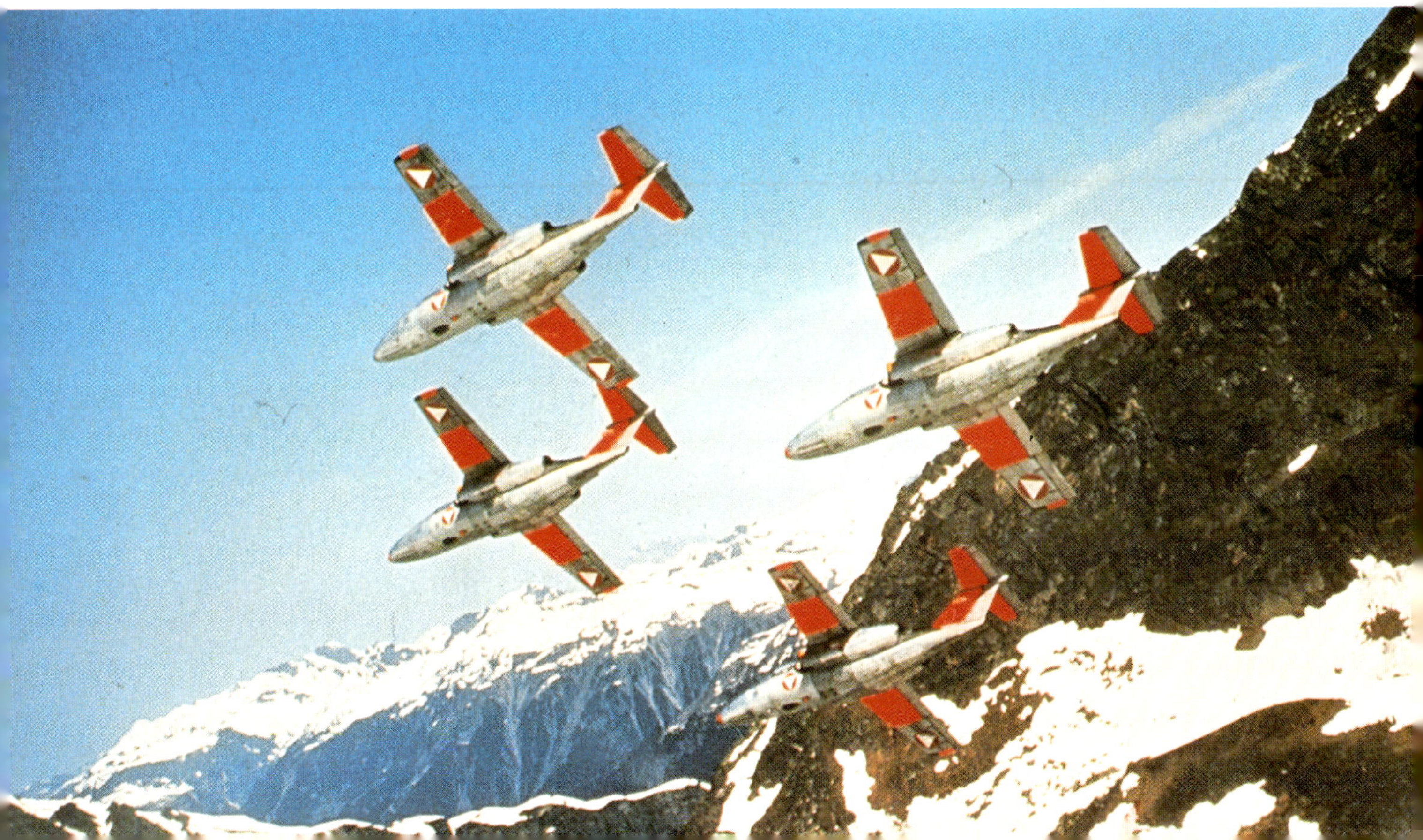

Above: SAAB 105 ÖEs of the Austrian Air Force *Silver Birds*, arriving at Greenham Common on 29 July, 1976 for the International Air Tattoo. (Adrian M. Balch)

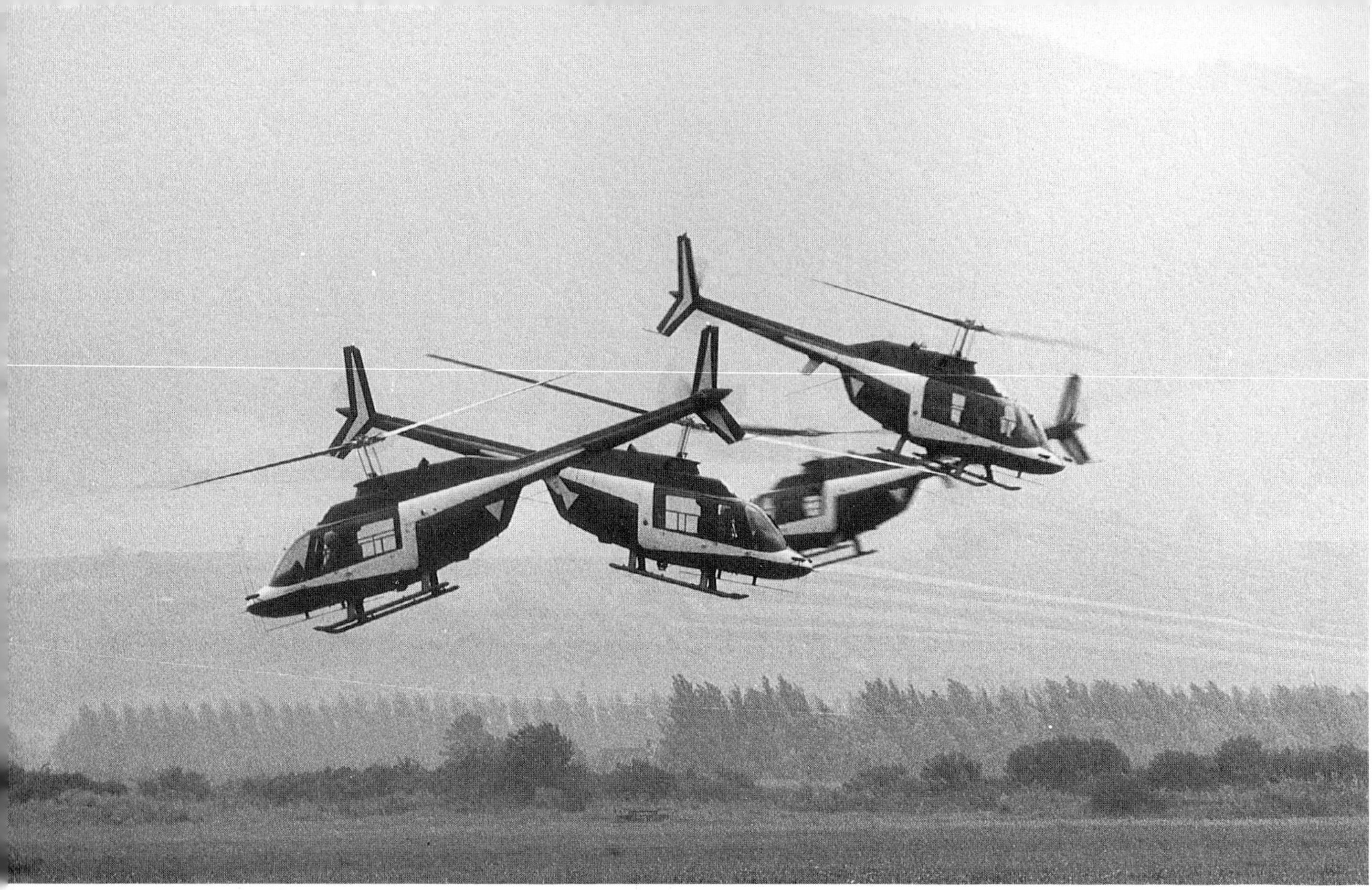

Above: A dramatic crossing by four JetRangers of the Austrian Army *Kleeblaat* team during 1975. Colour scheme is olive green and white. (Austrian Air Force).

1975-84: KARO AS ("Ace of Diamonds"), Graz/Thalerhof

This Austrian Air Force aerobatic team, flew four SAAB 105 ÖE trainers from 2 Staffel/jabogeschwader, based at Graz/Thalerhof. *KARO AS* flew their first public display on 12th July 1975, the aircraft retaining their standard training colours of silver and dayglo red. The team was originally led by Olt. Müller, who has taken the team to displays throughout Europe. At the 1977 International Air Tattoo at Greenham Common, *KARO AS* gained second place in the aerobatic competition and were awarded the Shell Trophy. They have made regular appearances in England ever since, until disbanding at the end of 1984.

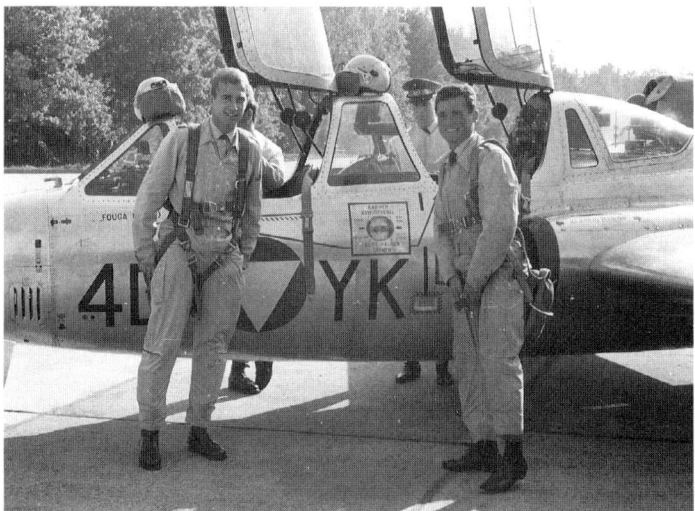

Above: Ostv Dietmar Schonherr (left) leader of the Austrian Air Force *Silver Birds* team with Fouga Magister '4D-YK' in 1966. (Austrian Air Force).

Below: Silver Birds Fouga Magister from the Austrian Air Force in 1966. (W. Hesz via R. Ward).

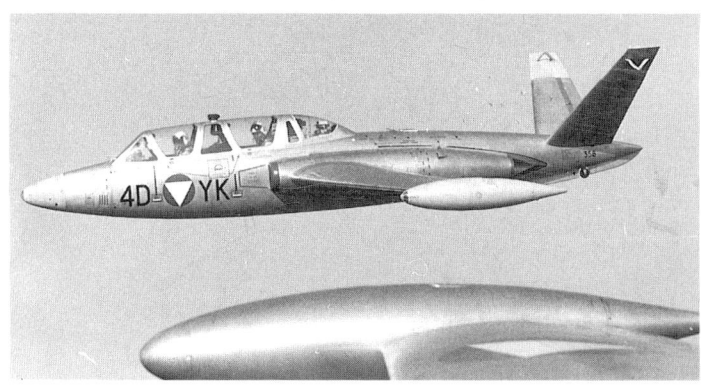

1975-to date: "Kleeblatt" helicopter team, Tulln/Langenlebn

This is a team of 4 Bell 206 JetRanger helicopters, which formed in 1975 during the 20th anniversary of the Austrian Army. Founded by Lt. Wolf-Dietrich Tesar, the *Kleeblatt* team presents a ballet of rhythmic movements to musical background, showing the mobility of helicopters in close formation. The frequent changes of velocity, and the fact that the rotor blades cause air turbulence, make flying in close formation more difficult, and demand the maximum of concentration and ability from the pilots. Based at Langenlebn in Lower Austria, *Kleeblatt* only performs at a few displays in Austria each year. Although they have been invited to perform in neighbouring countries, service reasons have prevented them from doing so. The team's JetRangers are painted olive green overall with a large white lightning flash down the fuselage. Codes of machines in team markings include: 3C-JF, 'G, 'H, 'J and 'L.

BELGIUM
Belgian Air Force

1957-76: "Les Diables Rouges/Rode Duivels/Red Devils", Brustem.

Before the Second World War, Belgium had several aerobatic teams flying Avro, Fiat, Firefly, Fox, Gladiator and Morane types. The aerobatic tradition was perpetuated in 1951 when 1 Wing at Bevekom formed the *Acrobobs* with their newly received Meteor F.8s under Captain Bobby Bladt. A year later, the team won an aerobatic competition at Lyon beating entries from several other countries.

In 1957, Major Bladt was at Chievres where five of the new Hunter F.6 aircraft of 7 Wing formed the *Rode Duivels/Diables Rouges* (Red Devils). The number of all-red Hunters increased to sixteen in 1959, but the ever-increasing danger of a multiple collision reduced this, in the next year, to just four plus one solo performer. The team's final performance with Hunters was on 4th October 1963, following which the team dissolved and 7 Wing disbanded. The team's red Hunters appeared at many European displays, including England, where they performed at RAF Gaydon's Battle of Britain Displays during September 1962 and 1963 and at Abingdon in 1963. The *Red Devil's* Hunters were red overall, with a white cheat line down the fuselage and the Belgian national colours of black/yellow/red under the wings, tailplanes and on the fin. A yellow rampant lion appeared on a black shield on the nose. For a short while, the tops of the wingtips were painted in small red/white checks. The team's Hunters 1957-63 included: IF-49, IF-62, IF-69, IF-70, IF-77, IF-78, IF-80, IF-93, IF-125, IF-131, IF-132, IF-137, IF-141 and IF-144.

In 1965, six red-painted Magisters of the VVS took over the role as the Belgian Air Force Aerobatic Team and thus the *Red Devils* were resurrected under the leadership of Major De Waelheyns. The first display was on 27th June 1965 and the team continued in this form until the end of the 1976 season, when the team disbanded once again, as funds could not be spared to keep the team going. In 1979, the Magister was withdrawn from service and replaced by the Alphajet. It is hoped the team will reform with this type, but no official

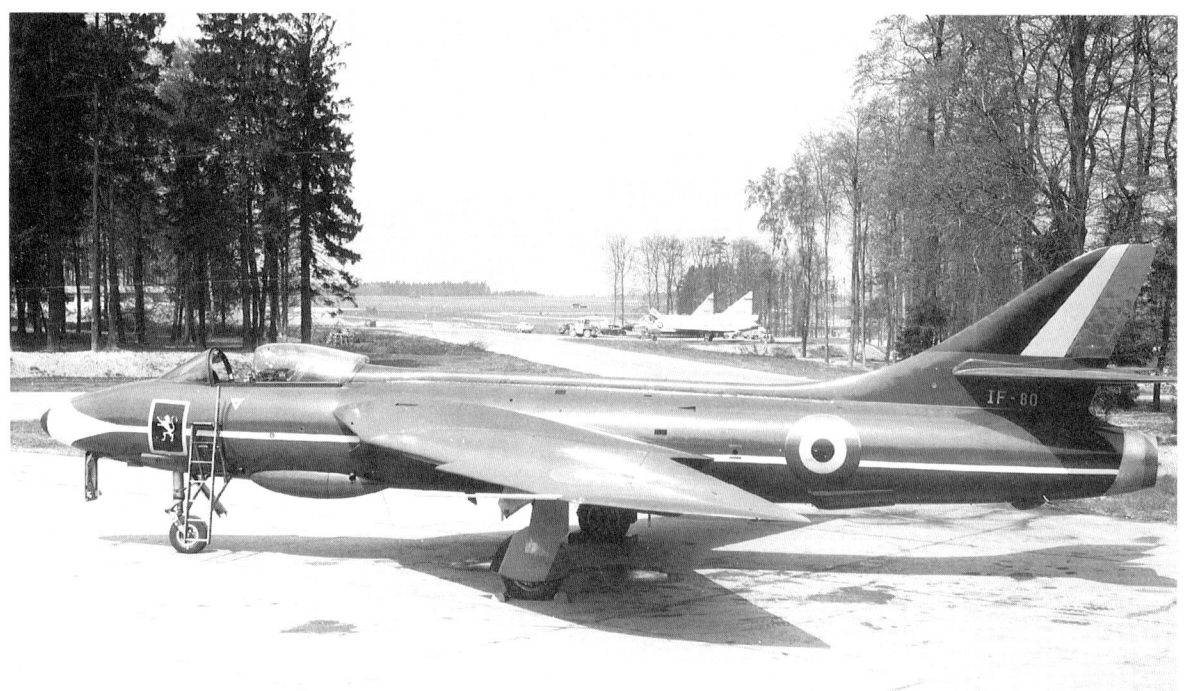

Above: Hunter F.6, IF-80, of the Belgian Air Force *Les Diables Rouges* team at Hahn, Germany in May 1960. (David W. Menard)

Fouga Magister, 275/MT18, of the Belgian Air Force *Les Diables Rouges* at the Paris Air Show in 1970. (Werner Gysin)

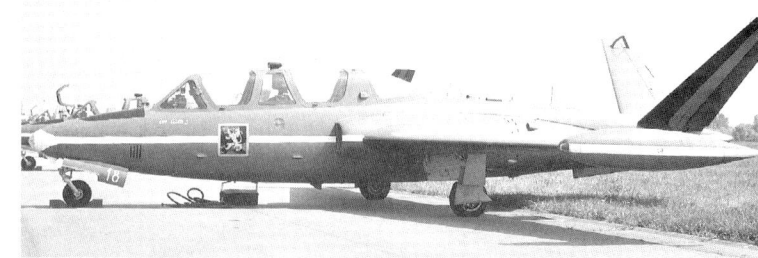

announcement has been made to this effect. The following Fouga Magisters operated in the team's colours 1965-76: 204/MT48, 259/MT2, 262/MT5, 263/MT6, 264/MT7, 265/MT8, 266/MT9, 268/MT11, 269/MT12, 272/MT15, 274/MT17, 275/MT18, 277/MT20, 278/MT21, 279/MT22, 280/MT23, 283/MT27, 284/MT27 (2nd), 288/MT31, 289/MT32, 290/MT33 and 314/MT39.

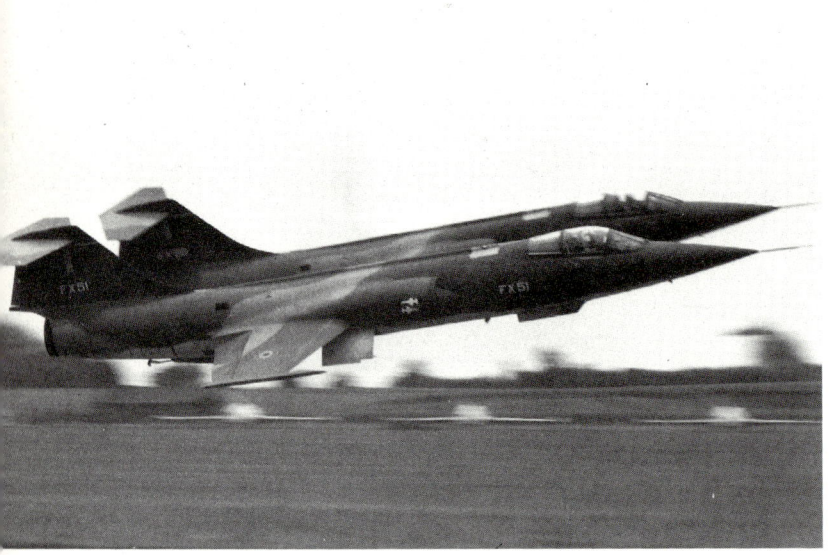

Above: The F-104G Starfighters of the *Slivers* on take-off. Note the insignia on the air intake. June 1971.
(A. Petelier via R. Ward)

Stampe SV.4c, 28, of the Belgian Air Force *Penguins* duo, after being refitted with a two-seater canopy. It is seen here at Beauvechain on 27 June 1970.
(Author's collection)

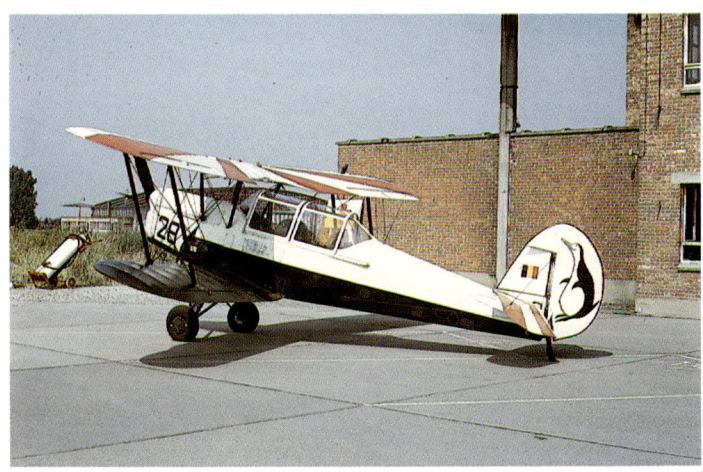

One of the Belgian Air Force's *Slivers* F-104G Starfighters seen taxying at Yeovilton on 21 September 1974. Note the team name on the intake and insignia on the pilot's helmet. (Adrian M. Balch)

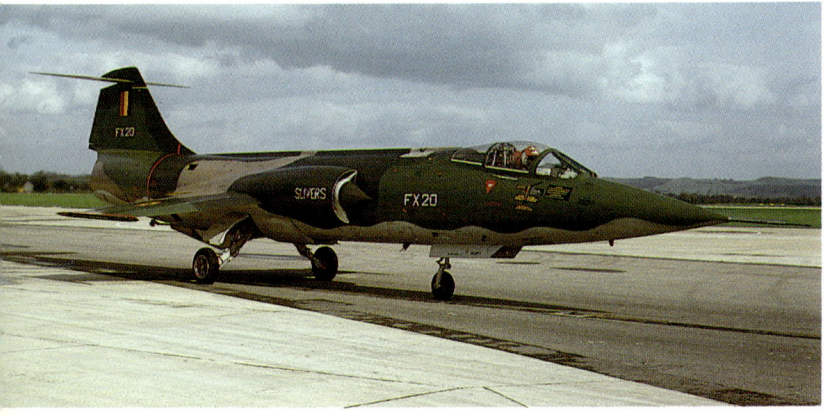

1968-75: 1 Wing, "The Slivers", Kleine-Brogel

The Slivers team of two F-104G Starfighters formed in 1 Wing during 1968 and gave their first public display at Bevekom on 14 May 1969. The duo were the official F-104G display team and regularly appeared at displays throughout Europe until they disbanded at the end of 1975. The pilots were Major Steve Nuyts and Adjutant Chef Palmer de Vlieger. Their display often started with each aircraft taking off from opposite ends of the runway simultaneously and crossing in the centre! The F-104Gs of *The Slivers* wore their standard camouflage of two-tone green and tan brown with light grey undersides. Two opposing F-104 silhouettes in white appeared on the intake during the 1971 season. This insignia was replaced by the team's name in white on the intakes. Belgian F-104Gs with the team's markings included: FX-20, FX-51, FX-68, FX-69 and FX-93.

1964-67: "The Penguins"/Les Manchots, Gossoncourt

This was another duo, which formed at Gossonourt in 1964 with two Stampe SV4 biplanes. The leader was Commander Pilot Jean Feyten, who was chief of the flight section at the Elementary Flying Training School. Training began in 1965 with the first display being at Brustem. The Stampes used by the team were converted to single-seaters for aerobatic purposes and the highlight of their display was back-to-back 'mirror' flying. The pair flew about twenty aerobatic manoeuvres and fifteen formation changes in twelve minutes. The team flew un-named until 1967, when *Les Manchots* (Penguins) was chosen as a humourous title and as the badge of the E.F.T.S. is a penguin. The two Stampes normally used were 'V18' and 'V28', which were appropriately painted in a black and white colour scheme, with the addition of a red sunburst design on top of the wings. However, 'V64' was used during 1966 in a black and yellow colour scheme. The team's second pilot was Flight Lieutenant H. Lambermont until 1966, when he was replaced by Captain Pilot Paul Chritiaens. *Les Manchots* disbanded at the end of the 1967 season and the Stampes were converted back to two-seaters.

1973-to date: "The Swallows", Goetsenhoven

When the Belgian Air Force received the SIAI-Marchetti SF-260M in 1970, several pilots began practising aerobatics and in 1972 Adjutant Serrien and Onder-Lieutenant Delacuvellerie performed at several displays, forming The Swallows the next year, with Serrien and Kapitein Fonderie. In 1975 the team changed with the return of Delacuvellerie and the addition of Adjutant Goussens. Captain Delacuvellerie led the team until 1979, when he was replaced by Captain Elleboudt from 1980. The team is based at Gossoncourt and uses three SF-260ms, all equipped to make smoke. The aircraft retain their green and brown camouflage with orange dayglo extremities and the Wing's penguin insignia on the fuselage. More recently, the team's name appears vertically up the rudder. SF-260Ms used by *The Swallows* include: ST-03, ST-07 ST-11, ST-14, ST-17, ST-25, ST-34 and ST-35.

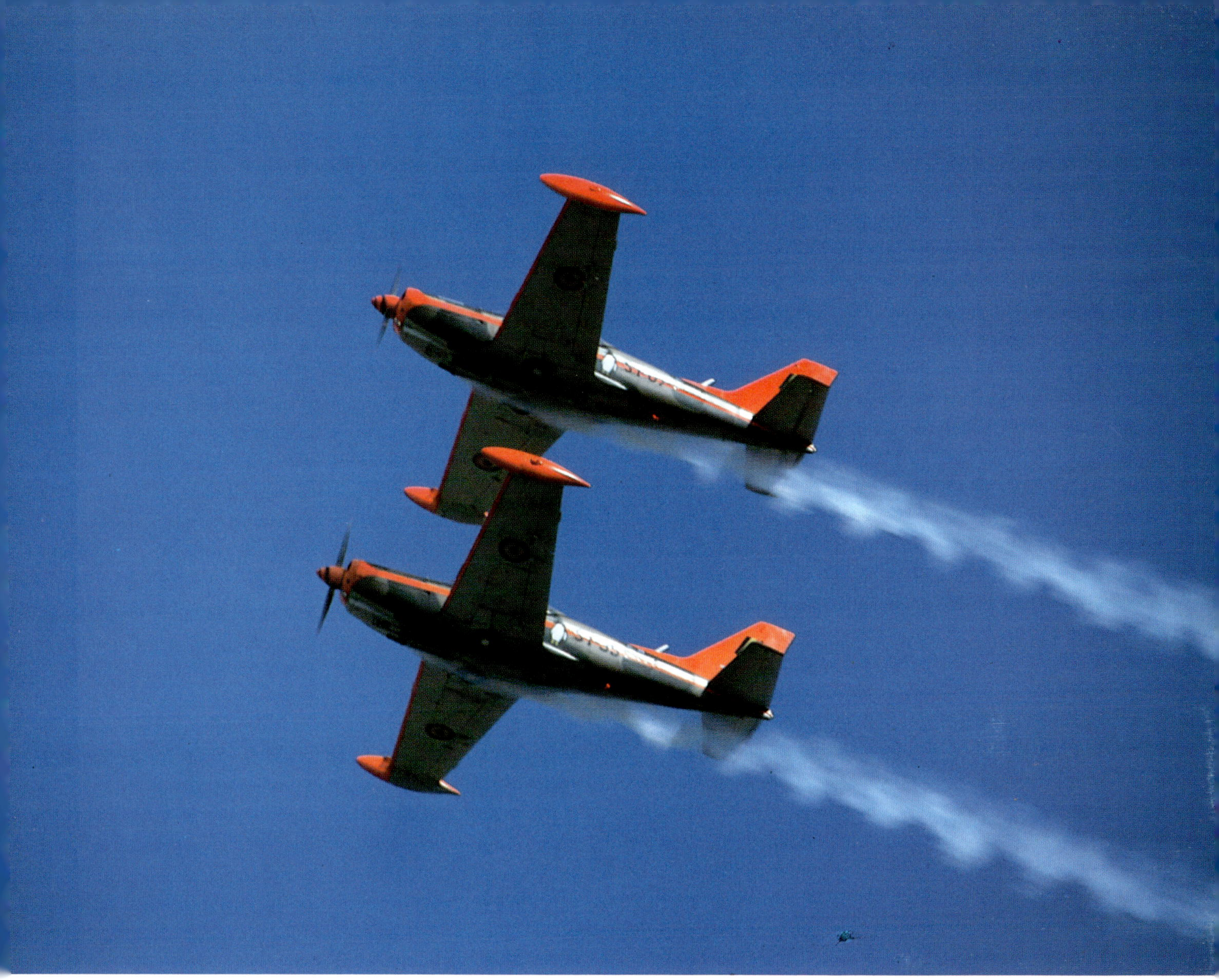

BELGIAN ARMY
1968-to date: "The Blue Bees", Werl Germany.

The Belgian Army had three squadron helicopter teams equipped with Alouettes by 1971. The 16th Squadron formed *The Red Pitch* in 1965, then the 17th Squadron formed *The Blue Bees* in 1968 and finally *The Larks* were formed by the 18th Squadron in 1970. In 1971, it was decided to disband two of the teams and retain *The Blue Bees* to represent the Belgian Army at displays throughout Europe.

The team's name comes from the squadron badge of 17 Smaldeel (Squadron), which is based at Werl and equipped with Alouette II and Alouette Astazou helicopters. The team flies six Alouettes, which retain the standard Belgian Army colour scheme of gloss olive drab with white lettering and the team badge on the front of the nose. The team pilots and servicing crews are all volunteers based at Werl, West Germany and the team's Alouettes are equipped with smoke canisters emitting red and blue smoke during their performance. Alouette IIs used by *The Blue Bees* include; OL-A42, OL-A48, OL-A54, OL-A60, OL-A62, OL-A64, OL-A68, OL-A70, OL-A73, and OL-A79, all of which appeared at Middle Wallop, England in July 1971 and '73. The 17th Squadron continued the team in 1972 which handed *The Blue Bees* over to the 16th Squadron in 1974. Then, in 1977, the honour was given to the 18th Squadron.

Above: SIAI Machetti SF-260s: ST-07 and ST-35 of the Belgian Air Force *Swallows* Team at Biggin Hill, 19 May, 1979. (Adrian M. Balch)

Below: Holding low on take-off are *Les Diables Rouges* (Red Devils) Fouga Magisters at Biggin Hill, 20 June, 1970. (Adrian M. Balch)

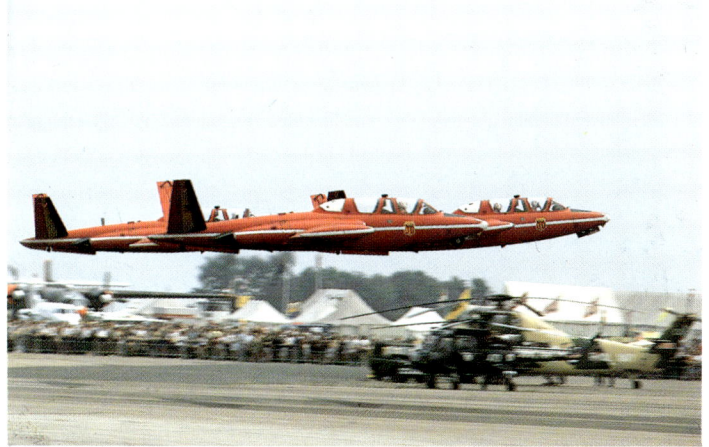

BRAZIL
Brazilian Air Force (Força Aerea Brasileira)

1952-to date: "Esquadrilha da Fumaça" (Smoke Squadron), Afonsos, then Sao Paulo

The *Esquadrilha da Fumaça* was formed in 1952 at Afonsos Base. A small group of instructors of the Escola de Aeronautica practised aerobatics in T-6 Texans during their spare time, partly for their own pleasure, and partly to demonstrate the proficiency of their instructors and machines to the pupils. They did so well that the Commandant of the School allowed them to give public displays. In May 1952, they made the first formation barrel roll performed in South America.

A quartet of T-6 Texans of the FAB *Esquadrilha da Fumaça* performing over Rio de Janeiro during the 1970s.
(Brazilian Air Force)

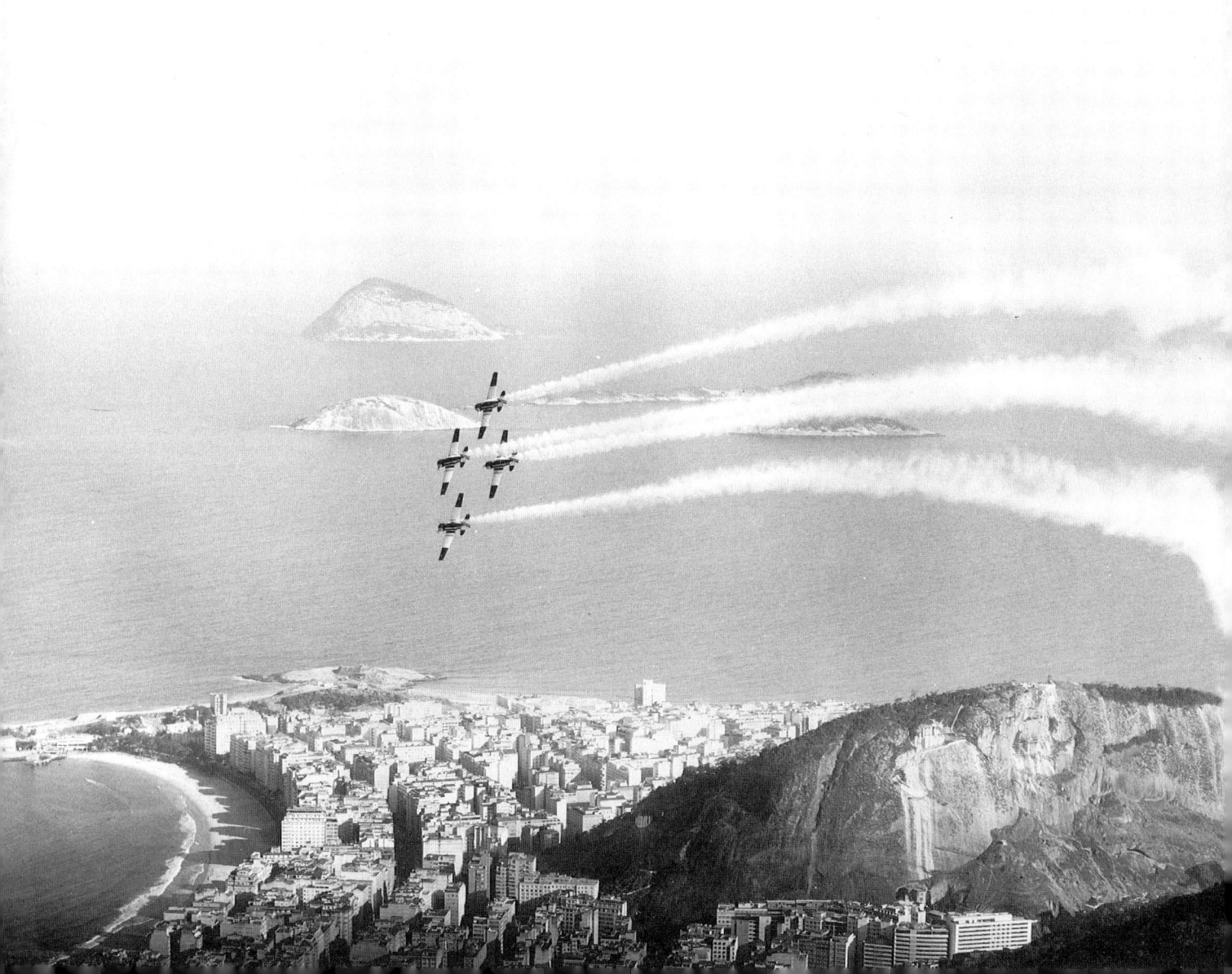

In 1953, the T-6 Texans were modified to make smoke by injecting oil into the exhaust from an oil tank located in the baggage compartment. In 1954, the Squadron moved from Afonsos to Megi-Mirim (Sao Paulo) with five aircraft. The team became very popular and acquired the name *Esquadrilha da Fumaça* (Smoke Squadron). In 1955, the aircraft were painted in their own scheme of red, white and dark blue. The team performed many shows, including the "Semana de Asa", when they performed over Copacabana. In December 1956, an accident killed two pilots in Salvador, but new pilots joined the team and the high morale of the squadron was not impaired. In 1958, pilots were posted to the squadron full-time and no longer had to be instructors. In May of that year, the squadron toured a number of South American countries. In 1963, a ministerial order created the Aerobatic Squadron as the official unit for aerobatic displays representing the Brazilian Air Force.

Pilots must be highly qualified to join the Squadron. They have to have not less than 1500 flying hours, of which 800 must have been spent as instructors, and must have three years' service as officers.

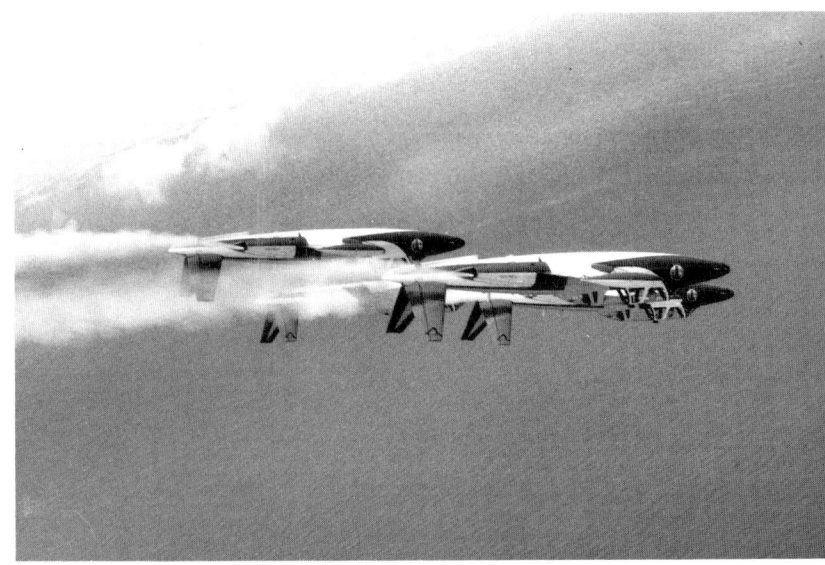

The Fouga Magisters of the FAB *Esquadrilha da Fumaça* at the top of a loop in 1969. (Brazilian Air Force)

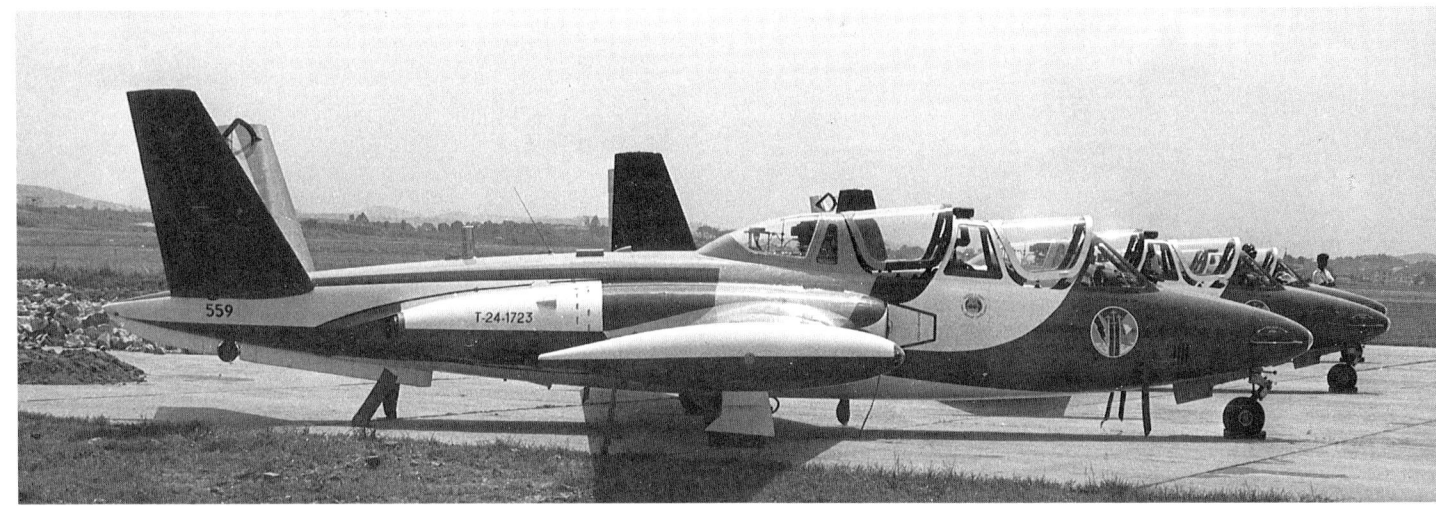

Above: Brazilian Air Force Magister, T24-1723 (c/n 559) of the *Esquadrilha da Fumaça* team in 1969. (via R. Ward)

Right: T27-1305, the first of six Tucanos for the *Esquadrilha da Fumaça* during flight testing from Sao José dos Campos in September 1983. Colour scheme is red with white and black trim. (Embraer).

In 1968, *Esquadrilha da Fumaça* re-equipped with seven Fouga CM-170 Super Magisters, known as the T24 in Brazilian Air Force service. The FAB acquired only seven of these aircraft, for the sole use of the aerobatic team. The team flew six in their routine, with one aircraft spare. Colour scheme was white, green, yellow and dark blue and all were equipped to make smoke. The team returned to the T-6 Texans in the early 1970s, when the Magisters were returned to France in part-exchange for Mirages. The *Smoke Squadron* disbanded at the end of 1977, but was reformed by Decree No.7739 of 22 October 1982, although it was a year before its new aircraft were received.

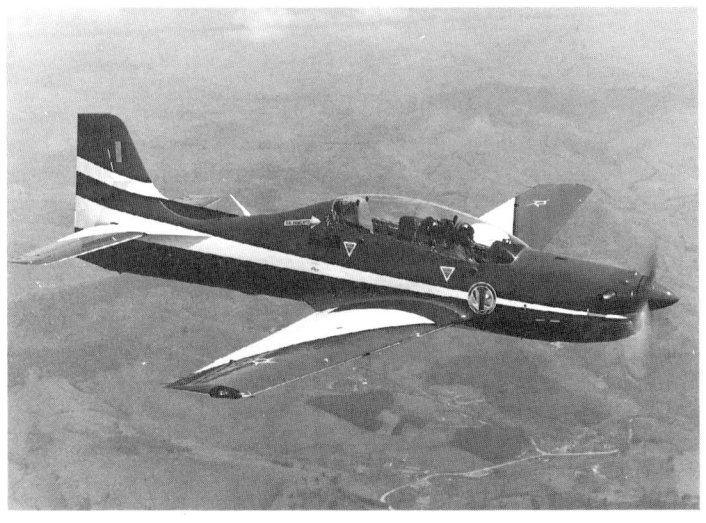

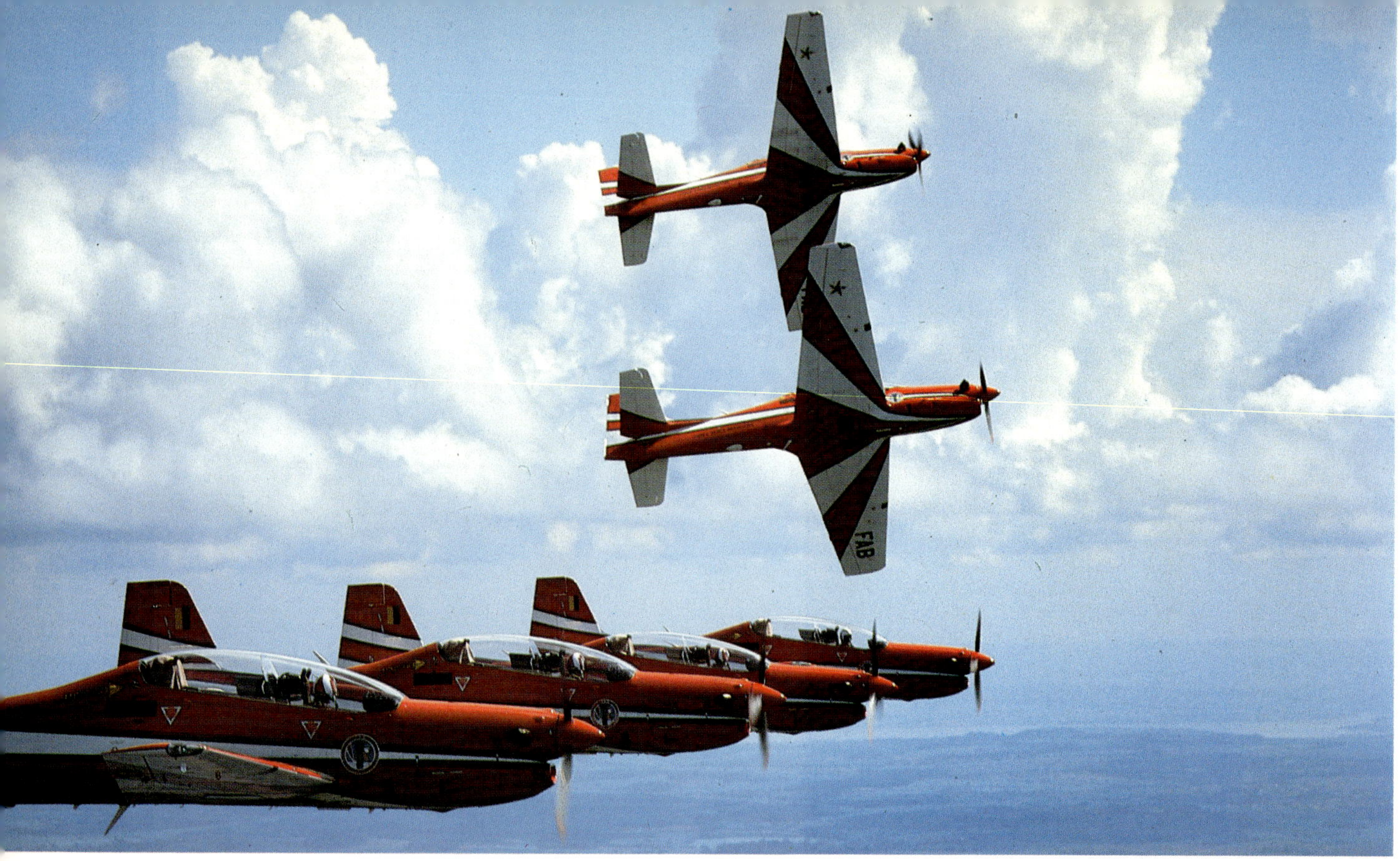

The 1984 Brazilian Air Force aerobatic team, *Esquadrilha da Fumaça*, with Embraer EM-312 Tucanos. These views show the underside and topside colour schemes to advantage. (Embraer)

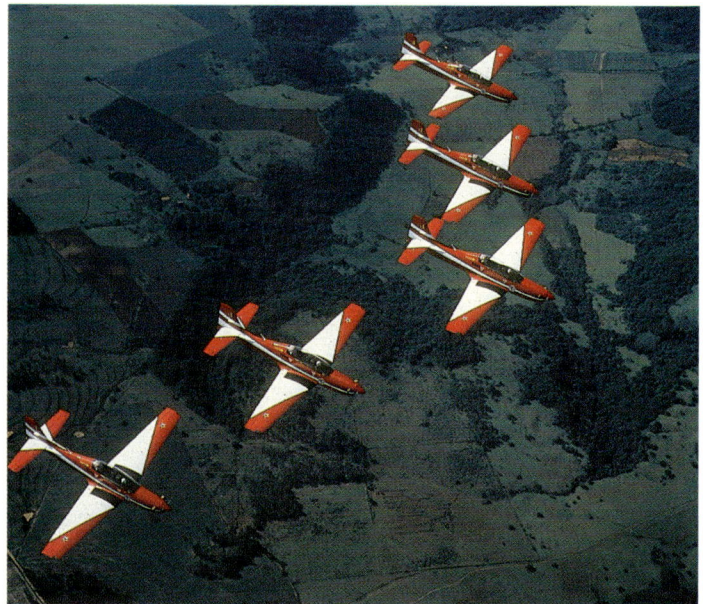

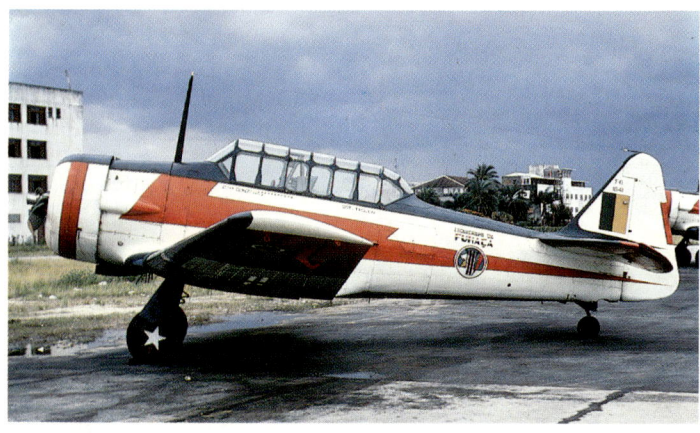

Bottom left: Brazilian Air Force T-6 Texan, 1641, of *Esquadrilha da Fumaça* at Santos Dumont, January, 1970. (via Werner Gysin)

Six Embraer EMB-312 Tucanos were delivered in October 1983 and the team began practising under the Command of Lieutenant-Colonel Geraldo Ribeiro Junior. The Tucanos are painted in a basically red colour scheme with white and black trim. One of the aircraft is T27-1305.

The first official demonstration tour abroad was made during March 2-11, 1984, when the team visited Chile to participate in an International Air Show at El Bosque, near Santiago.

The team made their first visit to Europe in August 1984, to carry out demonstrations in Portugal and Germany. Seven of the teams' Tucanos left their home base in Pirassununga on August 11, supported by a C-130H Hercules. They flew via Las Palmas to Lisbon for displays in Portugal, then flew via Paris-Le Bourget to Bonn for a display and arrived back in Brazil on September 2nd.

Over the years, no less than 22 T-6 Texans have been painted in the team's colours, from which six aircraft were drawn for each display. They were: 1243, 1275, 1390, 1427, 1455, 1467, 1482, 1500, 1508, 1539, 1542, 1550, 1551, 1559, 1600, 1612, 1631, 1641, 1643, 1646, 1658 and 1708. Some were written-off during their service and the rest retired or sold. '1390' is currently preserved at the Museu de Aeronautica, Sao Paulo.

The Fouga Magisters used by the team had the serials 1720-1726 (c/ns 556-560, 570, 571). During the 1970s, at least one Morane Saulnier MS-760 Paris was used as a support aircraft and was painted in the team's colours. The serial of the only known Paris was 2922.

CANADA
Royal Canadian Air Force/Canadian Armed Forces

1929-31: "The Siskins", Camp Borden

As their name implies, this team flew Armstrong-Whitworth Siskins and were the first RCAF aerobatic team to form, being established in 1929 by Group Captain E. A. McGowan. Based at Camp Borden, the 1930 team were trained by an RAF exchange officer, Flight Lieutenant F. V. Beamish, following which they made four appearances in the Autumn. *The Siskins* performed in the Trans-Canada Air Pageant in 1931 and at 26 air shows from Vancouver to Sydney, N.S. During that year, they were led by acting Squadron Leader R. W. Hewson, with pilots Flight Lieutenant W. I. Riddell, Flying Officers F. M. Gobeil, R. C. Hawtrey and E. A. McNab. *The Siskins* disbanded as a team at the end of 1931 after flying at a total of 55 locations in Canada and the U.S.A. Flying demonstrations were given in later years by those and other pilots, but never on a scale to equal the 1931 performances.

1949-50: "Blue Devils", St. Hubert

Members of 410 Squadron, St. Hubert, P.Q., flew silver Vampires with a blue stripe. Team leader was Flight Lieutenant D. C. Laubman, with Flight Lieutenants R. D. Schultz and J. A. O. Levesque, and Flying Officers W. R. Tew, W. H. Bliss and M. F. Doyle. Schultz and Tew specialised in solo aerobatics, and others in formation aerobatics.

Below: Line-up of CT-114 Tutors of the *Snowbirds,* 17 August, 1977 at Atlantic City, New Jersey.
(Stephen W. D. Wolf)

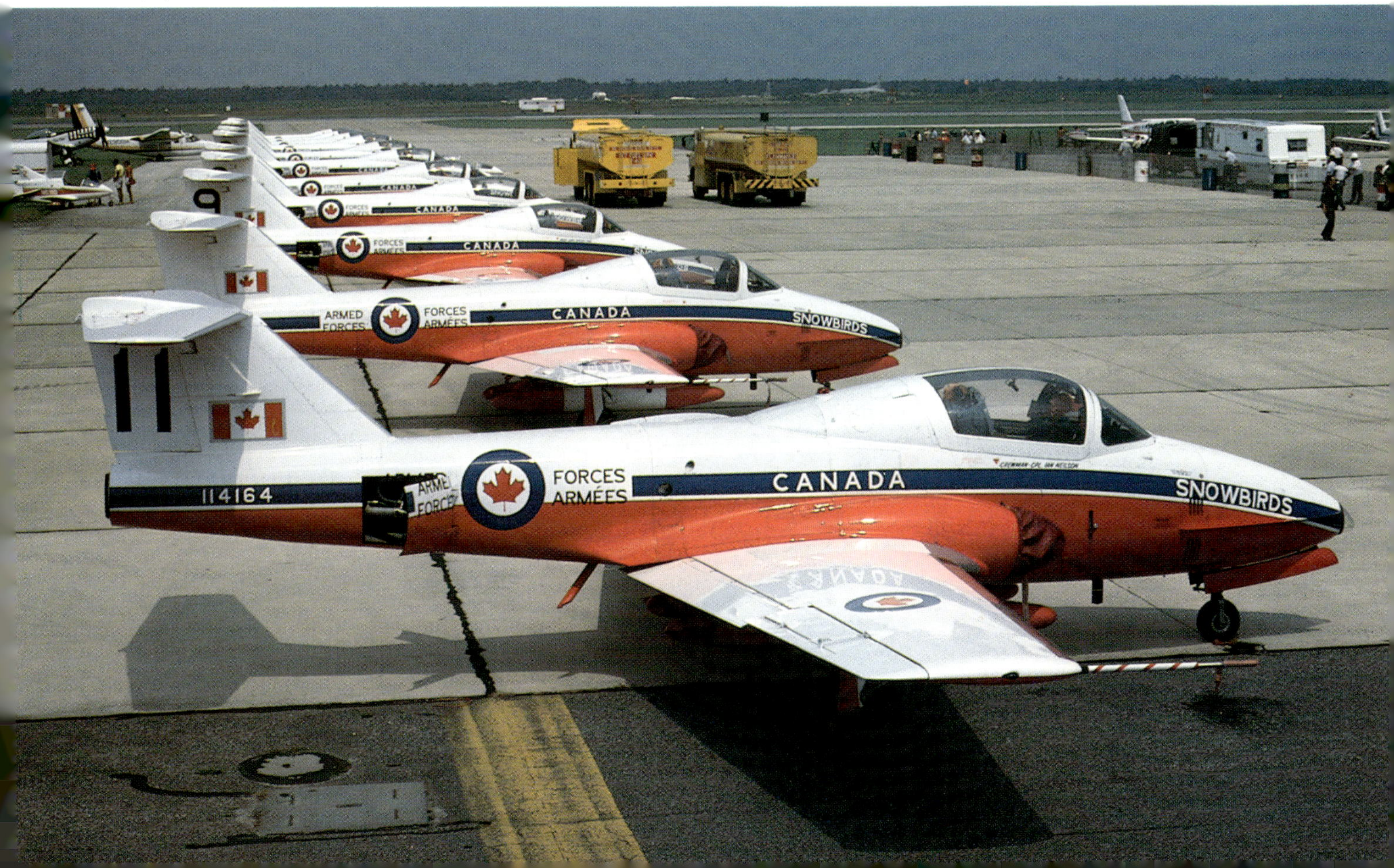

In 1950 the aerobatic team was expanded and became the "Air Defence Group Aerobatic Team". Pilots and aircraft were drawn from No. 410 and 421 Squadrons. Pilots from 410 Squadron were Flight Lieutenant Laubman (leader) and Flying Officers Doyle and Bliss. From 421 Squadron came Flying Officers Paisley, L. E. Spurr and F. W. Evans. The two sections of the team started off separately, but joined together in May of 1950, performing at such places as the Chicago Fair, USAF Convention in Boston and the CNE in Toronto. The team was disbanded on 11th September, 1950.

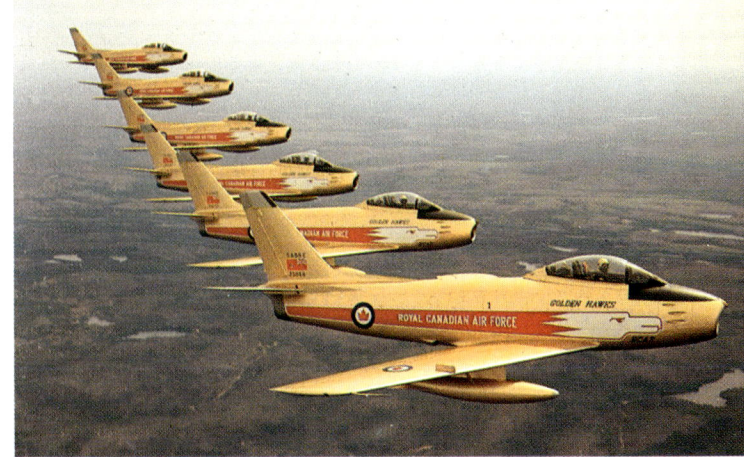

Above: Canadair Sabres of the *Golden Hawks* in 1959. Nearest aircraft is 23066. (RCAF)

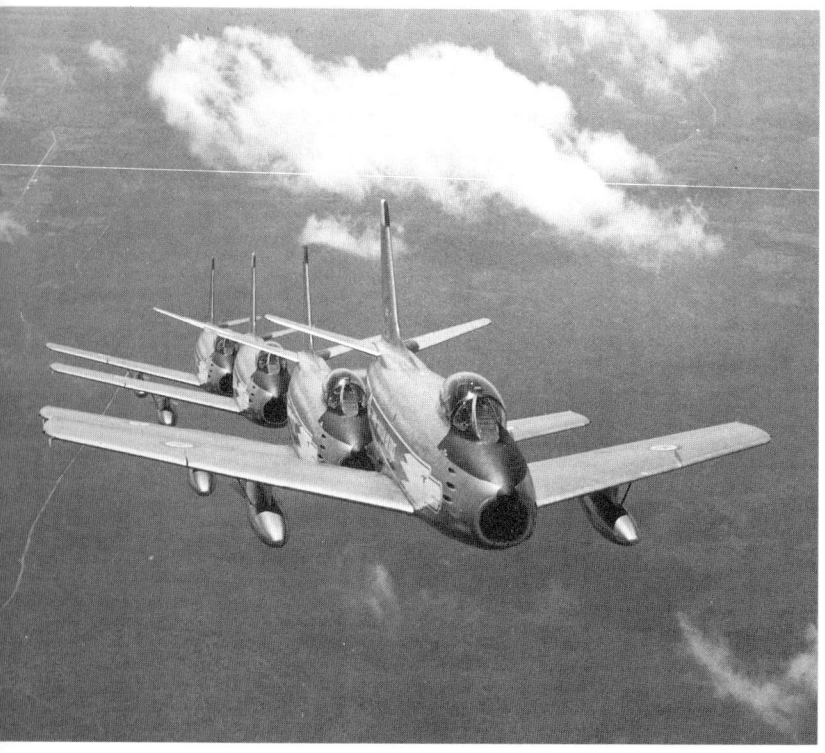

Canadair Sabre Mk.5s of the RCAF *Golden Hawks* in neat line-astern in 1959. (RCAF)

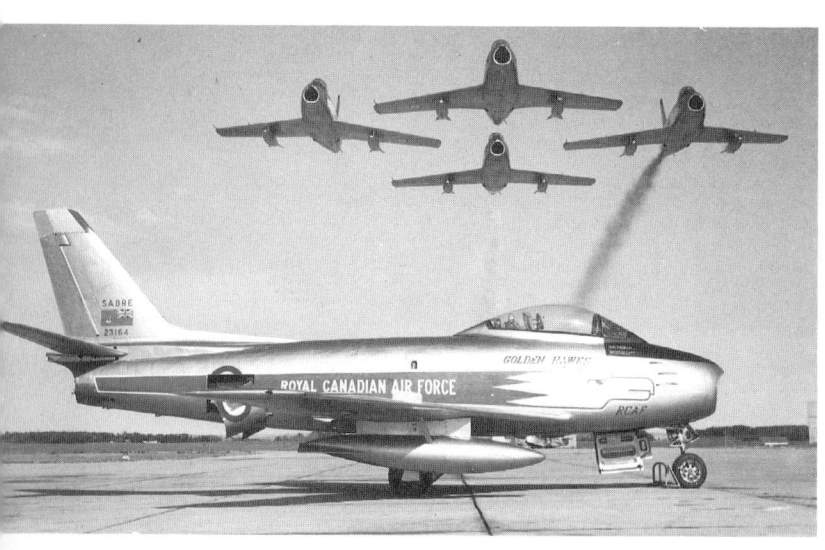

A quartet of Canadair Sabres of the RCAF *Golden Hawks* overflying 23164 in 1959. (RCAF via R. Ward)

1954: "Prairie Pacific Team", Cold Lake

During 1954, Western Canadian air show audiences were treated to aerial demonstrations by team members flying F-86 Sabres and T-33 Silver Stars.

Members of the team, flying Sabres, were Flying Officers G. F. Villeneuve (later to lead the *Golden Hawks*), Rod MacDonald, Fred Rudy, George Fulford and Art Maskell. Flying T-33s were Squadron Leader Lou Hill (leader), Flight Lieutenants Russ Scott, Alex Bowman and Flying Officer Jack Seaman. No special colour scheme was worn by the aircraft, as the team's machines were drawn from standard unit aircraft.

1954: No. 3 Fighter Wing, the "Fireballs", Soellingen, Germany

This team represented Canada and the RCAF at Air Shows throughout Europe.

The team comprised four Canadair Sabres, which were painted bright fire-engine red for a brief period. Members of the team were chosen from the Wing's three squadrons. They were Flight Lieutenant C. E. Keating (team leader), and Flying Officers S. E. Burrows, J. L. Frazer, E. R. Mace and the spare, Flying Officer C. A. Gripe, who later flew with the *Golden Hawks*.

1955: 1 Air Division, No. 2 Fighter Wing, "Sky Lancers", Grosentquin, France.

Another European RCAF team, the *Sky Lancers* were stationed at No. 2 Fighter Wing, Grostenquin, France. They participated in many International Air Shows throughout Europe during 1955. They took part in one of West Germany's first air shows following the lifting of the post-war ban on aviation in that country.

Flight Lieutenant Hannas was the team leader, with pilots Flying Officers L. M. Eisler, B. R. Campbell and G. C. E. Theriault. They flew the Canadair Sabre Mk.V, then in service with the Air Division in Europe. This team differed from others, in that in addition to giving aerobatic performances, they flew operationally with their squadrons. The Sabres retained their standard grey/green/blue camouflage with the addition of red and white trim. The fuselage had a red flash down the fuselage upon which the name *Sky Lancers* was painted in white-outlined blue script. One such painted aircraft was 23483.

1959-64: "Golden Hawks", Trenton, Ontario.

Originally formed in 1959 to help celebrate activities of the 35th Anniversary of the RCAF and the 50th Anniversary of Flight in Canada, the *Golden Hawks* went on to win international acclaim for their thrilling, perfectly-executed aerial manoeuvres.

Flying Canadair Sabres, the first team was commanded by Wing Commander J. F. Easton, and led by Squadron Leader F. G. Villeneuve with Flight Lieutenants E. J. Rozdeba, J. D. McCombe, R. H. Annis, G. J. Kerr and Flying Officers W. C. Stewart, J. T. Price and J. T. Holt. Public Relations Officer was Squadron Leader R. M. L. Bowdery, Flying Officer G. L. MacDonald was commentator, and engineering officer was Flight Lieutenant Ray Grandy, The *Golden Hawks* participated in 65 air shows and were viewed by 2½ million people.

The team was led again by Squadron Leader Villeneuve in 1960, with veterans Price, Annis, Steward, Rozdeba and McCombe. Flight Lieutenant D. V. Tinson also joined the team. That year, the team appeared in five shows in the United States.

A big change came in 1961 with Wing Commander J. F. Allan as Commanding Officer and Flight Lieutenant S. D. McCombe, promoted to Squadron Leader, appointed team leader. That year's team was composed of Flight Lieutenants E. Rozdeba, A. F. MacDonald, B. R. Campbell, L. S. Hubbard and S. L. Frazer and Flying Officer W. C. Stewart. Public Relations Officer was Flight Lieutenant L. G. Van Vliet and commentator was Flying Officer W. R. Dobson. The maintenance group was led by Flying Officer R. S. Perry. During the year they flew in 37 air shows, including one at the U.S. Naval Base at Pensacola, Florida.

For 1962, changes were minor, with Flight Lieutenant L. J. Hubbard being promoted to Squadron Leader and appointed team leader. Remaining were Flight Lieutenants Campbell, Frazer and MacDonald. The new pilots were Flight Lieutenants N. J. Garriock, G. E. Miller and E. J. McKeogh. The French commentator was Flight Lieutenant J. G. Boulet.

The *Golden Hawks* final year was 1963. Squadron Leader Hubbard once more led the team, with Flight Lieutenants Garriock and McKeogh. New pilots joining were Flight Lieutenants A. Young, C. B. Lang, D. J. Barker and L. W. Grip. Public Relations officer was Flight Lieutenant J. C. Giles, and Flight Lieutenant B. J. Lehans was commentator. Maintenance was led by Flight Lieutenant C. G. Peterson. The team closed their season in Montreal with their 317th public show. Although training started for another season, the team was disbanded on 28th February 1964.

Six Canadair Sabres were flown by the team, with four flying the main formations plus two solo performers. The aircraft were painted gold overall with a red and white Hawk's head and cheat line down the fuselage. During the 1962 season, the aircraft had individual fin numbers in black, 23651 being coded '1'. For the final season, 1963, these number codes were replaced by the letters 'GH' in red on the fins of all aircraft. Two Canadair T-33 Silver Stars were allocated to the team as support aircraft, being used by the commentator, engineering officer and P.R.O. The *Golden Hawks* Sabres included: 23066, 23073, 23164, 23424, 23457, 23487, 23649 and 23651. The two T-33s were 21500 and 21616.

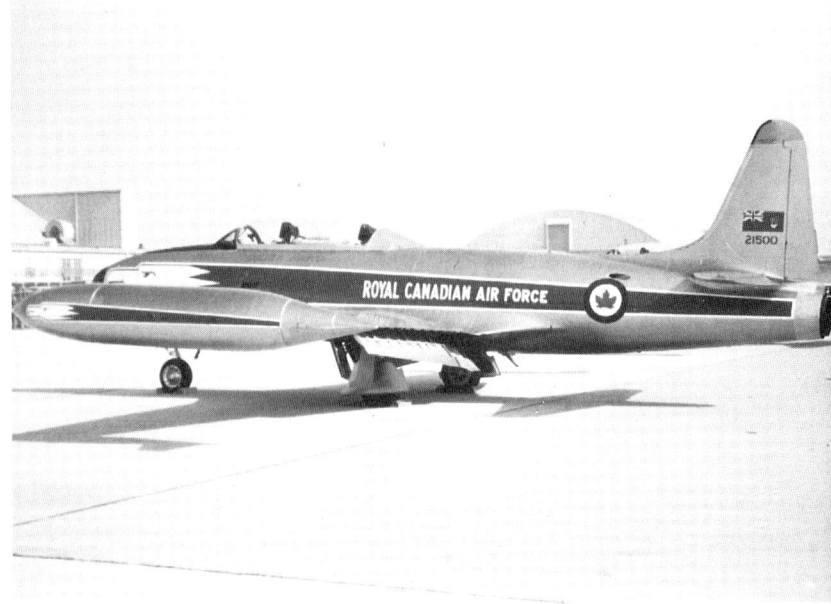

The RCAF *Golden Hawks* had two T-33s as support aircraft, including 21500, photographed in 1963. (Werner Gysin)

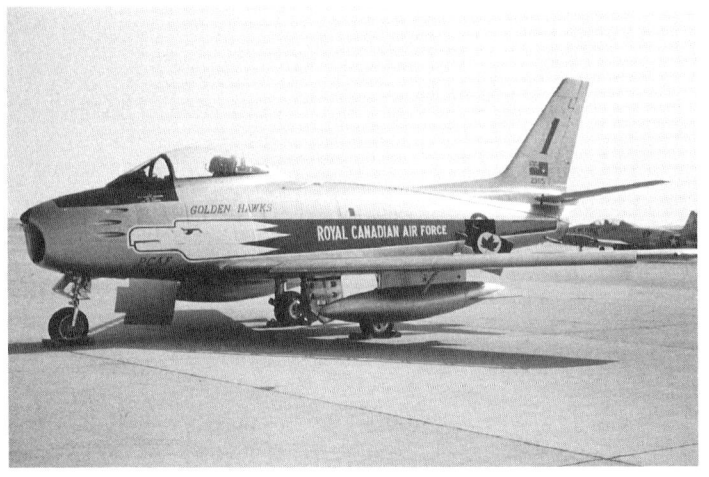

The RCAF *Golden Hawks* Sabres had number codes on their fins for a while. Here is 23651, the leader's aircraft, No. 1. (Werner Gysin)

Painted overall dayglo-red, 21057 was one of several T-33A Silver Stars flown by the *Red Knight*. Note Smoke-making pipe down the fuselage side. (R. W. Harrison via R. Ward)

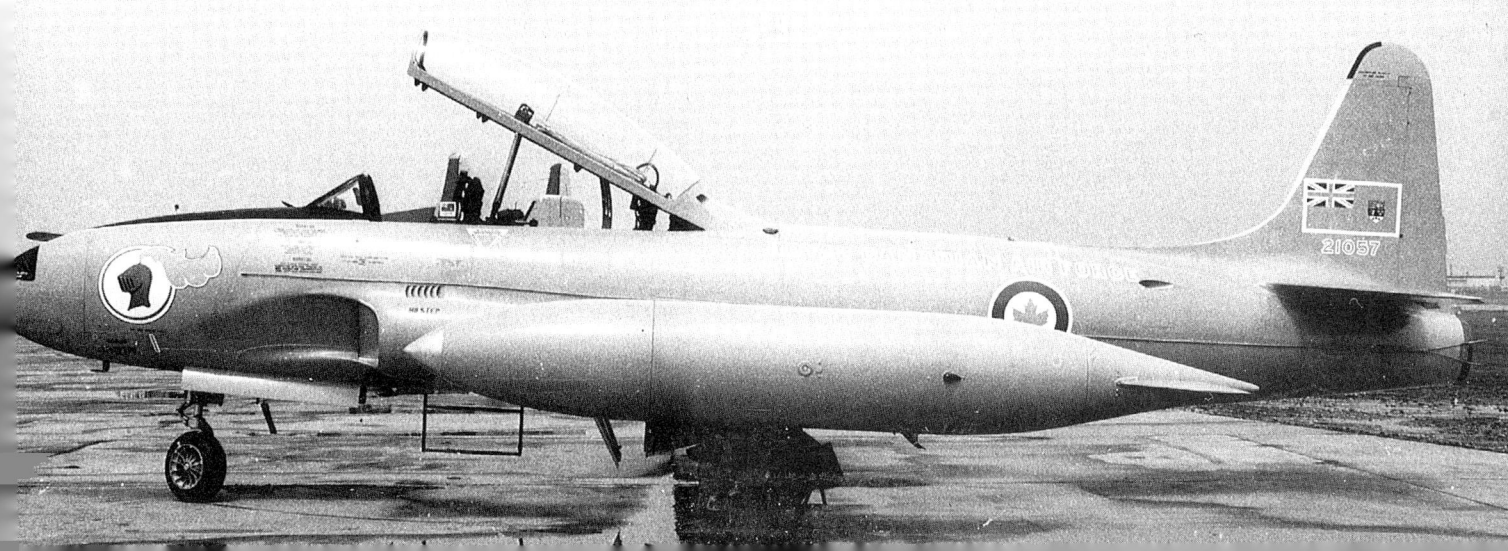

1959: "Gimli Smokers", Downsview

The *Gimli Smokers* were a precision formation team of four Canadair T-33s, which formed in 1959. The team was formed by Wing Commander K. C. Lett and performed before western audiences at Toronto's CNE and in Ottawa. They only flew for the one season and disbanded at the end of 1959.

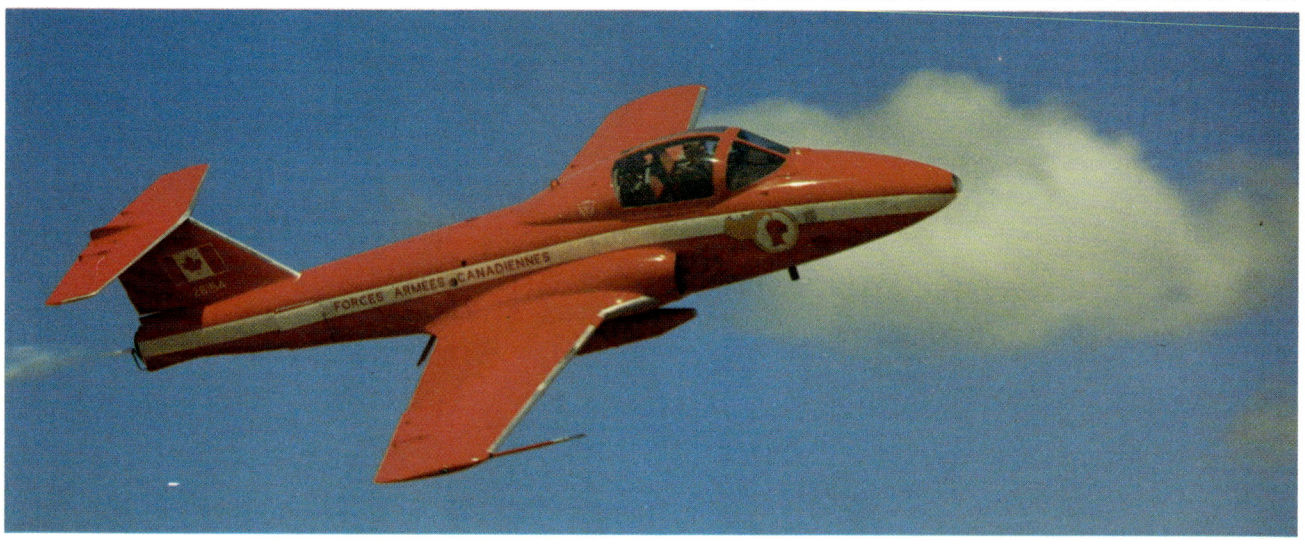

Above: The Red Knight flying Canadair Tutor, 26154, in 1968. (Canadair).

1959-1969: The "Red Knight", Portage La Prairie

This was not a team, but a solo aerobatic T-33 painted dayglo-red overall. The *Red Knight* originated at RCAF Station Portage La Prairie, Manitoba, in 1959, as Training Command's contribution to the 50th anniversary of powered flight in Canada.

One of the outstanding aspects of the demonstration was the ability of the *Red Knight* to confine his routine to the display area in spite of the relatively high speed of his flashing red T-33.

Red Knights who dazzled millions with their display of solo aerobatics were:

1959 — Flight Lieutenant Roy Windover; 1960 — Flight Lieutenant Bob Hallowell; 1961/2 — Flight Lieutenant Dave Barker; 1963 — Flight Lieutenant Bill Frazer (January-June) 1963 — Flight Lieutenant Bud Morin (June-August); 1963 — Flight Lieutenant Wayne MacLellan (August-March 64) 1964 — Flying Officer Slaughter with Flying Officer Tex Deagnon as alternate. 1965 — Flying Officer Tex Deagnon; 1966 — Flight Lieutenant Terry Hallett; 1967 — Flight Lieutenant "Jack" Waters with Flying Officer Rod Ellis as alternate; 1968 — Captain Dave Curran with Captain John Reid as alternate, 1969 — Lieutenant Bryan Alston with Captain Bob Cran as alternate. Several different T-33s were used over the years including 21057, 21630 and 21574. The latter was used during 1963 and wore the old-style fin flag, while 21630 had the current style insignia and was flown in 1967. The aircraft were dayglo-red overall and wore a nose insignia comprising a red (not dayglo) knight's head with a yellow plume, mounted on a white background. National insignia was outlined in white and varied slightly from year to year. The aircraft were equipped to make smoke and the T-33 was replaced by a Canadair CL-41A Tutor for the 1968 and '69 seasons. Only one aircraft was known to have been painted in the *Red Knight* colour scheme, being 26154, which differed from the T-33 in having a vermillion scheme overall, rather than dayglo-red. No CAF roundels were carried on the fuselage or wings. The same knight's head insignia appeared on the nose and a white cheat line ran down the fuselage side. On this was painted 'CANADIAN ARMED FORCES' on the port side and FORCES ARMÉES CANADIENNES' on the starboard. The current-style Canadian flag appeared on the fin with the serial number in white.

The *Red Knight* gave his last display at the end of the 1969 season.

1962-63 "Goldilocks", Moose Jaw
Goldilocks was a team of seven Harvards, formed in Moose Jaw in 1962 as a spoof on the famed *Golden Hawks*. The group appeared at many displays, including the Canadian National Exhibition, but Air Force Headquarters disapproved of the team's mounting fame and show-stealing antics. They ordered the name *Goldilocks* dropped and restricted performances to accredited air force shows. The team was disbanded at the end of 1963. The aircraft used were Harvards in the standard RCAF colour scheme of yellow overall with dayglo-red extremities. These Harvards included 20390, 20433, 20421 and 20449.

1967: "Golden Centennaires", Moose Jaw
Formed to help Canada celebrate its Centennial, the *Golden Centennaires* were to fly in 100 Centennial Year performances from coast to coast between April and October, 1967. The team started and finished their tour with opening and closing ceremonies at Expo 67 in Montreal.

The team flew six Canadair CL-41A Tutors with two spare aircraft and two supporting Canadair T-33A Silver Stars, all painted with gold upper surfaces, black undersides and red and white trim. No roundels were carried on the wings or fuselage. A gold and black-winged Maple Leaf insignia was carried on the nose.

The team was commanded by Wing Commander O. B. Philp and led by Squadron Leader C. B. Lang. Team pilots were Flight Lieutenants Tom Hinton, John Swallow, Russ Bennett, R. C. Dagenais, B. K. Doyle, Dave Barker, Bill Slaughter and Jim McKay. Throughout the year, they gave many thrilling performances before millions of Canadians and foreigners who visited Canada during Expo 67 year.

The air demonstration comprised more than just the Tutor show. The total package included the CF-104, piloted by Flight Lieutenant D. R. Serrao; the CF-101B piloted by Flight Lieutenant J. E. Miller. Two vintage AVRO 504K's were piloted by Flight Lieutenants G. Greff and G. Brown.

The group also included the *Red Knight* and his bright red T-33 Silver Star. The Public Information Officer was Squadron Leader L. J. Hubbard, ex-leader of the *Golden Hawks*, and Flight Lieutenant J. L. D. Gauthier as commentator. Flight Lieutenant C. D. Grant was the engineering officer.

The team was disbanded at the close of the Centennial celebrations in October 1967.

Only the 'last three' of the full serial number was carried by Tutors of the *Golden Centennaires*, the aircraft used being: 26122, '151, '154, '155, '163, '175, '179 and '180. The two T-33As were 21490 and 21592.

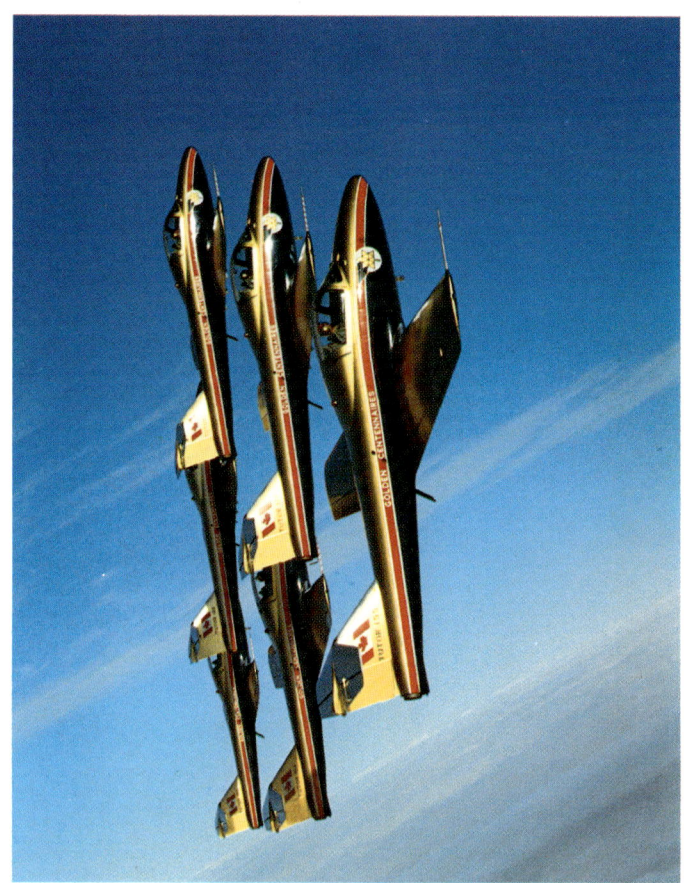

Above: Canadair Tutors of the RCAF *Golden Centennaires* in 1967. (Canadair).

Below: Canadair Tutors of the *Snowbirds* in 1982, showing the underside scheme. (Bill Johnson)

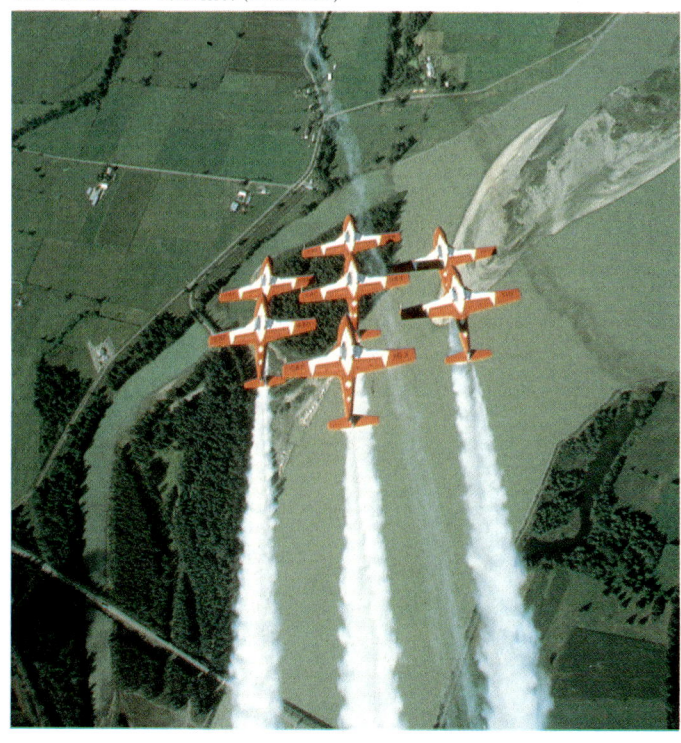

1971-to date: 431 (Air Demonstration) Squadron., "Snowbirds", Moose Jaw

The *Snowbirds* were formed in 1971 by flying instructors at CFB Moose Jaw for the 1972 airshow season. Eight white Tutors performed a 20-minute routine involving a seven-aircraft formation in various positions, interspaced by an aerobatic solo, all trailing white smoke.

The *Snowbirds* were founded by Colonel O. B. Philp, who was the ex-commanding officer of the *Golden Centennaires*. The 1972 team was led by Major Glen Younghusband and a team of volunteer instructor pilots and ground crew. The operation was conducted on a local, base level, and seven of the ex-*Centennaires* Tutors were utilised. The members of the 2 CF FTS Formation Team, as it was called, practised in the evenings after completing their flight instructor duties, and flew airshows at the weekends. During the 1971 season, the team performed 27 shows and made the first step towards Colonel Philp's ultimate dream of re-establishing a big-league Canadian Forces aerobatic team. In 1972, two solo pilots were added to the team and they participated in 25 shows during that season. That year a contest was held at the base elementary school to select a name for the team. The winning entry was, of course, the *Snowbirds*, an appropriate name for nine white aircraft with a winter home on the Canadian prairies. In 1973, Major George Miller became the *Snowbirds* leader and led the team in shows throughout Canada and the United States. 1974 saw clearance for the team to perform a fully aerobatic formation display, including formation changes during manoeuvres and the *Snowbirds* paint scheme was changed to the current red, white and blue design. During the '74 Northern Tour, the *Snowbirds* became the first North American formation aerobatic team to fly a show north of the Arctic Circle, when they performed at Inuvik, in the Yukon. At the end of the season, the team had flown 80 shows to an estimated audience of 2,000,000 people.

The 1975 season saw Major Denis Gauthier become team leader. One of the highlights of the 1975 season was another performance at Inuvik .... this time at midnight!

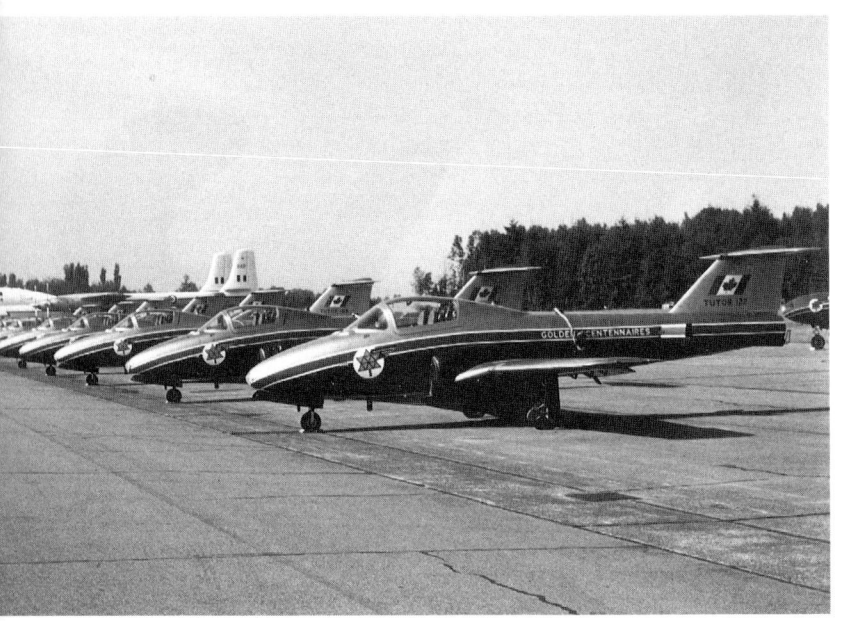

Specially formed for the RCAF's Centenary were the *Golden Centennaires* with Canadair Tutors, seen here lined up at Toronto in August 1967.
(Terry Waddington)

21592 was one of two Canadair T-33As used as support aircraft by the *Golden Centennaires* in 1967.
(via R. Ward)

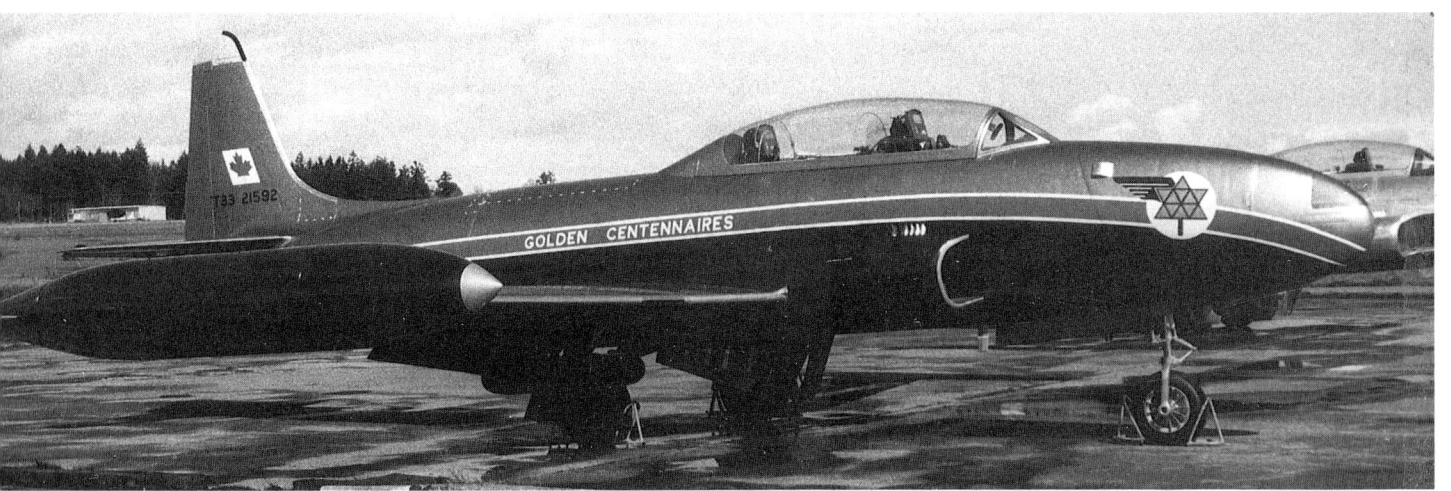

In 1976, the growing popularity of the team in the United States was reflected in the request for a performance at Philadelphia, on the 4th of July, as part of the American Bi-Centennial celebrations. In Canada, the team performed in the Summer Olympics ceremonies at both Montreal and Kingston.

Major Gord Wallis became Commanding Officer and Team Leader for the 1977-78 seasons, beginning a so-far unbroken tradition of former *Snowbirds* returning as leaders. In September 1977, the *Snowbirds* were finally made a permanent unit, with their official designation becoming The Canadian Forces Air Demonstration Team (CFADT). On 1st April 1978, the CFADT received squadron status. They were now designated 431 (Air Demonstration) Squadron. Under the direction of Major Tom Griffis, Squadron Commander and Team Leader for the 1979-80 seasons, the *Snowbirds* performance featured an expanded opening nine-plane sequence, and played to an estimated annual audience of over five million spectators, including huge 4th of July crowds at New York's Coney Island in 1980.

1981 marked the tenth anniversary of the *Snowbirds*, and 1982 was the final tour for Major Mike Murphy as Commanding Officer/Team Leader.

As the Canadian Forces permanent aerobatic team, the *Snowbirds* should continue in their present form until the Tutor is replaced.

The nine Tutors in the team wear a red, white and blue colour scheme with a stylised white bird motif under the wings and fuselage. Roundels are worn on the fuselage sides and above the wings only. 'CAF' and the 'last three' of the serial number appears under the wingtips. A large black aircraft identification number appears on the rudder, these not being permanent, as they are often changed when aircraft go in for maintenance. The following team aircraft, with codes, are known: 114003:6, 114032:2, 114043:4, 114114:3, 114118:8, 114122:9, 114147:2, 114151:1/8, 114152:3, 114155:5, 114164:11, 114178:1, 114055:9, 114105:7, 114163:5, 114030:6, 114177:4, 114036:2.

1980-to date: No. 3 CF-FTS, "Dragonflies", Portage la Prairie

This is a helicopter team of Bell CH-136 Kiowas, the Canadian military version of the Jet Ranger.

Pilots and aircraft are drawn from the Rotary Wing Squadron of 3 Canadian Forces Flying Training School at Canadian Forces Base, Portage la Prairie, Manitoba. They perform at Canadian Armed Forces Day celebrations held on the prairies.

All pilots are qualified flying instructors on the Kiowa helicopter and have had at least one operational helicopter tour in Canada. In addition, each pilot first qualifies on fixed-wing aircraft, before advancing to helicopters.

The pilots perform flypasts in flying formation as part of the air display. Spacing between helicopters is set at one rotor diameter (approximately 35 feet).

Colour scheme is the standard 3 CFFTS training scheme of yellow and olive green, one of the machines being serialled 136216.

One of the Bell CH-136 Kiowas used by 3 CFTS *Dragonflies* team, photographed in March 1980.
(F. T. Guthrie)

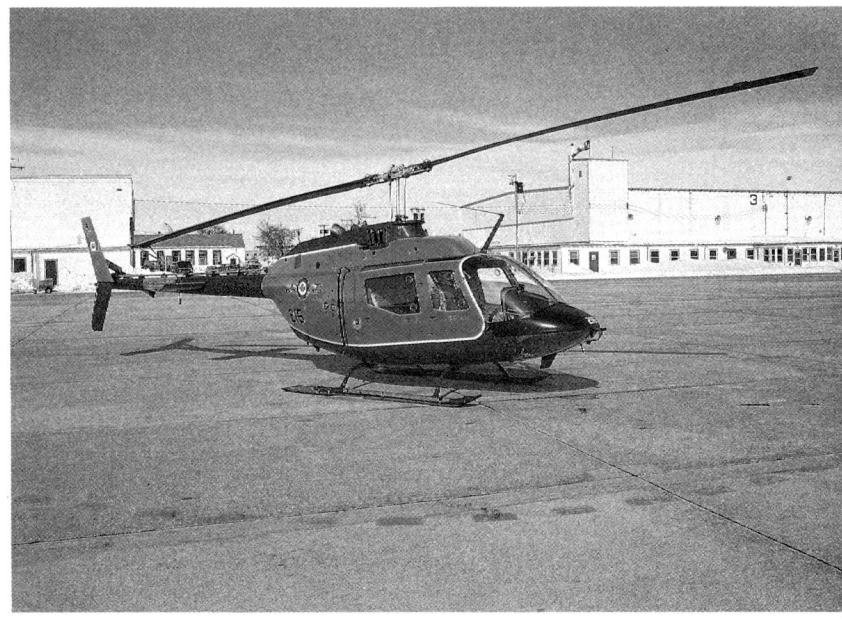

REPUBLIC OF CHINA
Chinese Nationalist Air Force

1954-to date: The "Thunder Tigers", Taipei

The *Thunder Tigers* aerobatic team made their appearance in the skies over Taiwan using four F-84G Thunderjets on 14 August, 1954 and immediately won recognition and praise all over the country. The team was formally established in December 1954, the night before the 7th Aeronautical Exhibition Week held in Manila, The Philippines. With continuing hard work and increased support, the team grew to nine aircraft, enabling them to make a 'diamond-nine' formation by 1957. In 1959, the team re-equipped with the F-86F Sabre and increased the number of planes from nine to twelve. They demonstrated their skills throughout Taiwan, Korea, Okinawa and the Philippines, as well as in Thailand, where they performed before the Thai Royal Family. The *Thunder Tigers* converted to the F-5A Freedom-Fighter in early 1967, then switched to the F-5E Tiger II in 1975, flying a team of nine with both versions. The Commander of the *Thunder Tigers* in 1983 was Liang Lüng and the team looks like continuing into the foreseeable future and participating in events throughout the Far East.

The *Thunder Tigers* F-84G Thunderjets were natural metal overall with national markings in six positions and white-blue striped rudder. The nose and fin-top was red, as was a lightning flash on the wing-tip tanks. The team's F-84Gs were: 52-3001, '006, '137, '201, '234, '021, '198, '014, '057 and '015. The 'last three' numbers appeared on the nose of each machine in black.

The team's F-86F Sabres were also natural metal overall, with a red or dark blue nose and a black/yellow checkered sash round the fuselage. The *Thunder Tigers* badge appeared on the fin on a purple disc. *Thunder Tigers* Sabres included: 373/51-13387, 430/55-5009, 392/52-5525 and 265/52-4438.

The F-5As were silver overall with the undersides painted in a similar scheme to that applied to the USAF *Thunderbirds* T-38A Talons. Due to its operational commitments, the current F-5Es retain their Vietnam-style green and tan-brown camouflage with pale grey undersides. Wing-tip tanks are red and serials of F-5As and F-5Es used by the team are unknown. Throughout its career, all types used by the *Thunder Tigers* have been equipped to make white smoke.

CNAF *Thunder Tigers* F-86F Sabre, 52-4438/F-86265 at Manila in 1960. Nose is red outlined in black and checks are black and yellow. (D. Kasulka via R. Ward).

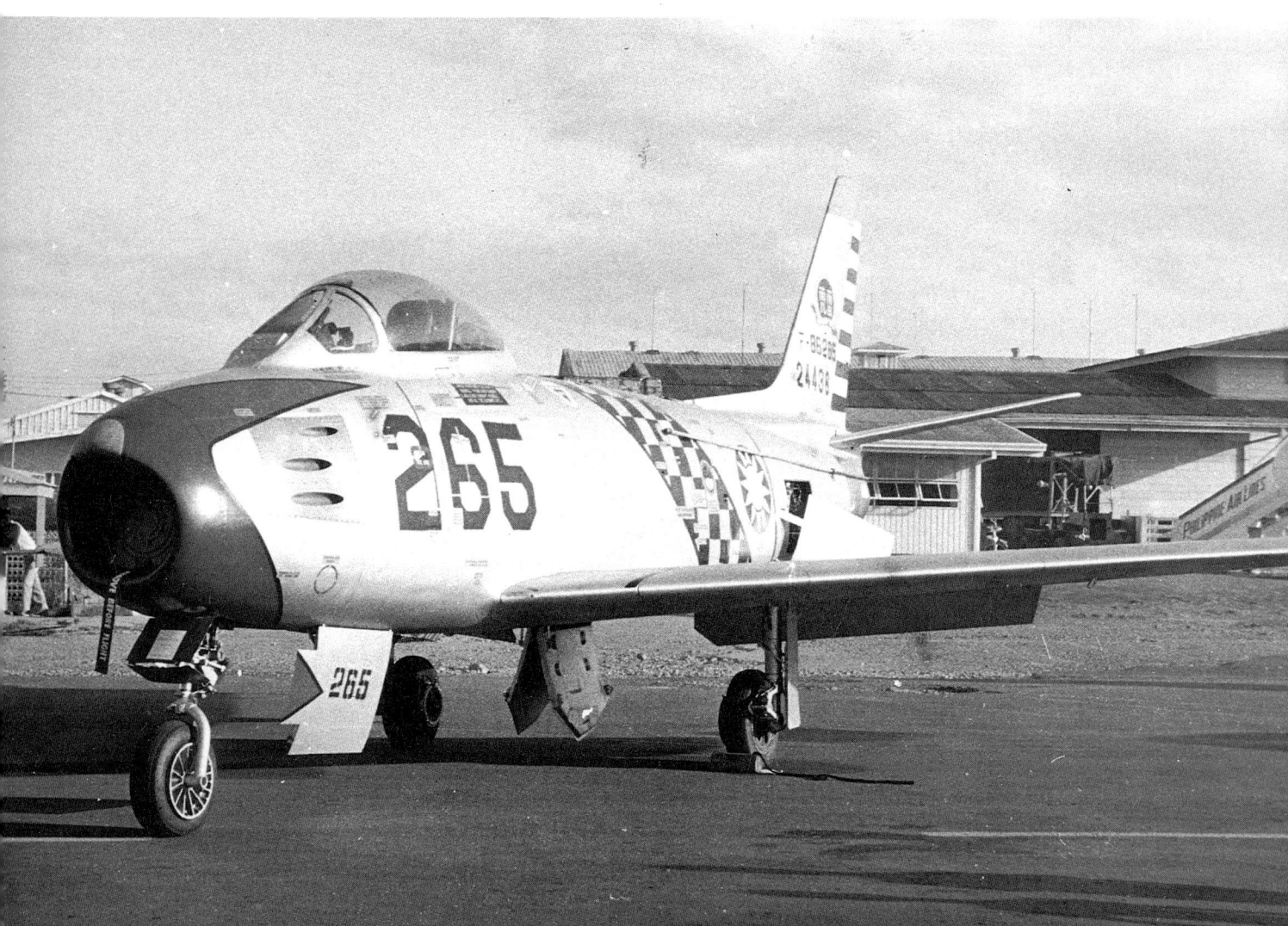

FINLAND
Finnish Air Force

1962-to date: "Jasska 4" team, Kauhava.
The Finnish Air Force formed an aerobatic team when Valmet-built Fouga Magisters were delivered to the Air Academy in 1962. Based at Kauhava, the team comprised four Magisters flown by staff instructors. The aircraft wore the standard overall natural metal colour scheme for the twenty years the team operated the Magister, with only dayglo orange panels on the extremities, providing a little extra colour from the mid-1970s. *Jasska 4* participated in the few air displays and at official occasions throughout Finland, the pilots practising during their spare time. The Fouga Magister was replaced by the British Aerospace Hawk T.51 during the early 1980s and *Jasska 4* converted to this type in 1983. The Hawks retain their standard camouflage of two-tone olive green and pale blue undersides. The team's Magisters were drawn from the batch serialled FM-1 to FM-82, replaced by Hawks serialled from HW-301 to HW-350.

FM-30, one of the Fouga Magisters operated by the Finnish Air Force *Jasska-4* team in 1976.
(Stephen W. D. Wolf)

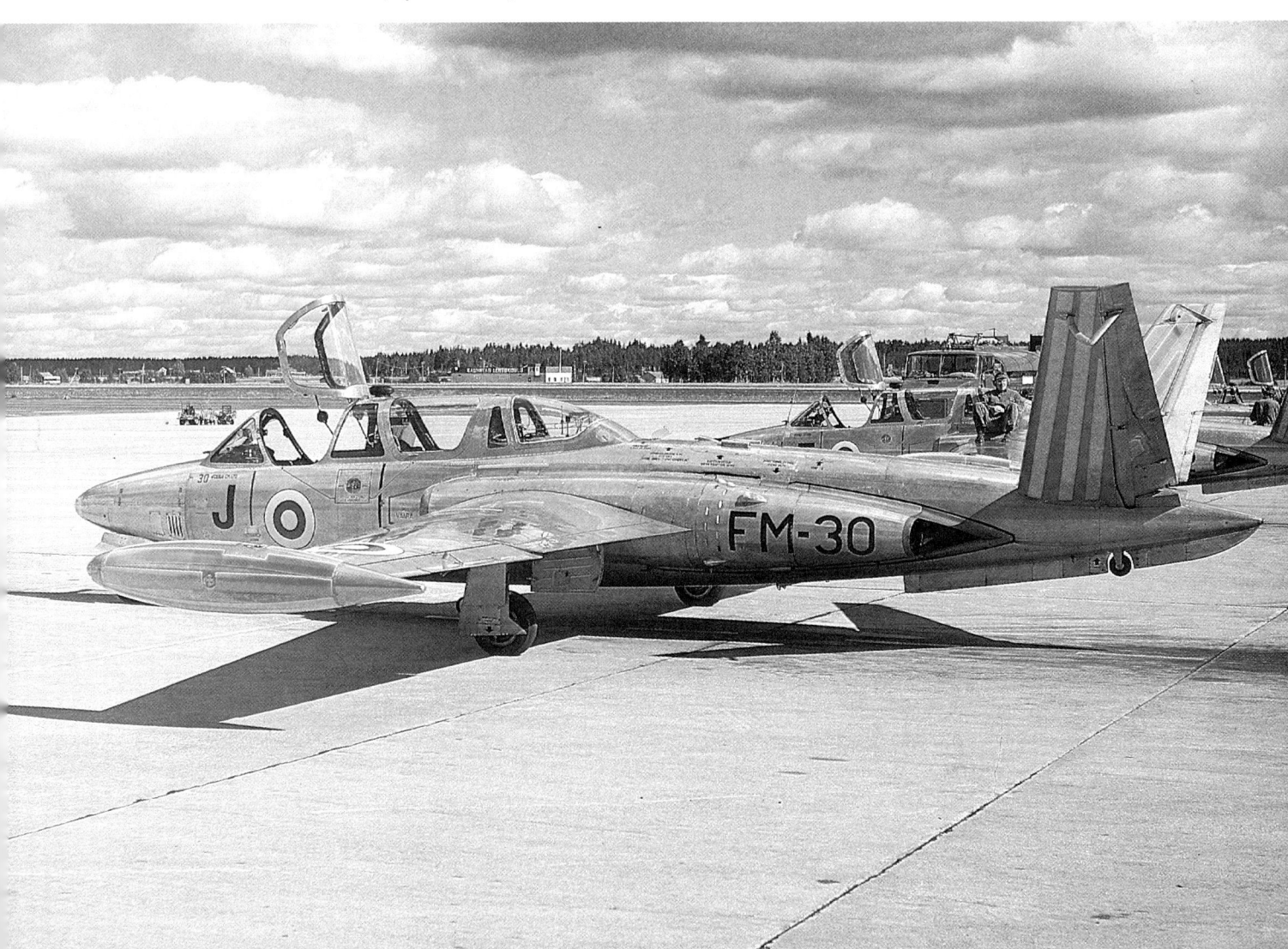

FRANCE
French Air Force

1953-to date: "La Patrouille de France", Salon-de-Provence

In 1931, the first French Air Force aerobatic team was formed at Étampes. The team was called *La Patrouille d'Étampes* and comprised three Morane 230s, being led by Capitaine Édouard Amouroux. From 1933 to 1939, Lieutenant Fleurquin led the team and during this period perfected the team, which participated at national and international shows with five aircraft.

In 1934, at Dijon, another aerobatic team was formed by 1/7 Escadre, called *La Patrouille Weiser*. Equipped with Morane 225 and SPAD 510 aircraft, the team performed 18 manoeuvres, some of which were in tied-together formations.

Right: Morane 225s of *La Patrouille Weiser* in 1934.
(Musée de l'Air)

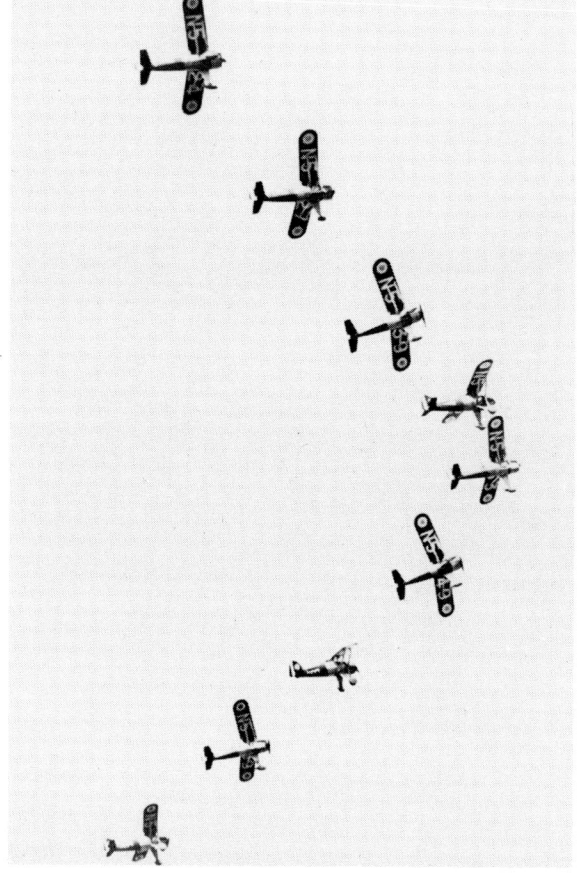

Below: Five Morane 230s of the French Air Force *Patrouille d'Etampes* at the top of a loop in 1939.
(French Air Force).

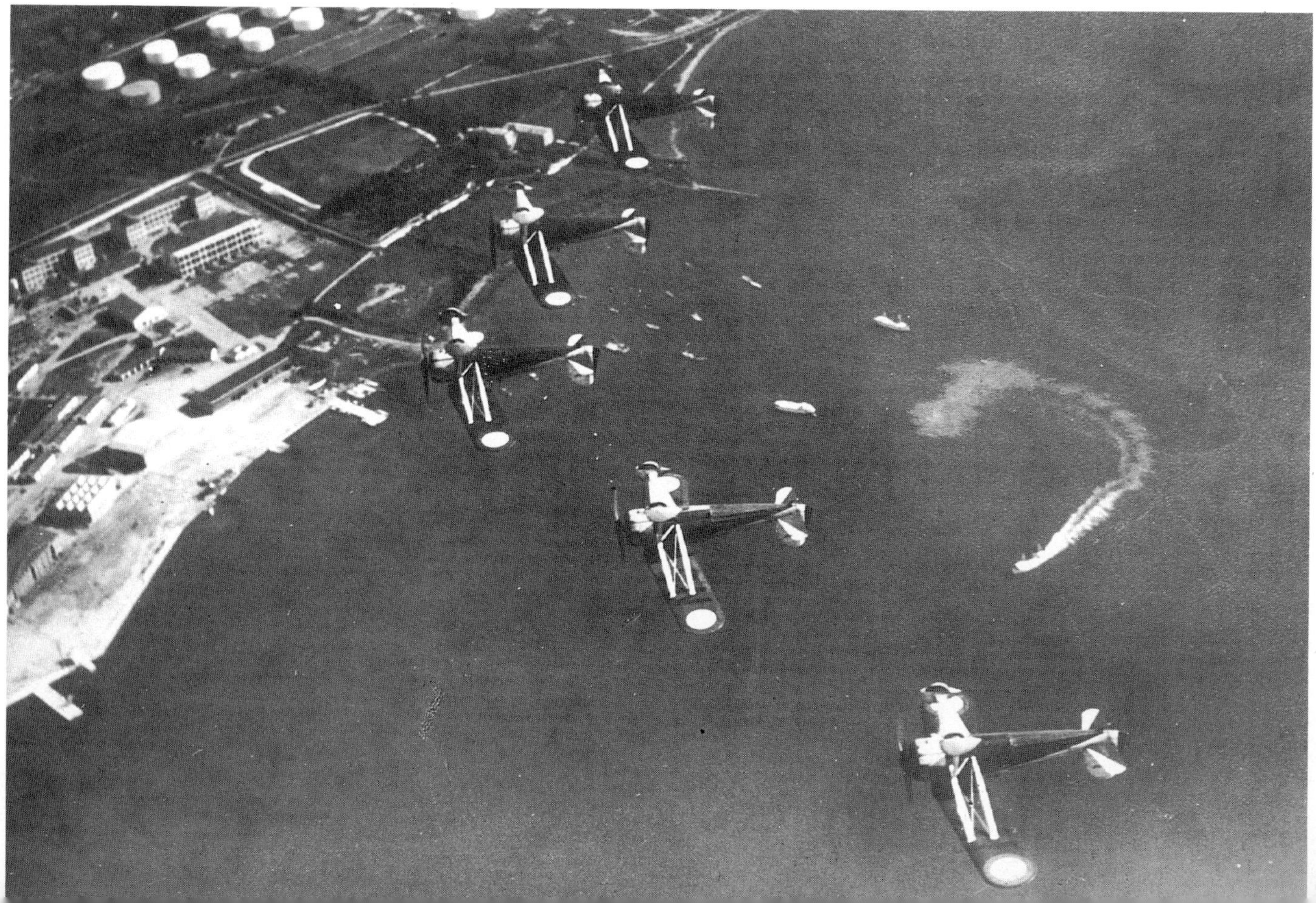

In 1937, *La Patrouille d'Étampes* moved to Salon-de-Provence and became the official team of L'Ecole de l'air. 1946 saw another move for the team, this time to Tours, where they were known as *La Patrouille de Tours*. 1947 saw a return to d'Étampes and the French Air Ministry nominated the team as the official aerobatic team of the French Air Force. In 1948, the team re-equipped with 12 Stampe SV4s and represented the French Air Force at events throughout Europe until 1953, when two jet fighter types were introduced into the Air Force. These were the F-84G Thunderjet and the Vampire, both of which were very suitable for aerobatics. In 1950, at Dijon, Commandant Gautier of 2 Escadre formed a team with Vampires. In 1951, there was also a team from 4 Escadre at Friedrichshafen led by Capitaine Marias. 1952 saw a team of three F-84G Thunderjets from 3 Escadre led by Commandante Delachenal at Reims. This team became the official aerobatic team of the French Air Force and in 1953, *La Patrouille de France* was born. Commandant Delachenal was given the honour of leading the first *La Patrouille de France*. In 1954, it was decided that the French Air Force's official aerobatic team should not only promote the Air Force, but also the French aircraft industry. Therefore, the team should only be equipped with French-built aircraft. The team's title was transferred to 2 Escadre, which operated Dassault Ouragans from Dijon.

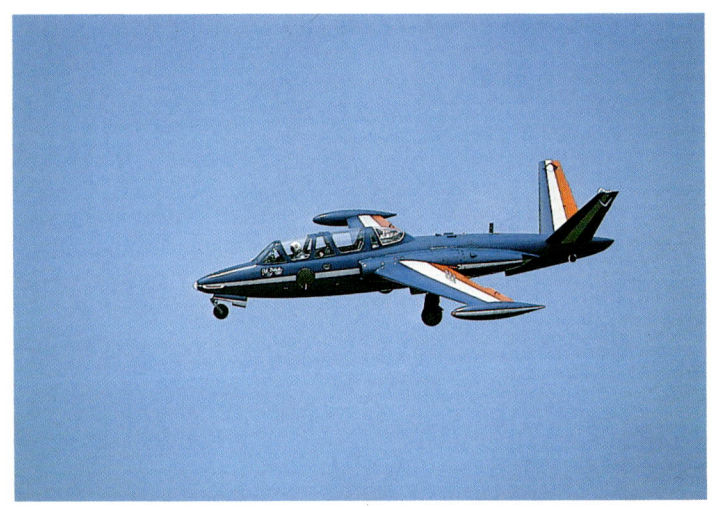

A Fouga Magister of *La Patrouille de France* in the later blue colour scheme landing at Greenham Common, 29 July 1976. (Adrian M. Balch)

Below: Fouga Magisters of *La Patrouille de France* at Biggin Hill, 21 May 1972. (Adrian M. Balch)

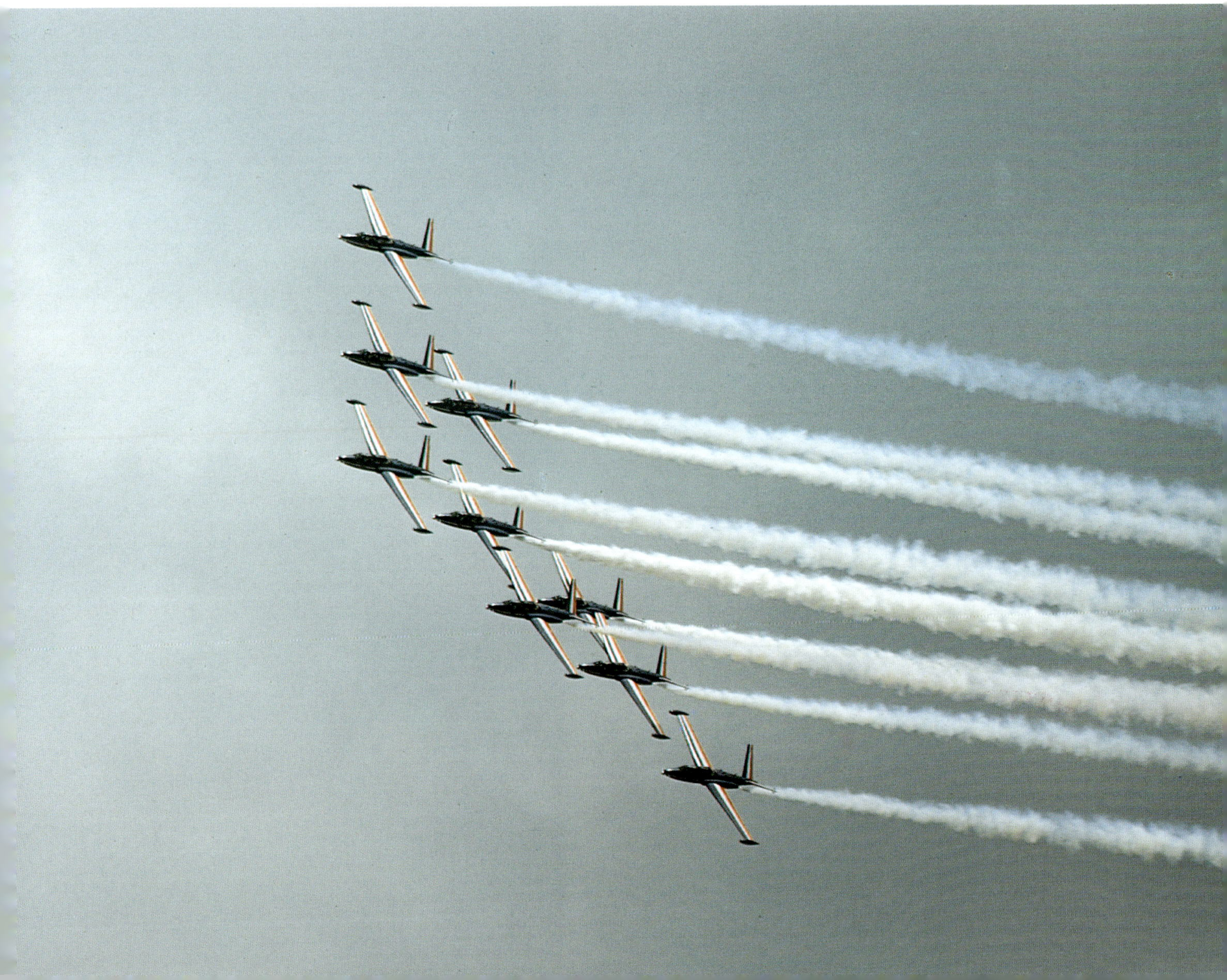

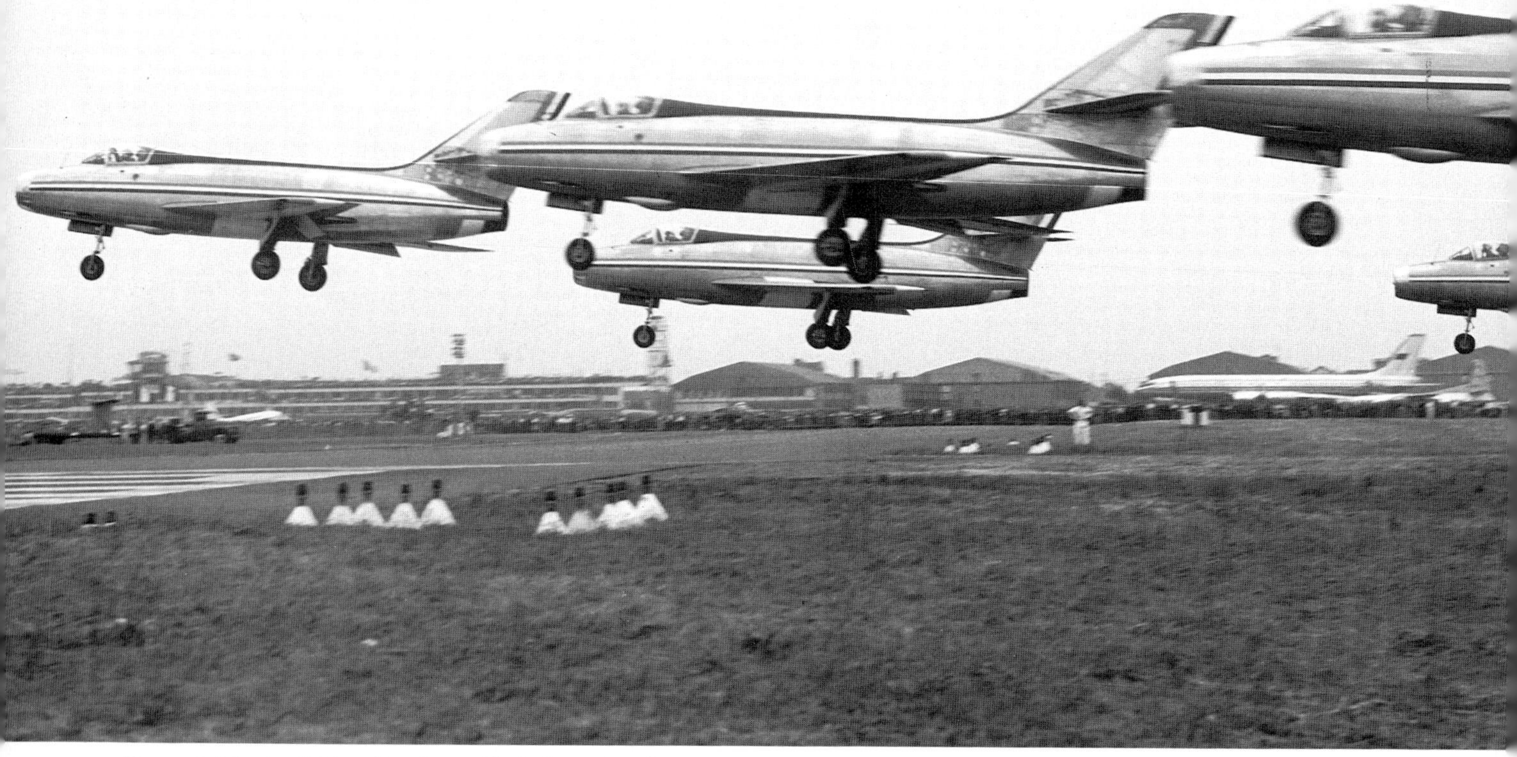

Dassault Mystère IVAs of *La Patrouille de France* landing at Le Bourget during the 1963 Paris Air Show. (French Air Force).

Below: 363:UD heads a line-up of Fouga Magisters of the 1965 French Air Force *La Patrouille de France* team with supporting Noratlas behind. (Peter R. March).

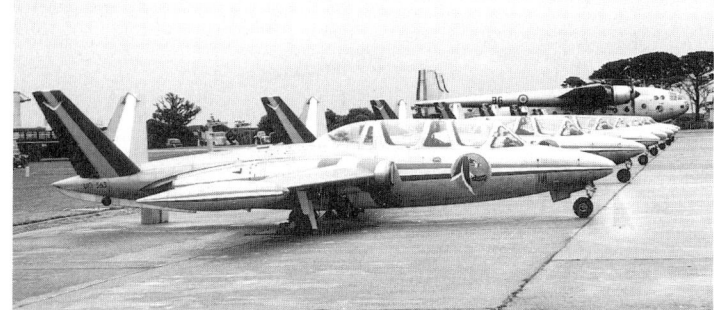

Below: Fouga Magisters of *La Patrouille de France* in the later dark blue colour scheme worn from 1971 to 1980. (French Air Force)

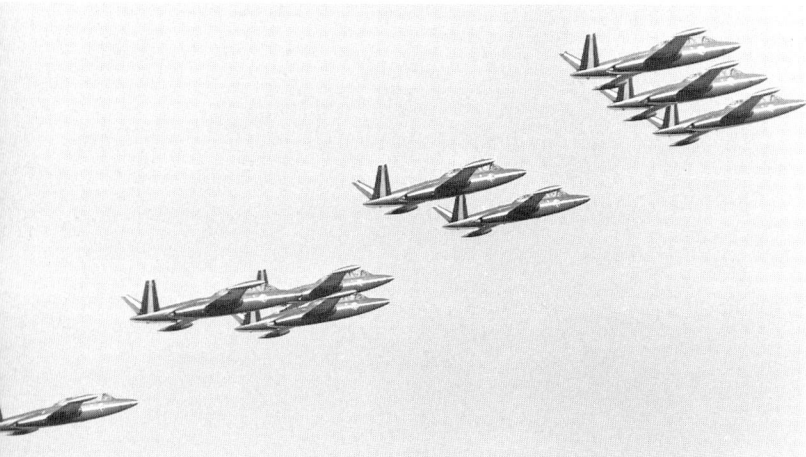

From 1955 to 1963, four squadrons were given the title *La Patrouille de France* in succession. 12 Escadre at Cambrai were the official team with Ouragans in 1955 and with Mystère IVAs in 1956. 4 Escadre held the title in 1956 with Ouragans at Bremgarten, then 2 Escadre at Dijon from 1957 to '61, with Mystère IVAs, flying from seven to twelve aircraft. 7 Escadre at Nancy became *La Patrouille de France* in 1962 and 1963 with seven Mystère IVAs continuing the tradition of the team using French equipment.

In January 1964, due to economy measures, it was decided that *La Patrouille de France* could no longer be represented by fighter aircraft, which were expensive to operate and were needed for other duties. L'École de l'Air, situated at Salon-de-Provence since 1937, was once the home of *La Patrouille d'Étampes* and so it was decided that the team would now fly training aircraft from the School. The French Air Force had operated the Fouga Magister since 1957 and were pleased with the aerobatic qualities of the type. So, in 1964, *La Patrouille de France* came under L'Ecole de l'Air and re-equipped with Fouga Magisters, first six, nine, then eleven aircraft. The aircraft were basically in a natural metal scheme with French tricoloured wings and tails. The fuselage had tricoloured cheat lines, upon which a large badge of L'Ecole de l'Air was painted. In 1971, the natural metal areas were painted dark blue and the team's own badge appeared on the port side of the nose, while that of *L'Ecole de l'Air* appeared on the starboard side of the nose in black and silver stylised form. With eleven Magisters, the team continued in this form until its last display with the Magister on 16th September 1980 at Salon. At this point, the Magisters had flown a total of 60,300 hours, performed 810 displays and had been seen by 20 million spectators.

In 1981, *La Patrouille de France* re-equipped with seven Alphajets, which increased to eight from 1982 to date. The whole aircraft are painted in French blue, white and red tricolours and, like the Magisters, wear the team's badge on the port side of the nose and the badge of L'Ecole de l'Air on the starboard. The aircraft use white or coloured smoke, as required.

Fouga CM170 Magisters used by *La Patrouille de France* 1964-80: 315: FTF-UB, 351:FTF-UG, 352:FTF-UA, 353:FTF-UF, 362:FTF-UG, 363:FTF-UD, 374:FTF-UE, 454:FTF-UH, 455:FTF-UI, 457:FTF-UE, 458:FTF-UF, 487:FTF-UA, 488:FTF-UD, 491:FTF-UB, 492:FTF-UG, 493:FTF:-UJ, 494:FTF-UK, 527:FTF-VA, 529:FTF-VB, 534:FTF-VC, 535:FTF-VD, 536:FTF-VE/F, 541:FTF-VG/VC, 542:FTF-VH, 543:FTF-VI, 544:FTF-VJ, 545:FTF-VK, 546:FTF-VL, 561:FTF-VM, 565:FTF-VP, 576:FTF-VN, 563:FTF-VF, 564:FTF-VO, 562:FTF-VI, 533:FTF-VQ, 538:FTF-VR

Alphajets use by *La Patrouille de France* 1981 to date:
E51/F-TERA/4, E52/F-TERB/6, E53/F-TERC/O, E55/F-TERE/4, E56/F-TERF/8, E57/F-TERG/2, E58/F-TERH/7, E59/F-TERH/7, E59/F-TERI/5, E61/F-TERJ/8, E62/F-TERL/1, E107/F-TERK/3.

The fin codes were applied from 1983, but may change during maintenance. The above list is how the team stood during the 1983-84 seasons.

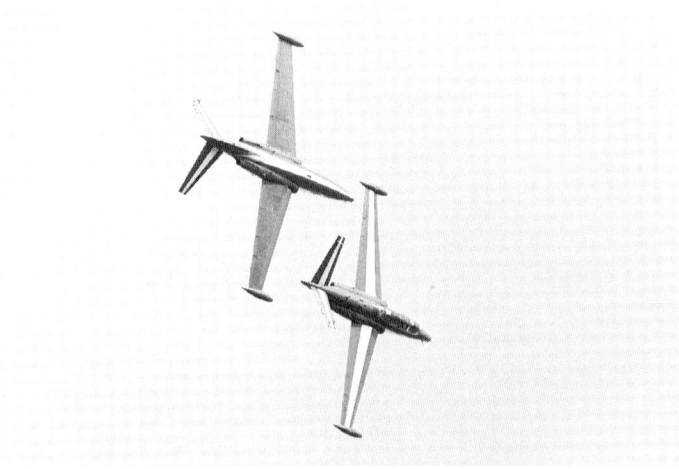

Top: 'Mirror' formation by a pair of Fouga Magisters of *La Patrouille de France.* Note undersides of wings are plain dark blue, while French blue/white/red stripes adorn all tail surfaces and topsides of wings. (French Air Force)

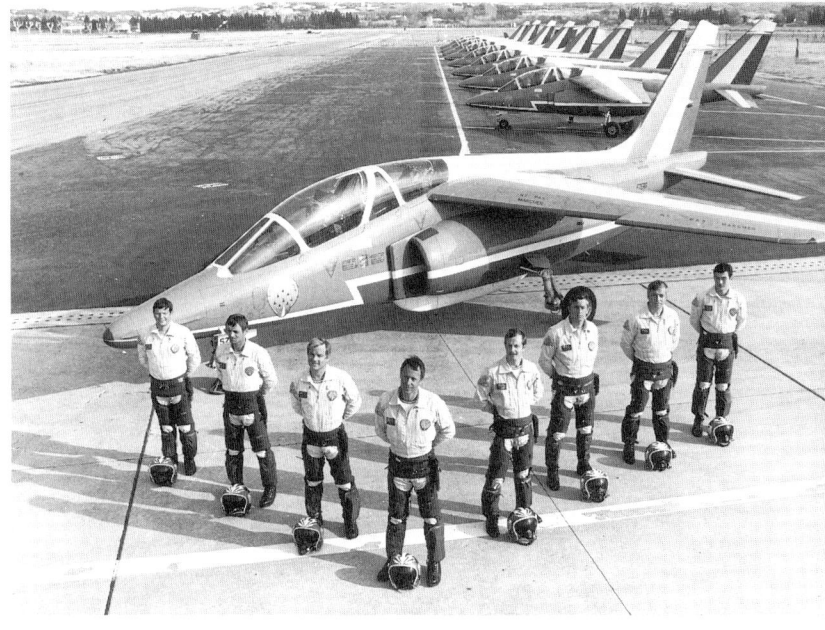

Right: The 1983 *La Patrouille de France* team pose in front of Alpha-jet, 57/F-TERG, at Salon de Provence. (French Air Force)

Below: 'Echelon-Right' formation by Alpha-jets of the current *La Patrouille de France* team, photographed in 1982. (French Air Force)

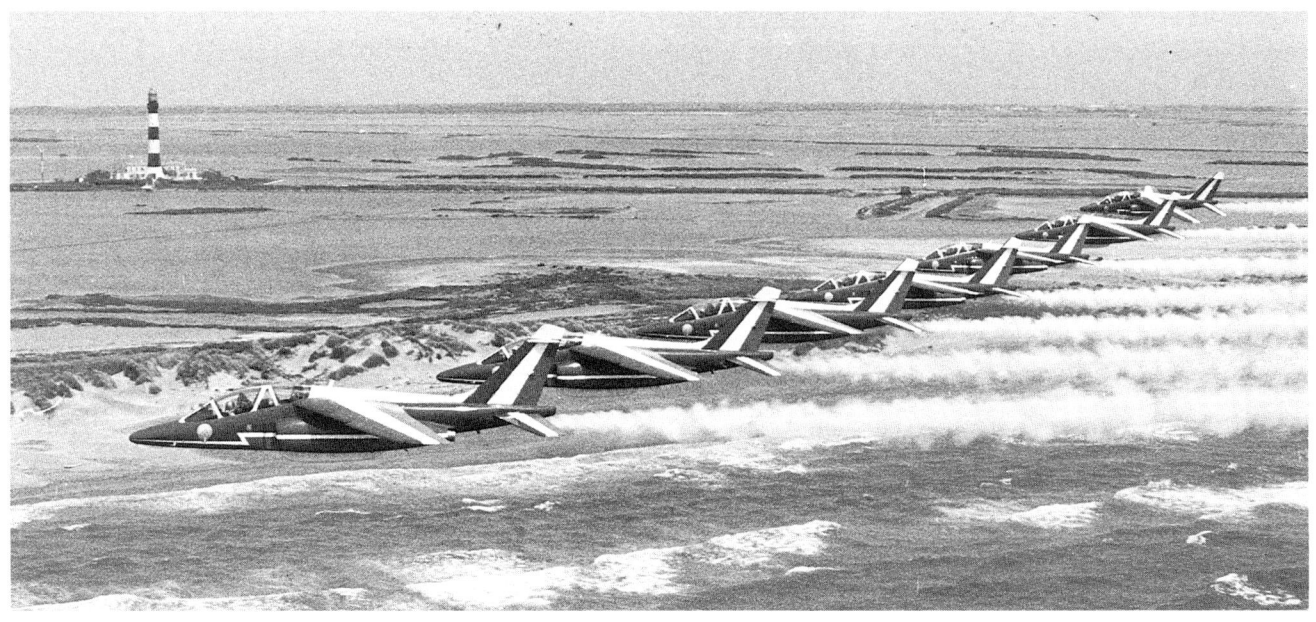

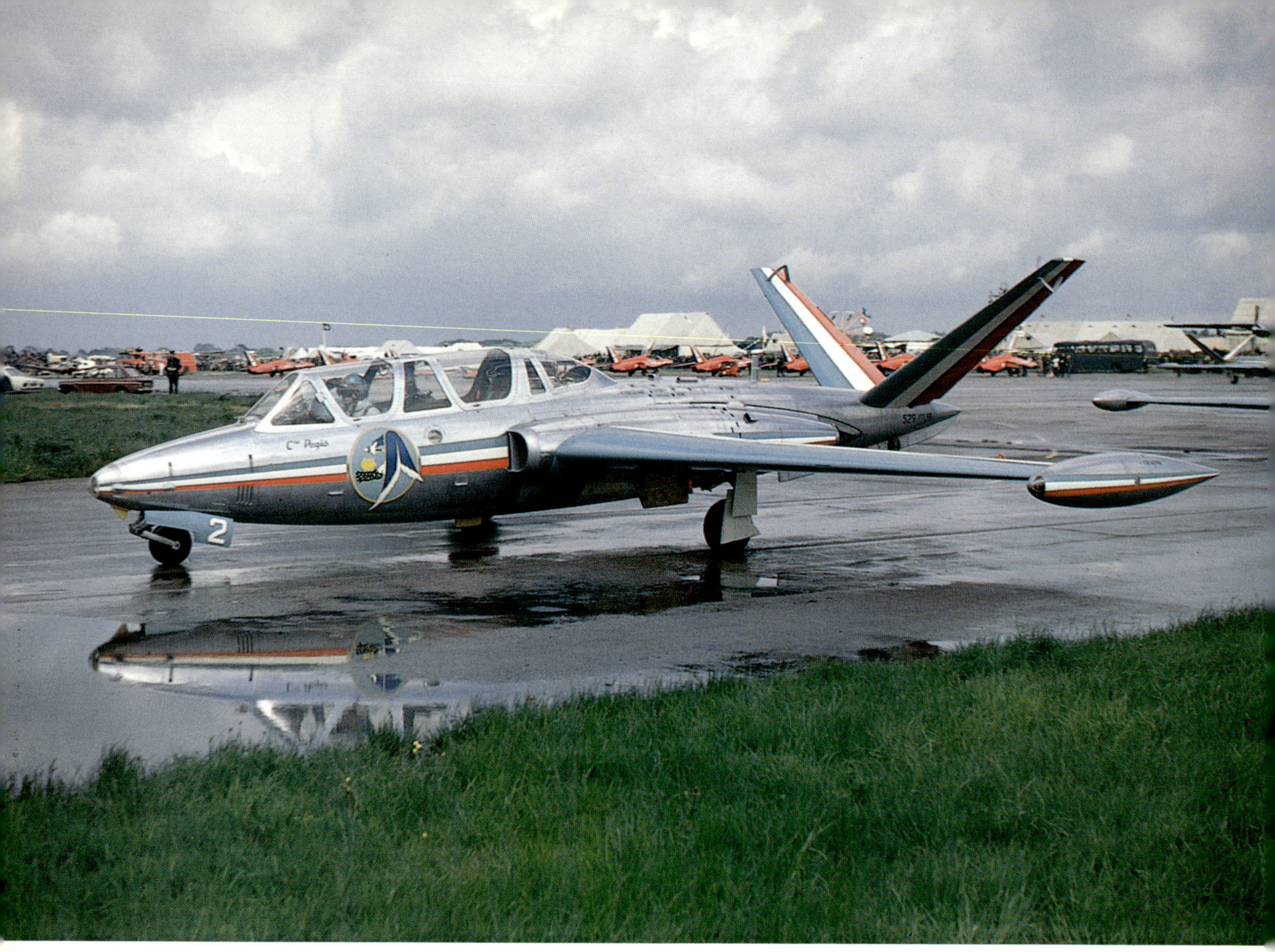

Above: Fouga Magister, 529/FTF-VB, of *La Patrouille de France* seen taxying in at rain-soaked Biggin Hill, Kent, on 18 May 1969 during the Air Fair. Note *Red Arrows* Gnats in the background. (Adrian M. Balch)

Below: E56/F-TERF heads the line-up of *La Patrouille de France* Alphajets at Greenham Common on 28 June 1981. Note silver and black Ecole de l'Air badge appears starboard side only. (Stephen W. D. Wolf)

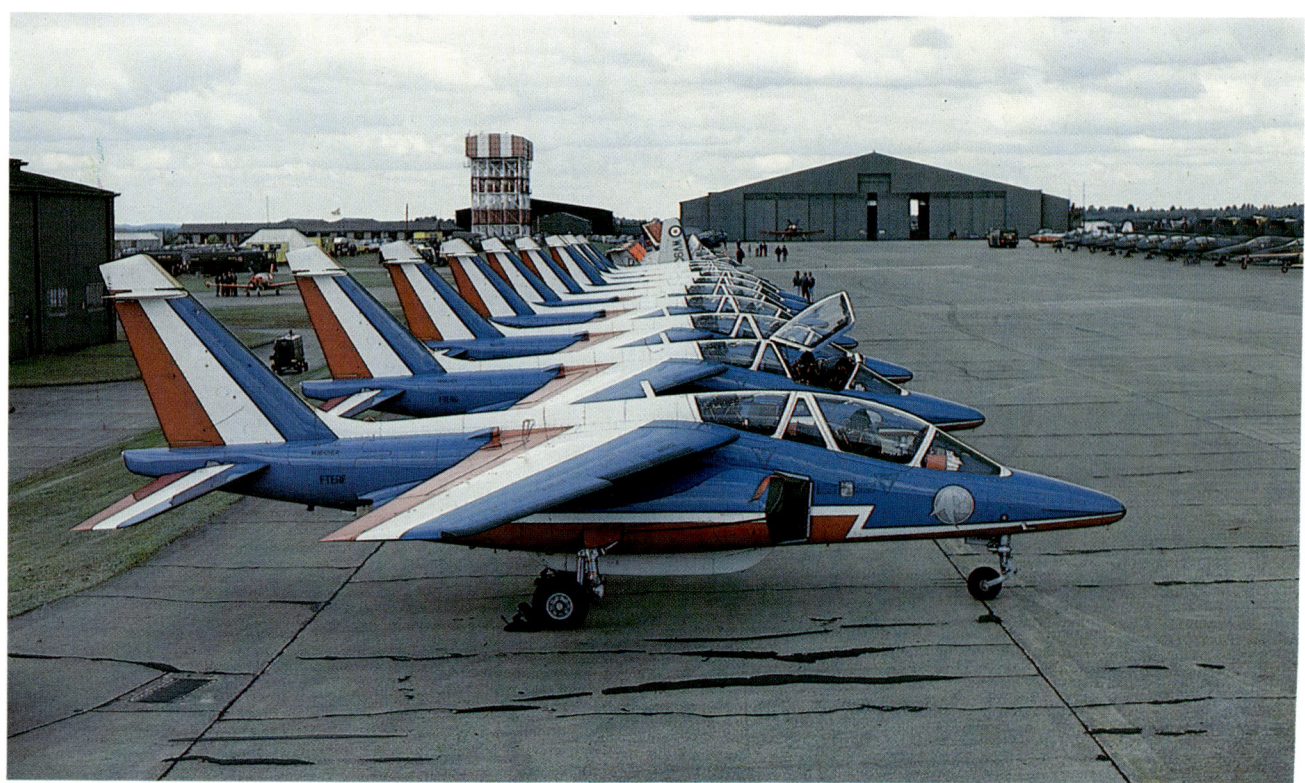

GERMANY – (Federal Republic)
Federal German Air Force — Luftwaffe

Having been heavily involved in two world wars, the German Air Force did not have the time or equipment for aerobatic teams. However, once they had fully re-equipped the Air Force after WWII, several squadron teams were formed in the late 1950s and early '60s.

In 1961, FFS-B (Flugzeugführerschule) at Fürstenfeldbruck, formed a team of four Lockheed T-33As called the *Stocker-team* after their leader. There were four aircraft plus a solo, all equipped to make smoke, which participated in displays during 1961 and '62. The aircraft were natural metal with the undersurfaces being painted in a sunburst scheme of the German national colours — black, red and yellow. One of their T-33s was coded 'AB-748'.

Around the same time, 2/FF-S had a team of four Focke-Wulf-built Piaggio P-149D trainers operating from Diepholz. The aircraft were in the, then, standard training colours of yellow and dayglo, apart from the leader's aircraft, which sported a basically natural metal finish with dayglo-orange fuselage and yellow cheat-line. The underside of the wings was finished in a silver and orange sunburst scheme. This P-149 was coded 'AS-471'.

Meanwhile, over at Landsberg, a team of Fouga Magisters was being formed by FFS-A during 1962. The colour scheme was natural metal overall, with the tail-fins and wingtip tanks painted in German tricolours. A red lightning flash adorned the fuselage and red trim appeared on the wings. One of the team's aircraft was coded 'AA-011'.

Below: The ill-fated team of four F-104F two-seater Starfighters from the German Air Force's WS-10. They are shown here during a display in 1961, but put an end to German display teams after a disastrous accident in 1962. Codes of these aircraft are (left to right). BB+380, BB+386, BB+377, and BB+387.
(Werner Gysin).

A team of four F-104F two-seat Starfighters was formed by WS-10 in 1961 and continued into 1962 until there was a disasterous accident with this team and all aerobatic flying was banned. Since then, there have been no German Air Force aerobatic teams, which is a pity, as this is one of the few European countries that doesn't have an official team to represent its air force at displays.

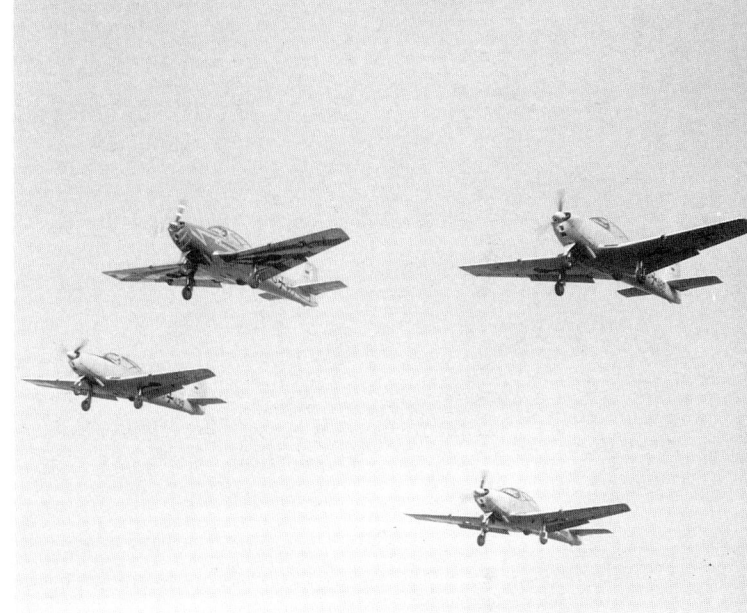

Above: A team of German Air Force P-149D trainers from 2/FFS-S performing at Fürstenfeldbruck in 1961. The aircraft are yellow and orange dayglo, apart from the leader's machine, which is silver and orange dayglo. Codes are AS+471 (leader), AS+439, AS+460 and AS+499. (Werner Gysin).

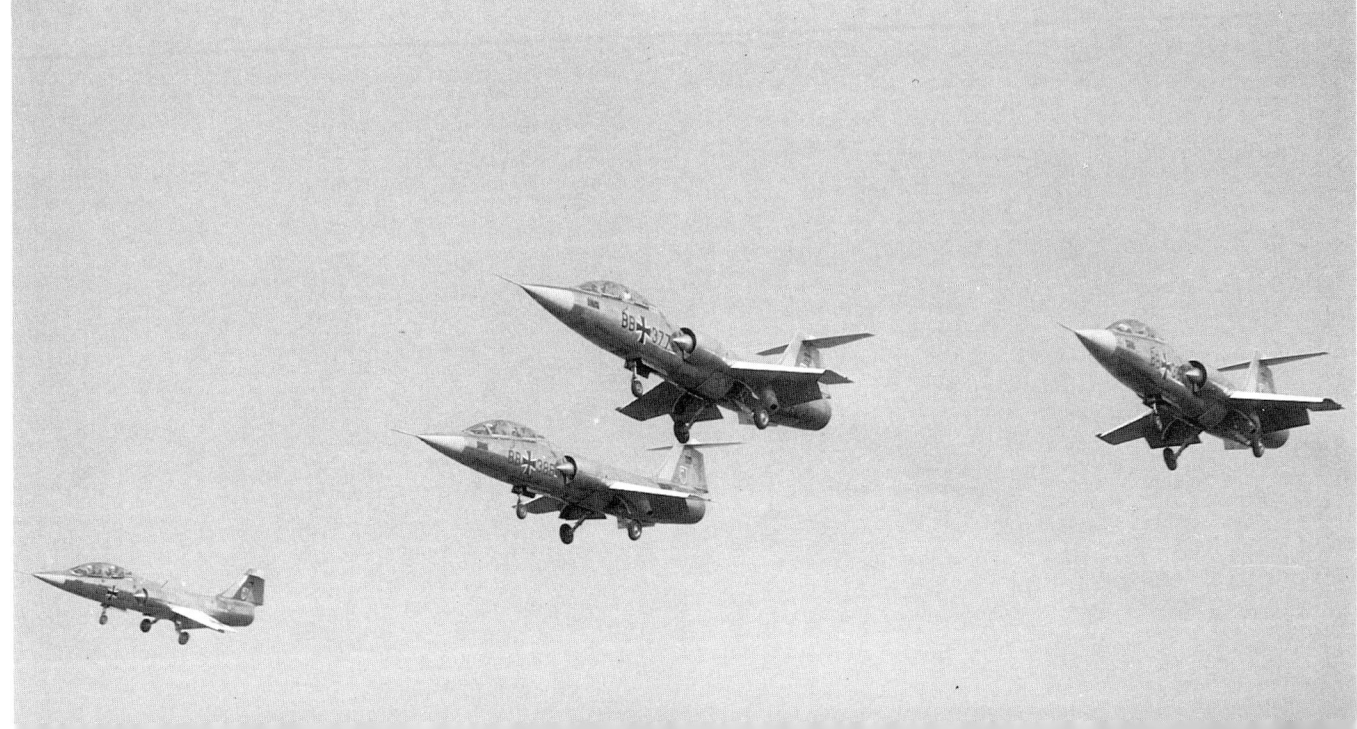

GREAT BRITAIN
The Royal Air Force

Aerobatics have always played a prominent part in Royal Air Force pilot training. They are not performed merely to provide a spectacle for the public, but are an essential step in the making of a pilot, giving him complete confidence in himself and his aircraft. Formation aerobatics give him the added factor of confidence in his leader and other members of the team. In the biplane era, aerobatics were also an important part of air fighting.

Since the first RAF Pageant at Hendon in 1920, formation aerobatics by the old biplanes left over from the First World War have gradually been supplanted by bigger formations and faster aircraft and flying even closer together. The aerobatic displays of the Central Flying School and other RAF units were eagerly awaited items in the Hendon programme and other shows. At the first displays, the CFS provided five Sopwith Snipes, which looped and rolled in formation, all in perfect unison and flew inverted — some of the finest formation flying that had been seen anywhere, laying the foundation for the international reputation which was subsequently established. In 1921, the CFS team of Snipes was led by Squadron Leader C. Draper.

1922 and '23 saw a team of five SE5As from the Royal Aircraft Establishment led by Flight Lieutenant P. W. S. Bulman, who actually had the team spinning in formation!

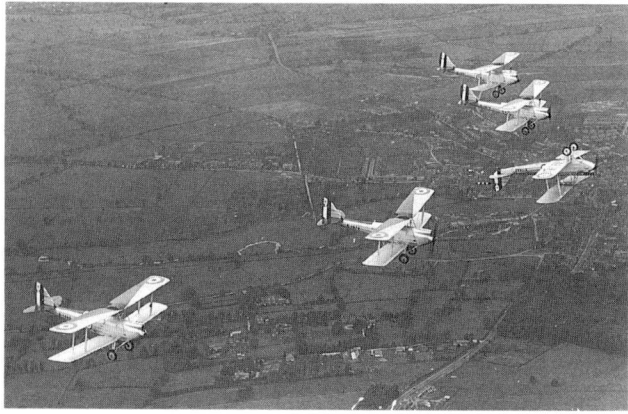

The CFS returned with a team of five Sopwith Snipes in 1924, led by Flight Lieutenant H. H. Down and in 1926, the RAF had a team of nine Gloster Grebes provided by No. 25 Squadron in three formations of three. This team was led by Squadron Leader A. H. Peck, and instructions were given from the ground by wireless and were broadcast so the public could hear them. In 1927, a lighter note was introduced by Siskins of No. 41 Squadron, led by Squadron Leader F. Sowrey. Formation changes and aerobatics were done to the accompaniment of relayed music. That year saw the first of the CFS Genet Moth teams, five being led by Flight Lieutenant D. Greig. New items were introduced, including an outside half-loop, or bunt, and the formation spin was revived.

1928 saw a duo of Avro 504Ks from No. 2 Flying Training School, led by Flying Officer C. H. G. Brembridge, while a second duo of CFS Genet Moths was led by Flying Officer D. A. Boyle.

In 1929, two Gloster Grebes of the Aeroplane and Armament Experimental Establishment, Martlesham, gave a synchronised performance at the Hendon display, and added to the effect of their show by trailing smoke. This duo was led by Flight Lieutenant J. Bradbury and 1929 saw a trio of CFS Genet Moths led by Flight Lieutenant J. S. Chick. The RAF had five display teams in 1930, among which Flight Lieutenant Chick returned with a team of five Gipsy Moths from the Central Flying School. A pair of Siskins from No. 56 Squadron performed synchronised aerobatics led by Flying Officer C. K. Turner-Hughes, while No. 23 Squadron gave a similar display with two Gloster Gamecocks led by Flying Officer McKenna. During 1930, an innovation was provided by No. 43 Squadron, which flew nine Siskins in flights of three with their wings linked by easily breakable cords. Led by Squadron Leader C. N. Lowe, it was a point of pride for the aircraft to land with the cord intact. This year also saw a team of three Grebes at the Hendon display, which were led by Flight Lieutenant D. M. Fleming from the A. & A.E.E. and which trailed coloured smoke to enhance their display.

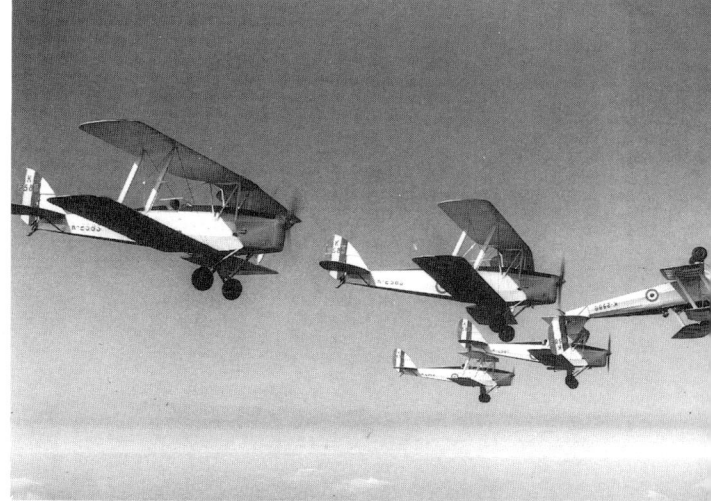

Above: 1932: Tiger Moths of the C.F.S. team, led by Flt. Lt. P. McG. Watt. (Charles E. Brown/RAF Museum).

Above left: Flt. Lt. Embry (inverted) leading the 1931 C.F.S. team of five red and silver Gipsy Moths. (Flight International).

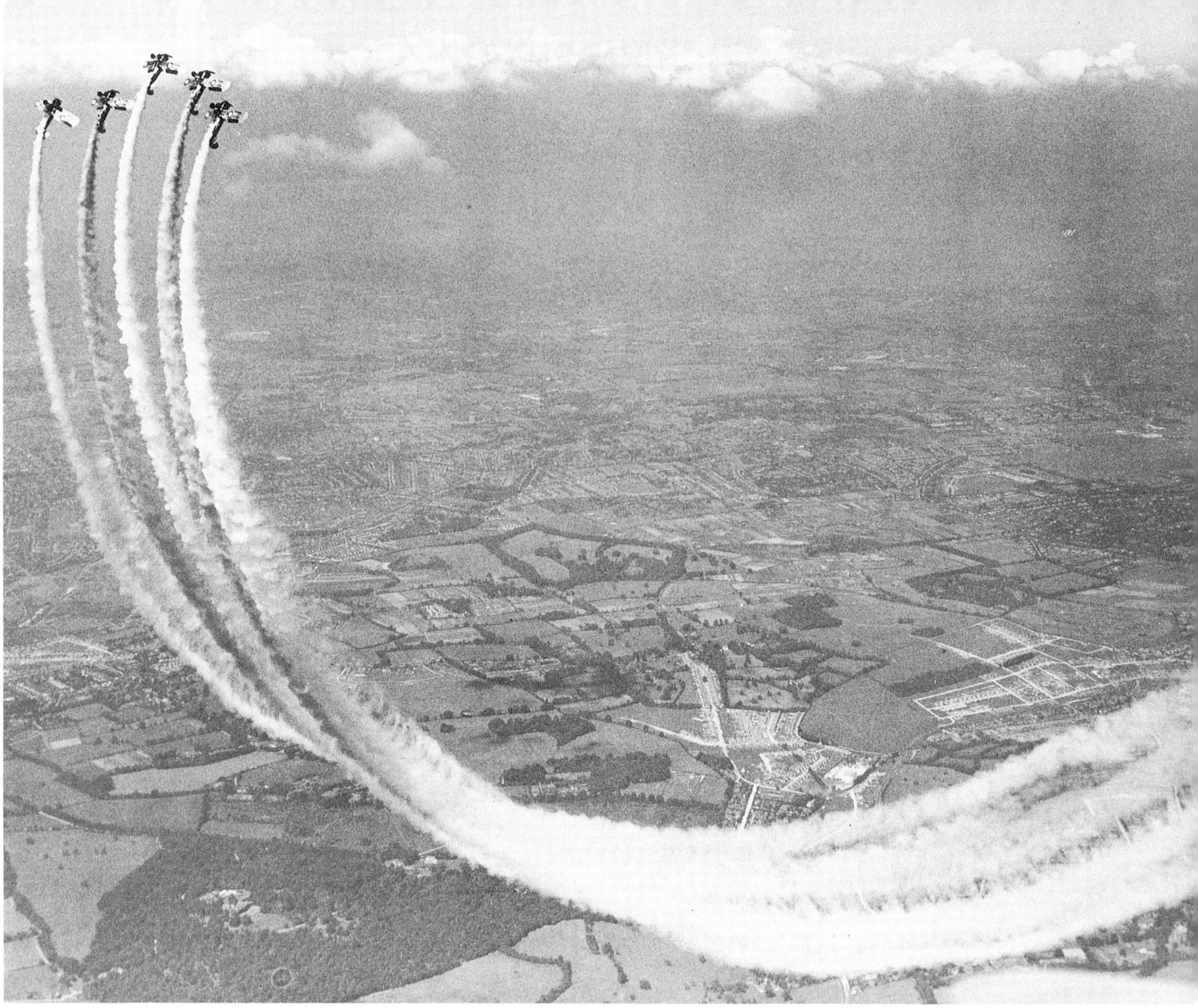

Hawker Furies came into the aerobatics scene in 1931, with a team of three from No. 43 Squadron, led by Flight Lieutenant E. T. Carpenter. That year, the CFS team of five silver Gipsy Moths had red markings on the upper surfaces of the wings, tailplanes and fuselage, so that the spectators could readily see when the aircraft were inverted. Led by Flight Lieutenant B. E. Embry, the Gipsy Moths thus painted included K1878, K1879, K1881, (leader's a/c) and K1883. Flight Lieutenant H. M. Day took over the leadership of No. 23 Squadron's Gamecock duo for the 1931 season.

In 1932, the CFS team comprised five Tiger Moths, which had red and white checkered upper surfaces to the wings and tailplanes. Flying from RAF Wittering, the team was led by Flight Lieutenant P. McG. Watt and the Tiger Moths specially painted included K2583, K2584, K2585, K2586 and K2587. Also in 1932, three Bulldogs from Martlesham appeared for the first time trailing smoke, executing a neat "Prince of Wales feathers" in which the leader, Flight Lieutenant J. Moir, looped and the wing-men half-rolled to either side. No. 1 Squadron had teams with two and three Hawker Furies during 1932 and '33, while No. 25 Squadron revived the tied-together drill in 1933 with nine Furies linked together for the take-off and first part of their display. Led by Squadron Leader A. L. Paxton, the team then deliberately broke into tied flights of three and landed with the remaining cords intact.

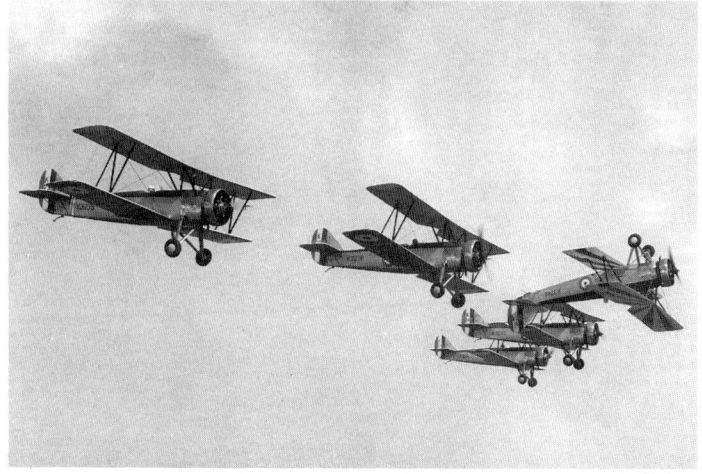

Above: 1933: Avro Tutors of the C.F.S. team led by Flt. Lt. H. A. Constantine. (Charles E. Brown/RAF Museum).

Top: Bristol Bulldog IIAs of No. 19 Squadron, Royal Air Force, going up into a loop with smoke on, while practising for the 1932 Hendon Air Pageant.
(British Aerospace).

35

Bottom: Gloster Gladiators of No. 87 Squadron from Debden in 'tied-together' formation over Villacoublay, France, in 1938. (Charles E. Brown/RAF Museum).

Below: The 1934 C.F.S. team of Avro Tutors led by Flt. Lt. Waghorn showing the red and white wing markings. (Flight International).

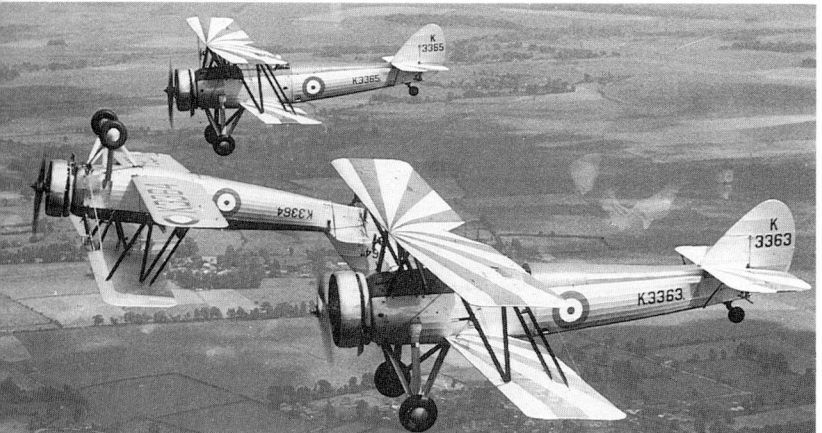

In 1933, the Central Flying School had a team of five Avro Tutors, led by Flight Lieutenant H. A. Constantine, which had their wing and tailplane upper surfaces painted in a red and white 'sunburst' scheme, to show when they were inverted — which was most of the time! The team stayed together for three years and the aircraft specially painted included K3238, K3239, K3240, K3241, K3242, K3363, K3364 and K3365, all being based at Wittering. Apart from the wings and tailplanes, the aircraft were silver overall with the addition of red to the top of the fuselage. For the 1934 season, this team was reduced to three Tutors, led by Flight Lieutenant D. J. Waghorn.

During 1934, there were two Fury teams comprising No. 1 Squadron's pair, while No. 43 Squadron had a team of six aircraft. Bulldogs were a very popular aerobatic mount and the 1934 Hendon display included No. 19 Squadron's five-aircraft team, led by Flight Lieutenant H. Broadhurst, who continued to lead this squadron's team when they re-equipped with Gloster Gauntlets in 1936.

Formation changes during loops were a noteworthy feature of No. 25 Squadron's three-Fury formation of 1935, a performance extrapolated by No. 1 Squadron in 1937 when a fourth aircraft was added 'in the box', flying just far enough below the leader to avoid his slipstream. Led by Flight Lieutenant E. M. Donaldson, this team carried out spectacular displays at low-level, with subtle formation changes, given at Hendon, Zurich and elsewhere. The leader's aircraft was K5673, while the other three Furies often comprised K2881, K2043 and K2039.

With the introduction of monoplanes to the RAF and changes in air tactics, it became no longer necessary to teach aerobatics as part of air fighting, although they still formed, as they form today, part of training to induce in the pilot absolute confidence in his aircraft and enable him to master it in any situation. The RAF reached the peak of perfection with biplane aerobatics, the last biplane teams consisting of two trios of Gauntlets from Nos. 17 and 151 Squadrons in 1938, together with a trio of Gladiators from No. 87 Squadron. The latter team revived the tied-together display using K8027 (Sqn. Ldr's. aircraft), K7967 and K7972. Also in 1938, No. 43 Squadron had a team of six Furies led by Pilot Officer F. Rosier.

The Second World War deprived spectators from seeing many interesting types of aircraft in formation aerobatics, but in 1947 the RAF's first jet team of three Vampires, led by Squadron Leader M. Lyne, was provided by the Odiham Fighter Wing. In 1948 No. 54 Squadron, led by Squadron Leader R. W. Oxspring, demonstrated its team of six Vampires before a highly appreciative audience in the USA and Canada.

Vampires were flown by the teams up to 1950, by which time No. 72 Squadron, led by Squadron Leader D. Kingaby, was flying seven aircraft. No. 54 Squadron, led by Flight Lieutenant H. Bennett, provided a five-Vampire team, the first RAF jet formation team to trail smoke. This team participated in the 1950 Farnborough Air Show.

Meteor teams began coming in after the Vampires, which included No. 600 Squadron, who had a team of six led by Flight Lieutenant K. N. Haselwood. No. 64 Squadron had a team of five Meteors from 1952 to '54 led by Flight Lieutenant H. Bennett and this was one of several teams flying at the time. 1952 saw the first team to be officially given a name. From here on, each team has been given its own heading.

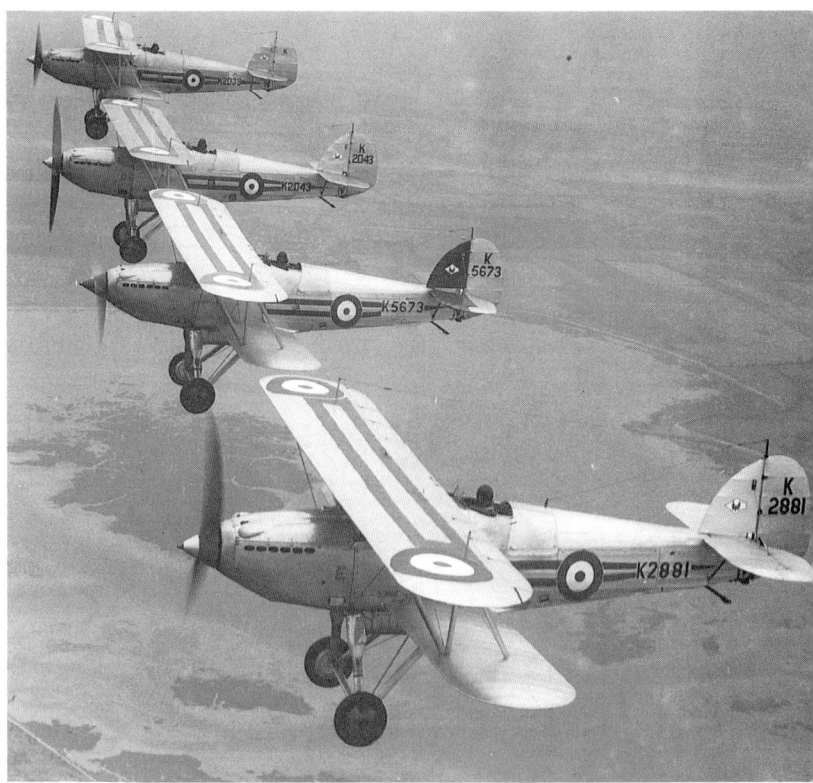

Top: 1937: The four-Fury formation of No. 1 Squadron, led by Flight Lieutenant E. M. Donaldson. (RAF Museum/Charles E. Brown)

Right: One of the first Royal Air Force jet aerobatic teams was provided by No. 54 Squadron in 1948 with five Vampires. They were the first RAF jet team to trail smoke and are seen here performing at Farnborough in Sept. 1950. (Flight International).

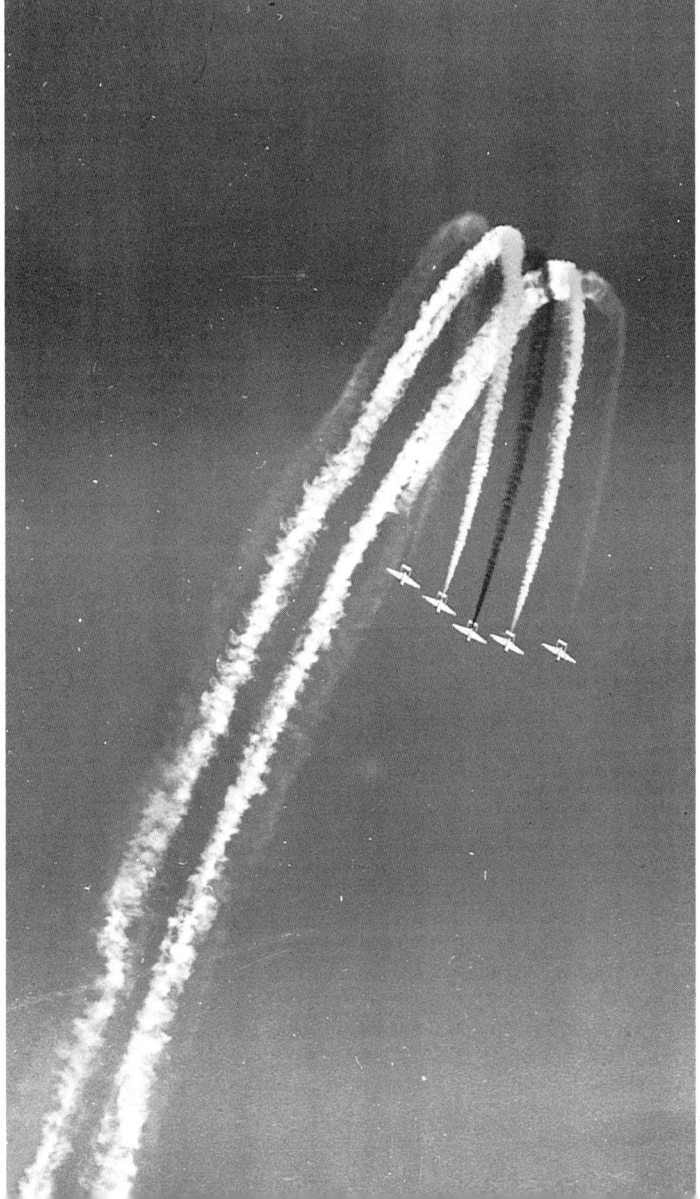

1952: Central Flying School, "The Meteorites", RAF Little Rissington, Gloucestershire.

This was the first RAF team to be given a name, flying four Meteor T.7s from Little Rissington, Gloucestershire. Led by Flight Lieutenant C. R. Gordon during 1952, the Meteors were in the standard training colour scheme of silver overall, before yellow training bands were added to the wings and fuselage. The aircraft used were usually drawn from WA615, WA691, WF852, WH241 and WG962. The team was disbanded after the 1953 season.

Squadron Leader H. Bennett led No. 64 Squadron's team of five Meteor F.8s in 1953 and 1954, and in 1955 the first Hunter aerobatic team appeared when No. 54 Squadron had a four-aircraft formation.

1956: No. 54 Squadron, "The Black Knights", RAF Odiham, Hampshire.

After flying a season of displays un-named, the pilots of No. 54 Squadron's team were given black flying suits and thus the team were called *The Black Knights*. Flying four Hunter F.1 fighters, the team was led by Captain R. G. Immig — a USAF exchange officer. The aircraft retained their standard camouflage colours of gloss grey and green camouflage with silver undersurfaces. The squadron's blue/yellow checks appeared on the nose and the leader's aircraft had a blue fin with a yellow lightning flash through the fin flash. The 'slot' aircraft had the tail colours reversed, being yellow with a blue lightning flash. These tail markings were not thought to be specially applied for the team, as they denoted Flight Commanders' aircraft. Aircraft used were usually WW636, WT659, WT696 and WT692.

Opposite: Hunter F.1s of No. 54 Squadron, *The Black Knights* in 1956. Note lead aircraft (WW636) has dark blue fin with yellow lightning flash and rear aircraft (WT692) has reverse scheme on fin. (H.S.A.).

Below: The Meteorites — Meteor T.7s, WH241 and WA691 with Flt. Lt. C. R. Gordon inverted in WF852 leading this C.F.S. team in 1952. (M.o.D.).

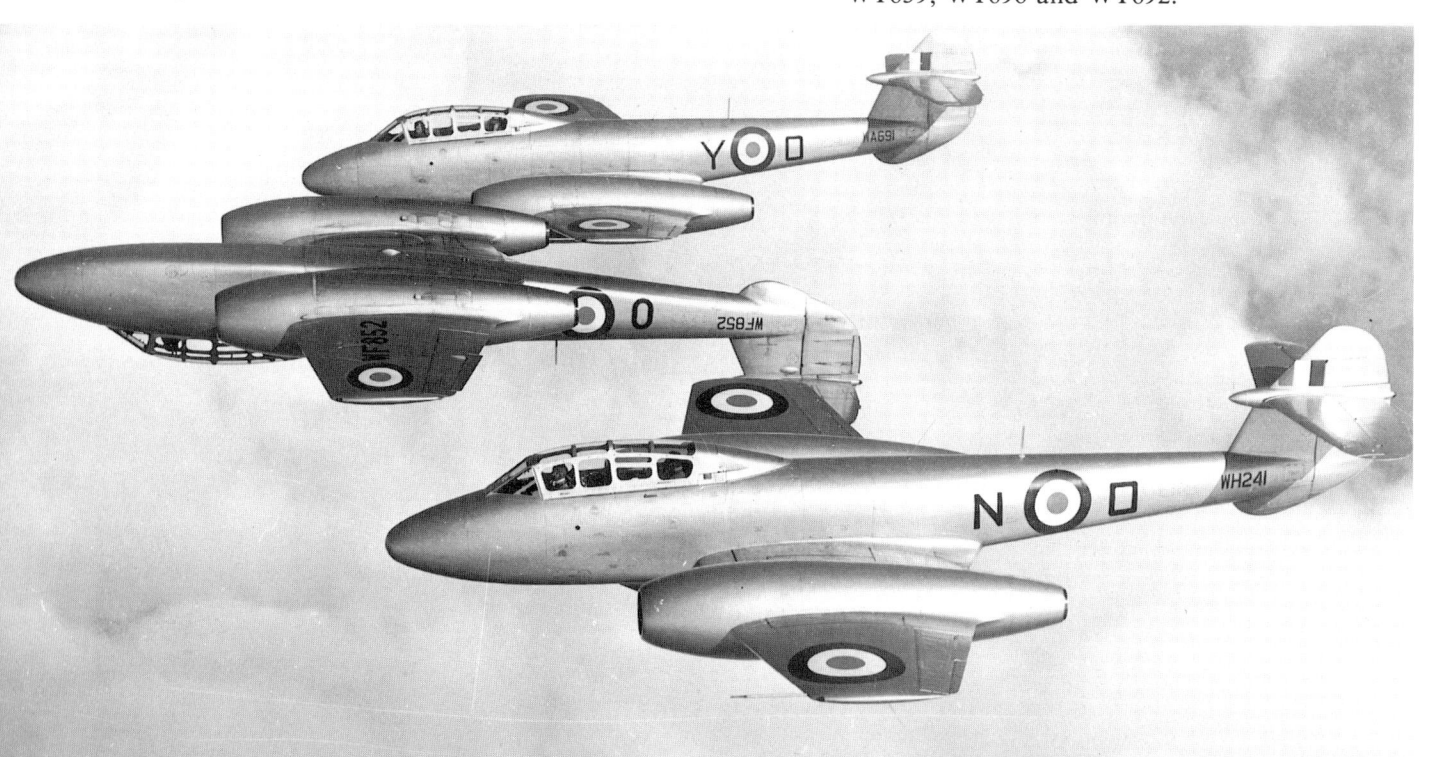

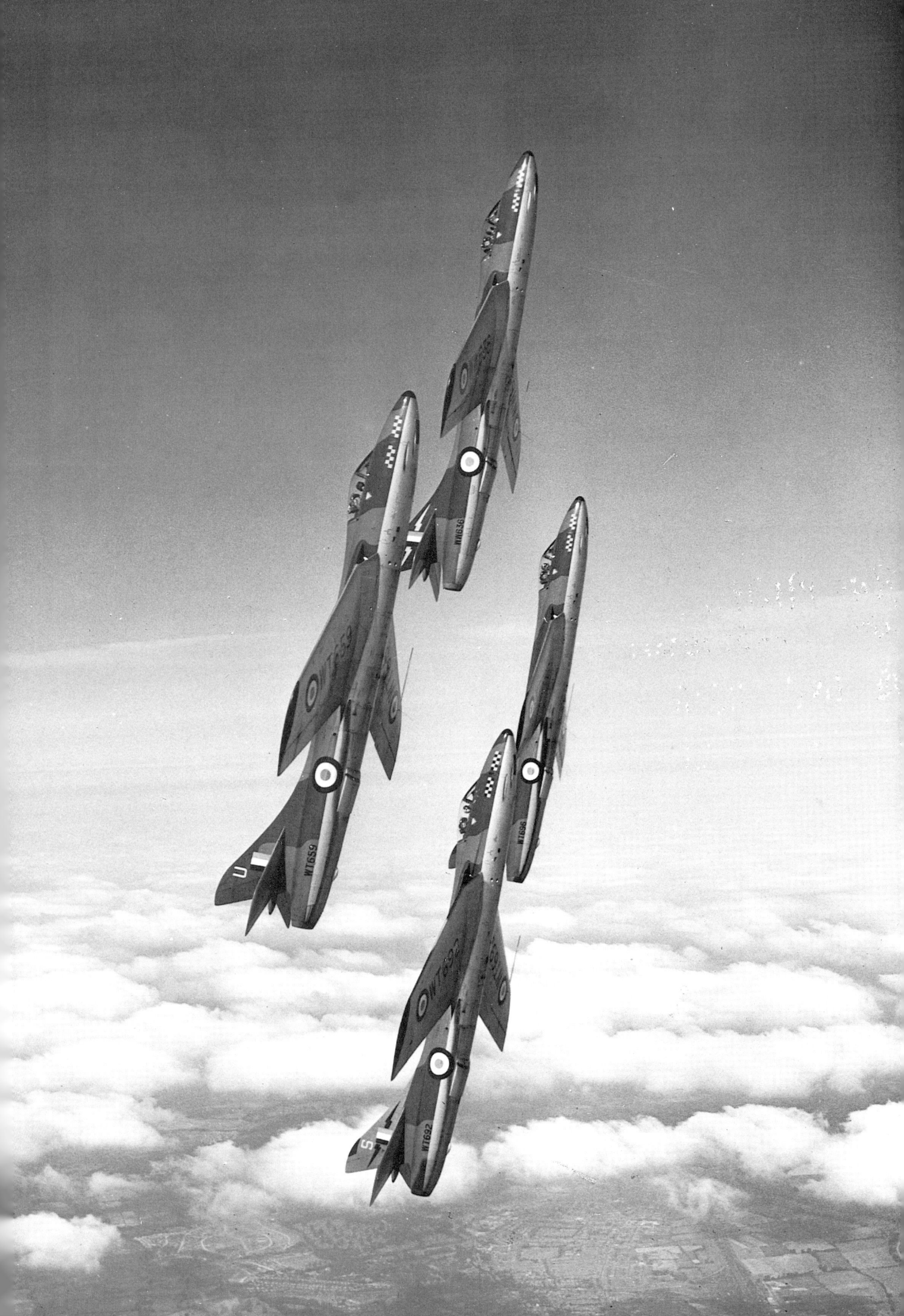

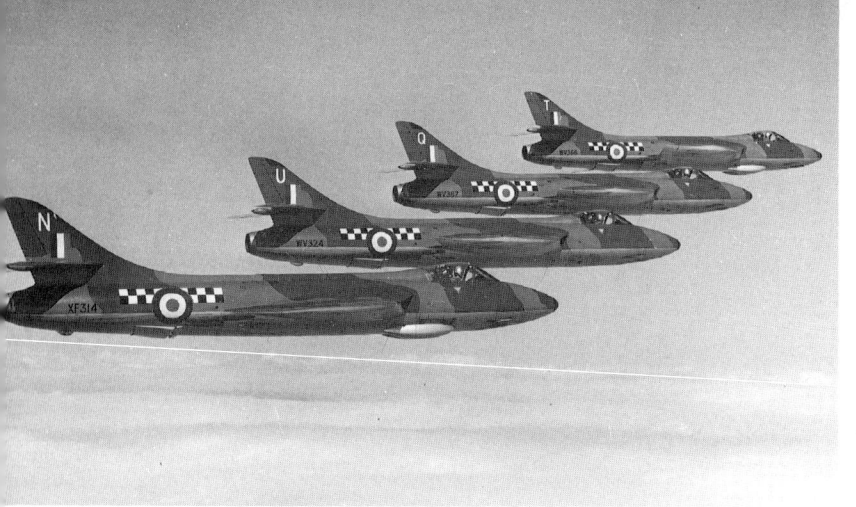

Above: The Fighting Cocks — Hunter F.1s of No. 43 Squadron, led by Flt. Lt. P. Bairsto from Leuchars in 1956. (M.o.D.).

1956: No. 43 Squadron, "The Fighting Cocks", RAF Leuchars, Fife.

1956 also saw the introduction of No. 111 Squadron's team, four Hunters being led by Squadron Leader R. L. Topp, and of No. 43 Squadron's *The Fighting Cocks,* led by Flight Lieutenant P. Bairsto. Both teams used aircraft painted in standard camouflage colours, *The Fighting Cocks* wearing No. 43 Squadron's black/white checks on the rear fuselage. The team's name was derived from the squadron badge, which depicts a fighting cockerel and the four aircraft were not specially picked from the squadron's allocation.

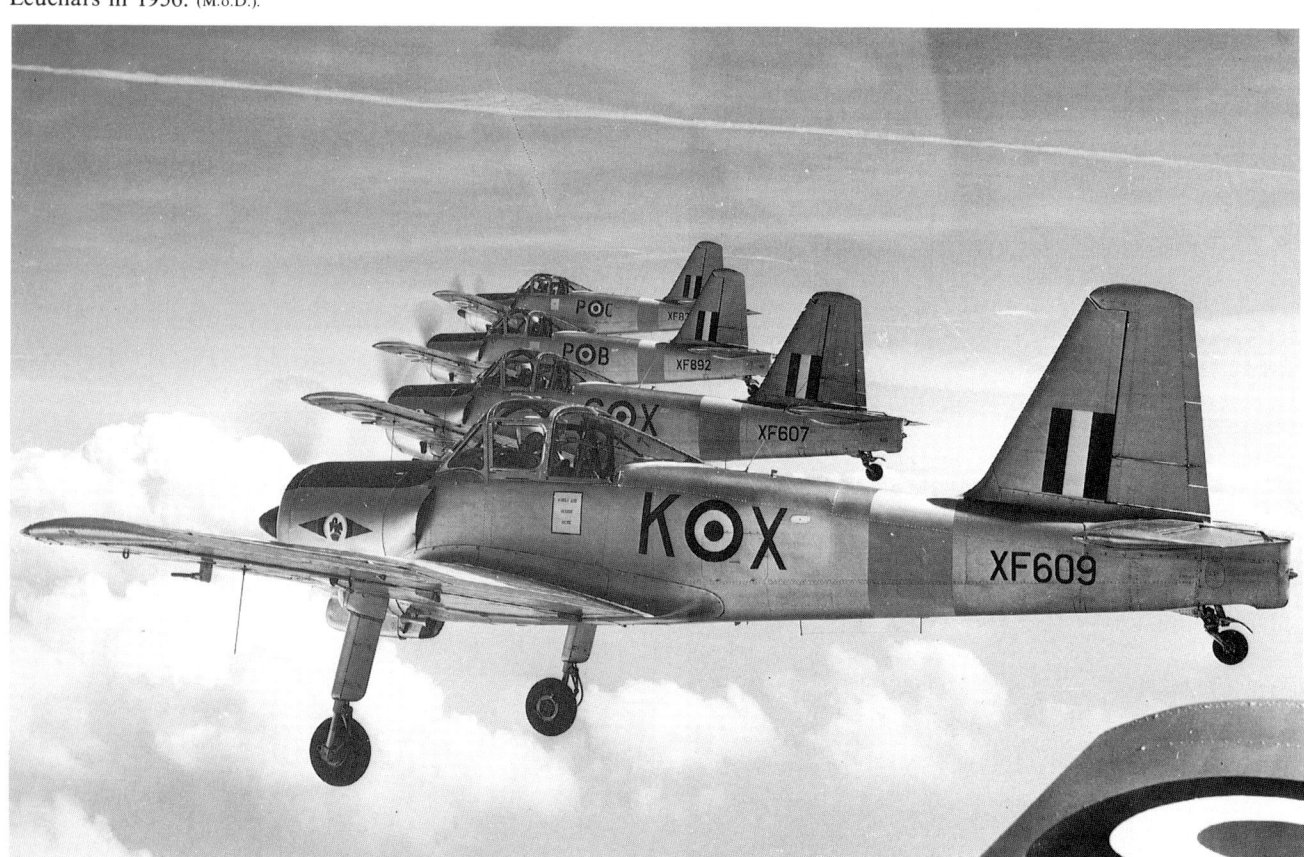

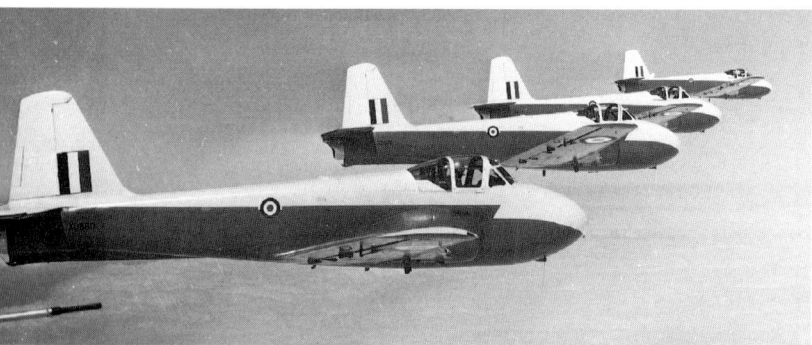

Above: The Sparrows were equipped with four Jet Provost T.1s in 1958, led by Flt. Lt. N. H. Griffin of C.F.S. Nearest aircraft is XD680. (M.o.D.).

Above Middle: The Sparrows — four C.F.S. Hunting Provost T.1s led by Flt. Lt. J. H. Kingsbury from Little Rissington in 1957. (M.o.D.).

1957: Central Flying School, "The Sparrows", RAF Little Rissington, Gloucestershire.

The CFS continued to form teams and in 1957 *The Sparrows* flew four Hunting Provosts led by Flight Lieutenant J. H. Kingsbury. This team participated in the 1957 SBAC display at Farnborough and used four aircraft drawn from: XF607, XF609, XF837, XF892 and XF895. The colour scheme was silver overall with standard yellow training bands on wings and fuselage.

The following year, 1958, the team re-equipped with the long-undercarriaged Jet Provost T.1 and were led by Flight Lieutenant N. H. Griffin, both teams flying from Little Rissington, Gloucestershire. Colour scheme was white upper surfaces and red undersides, divided by a thin pale blue cheat line. Serial numbers appeared in minuscule black numerals on the rear fuselage only, the aircraft being drawn from XD675 to XD680.

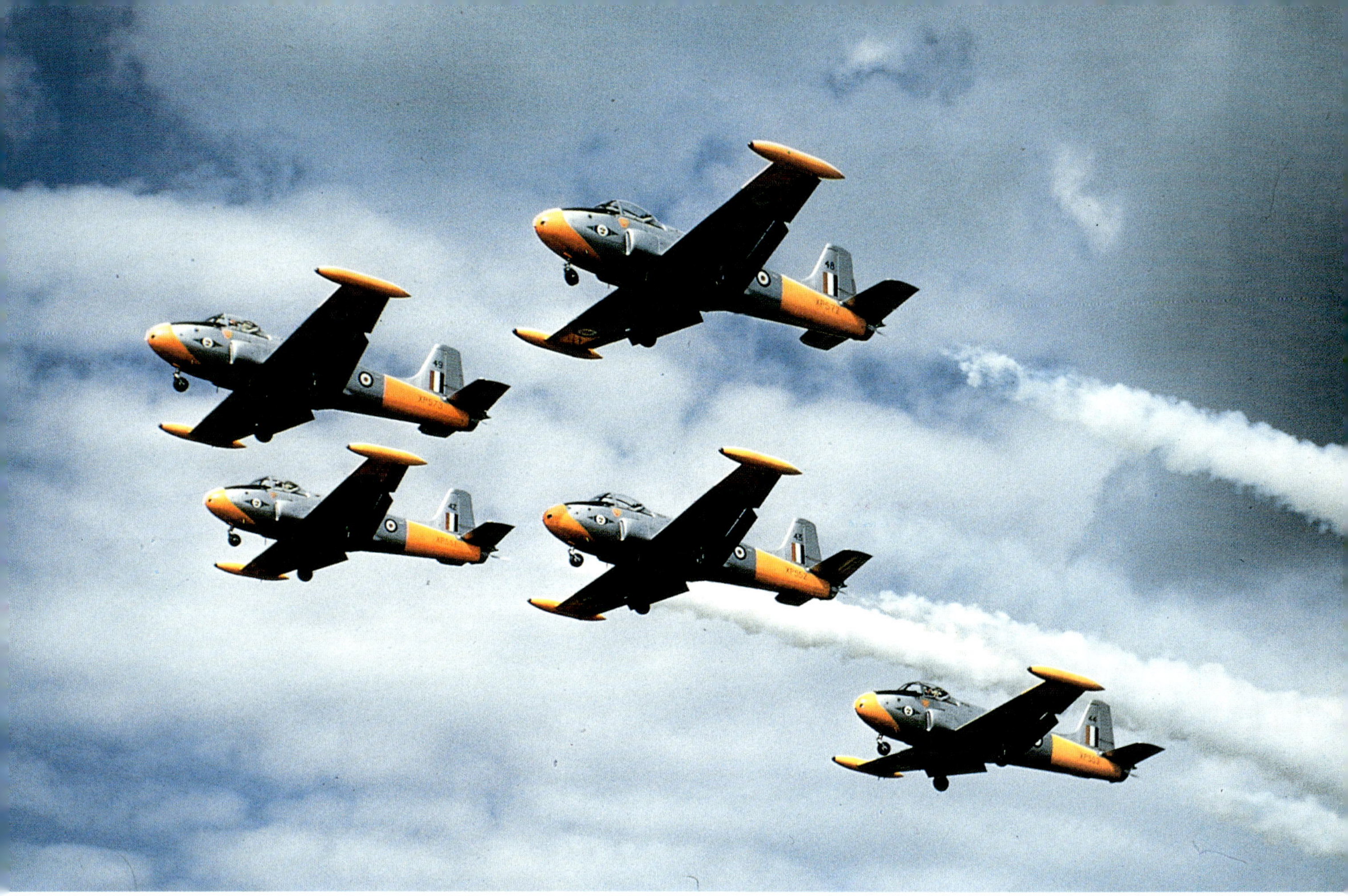

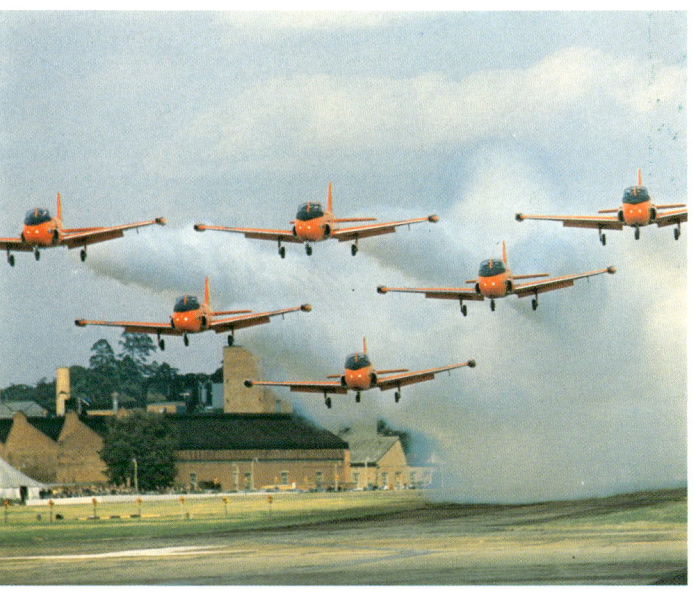

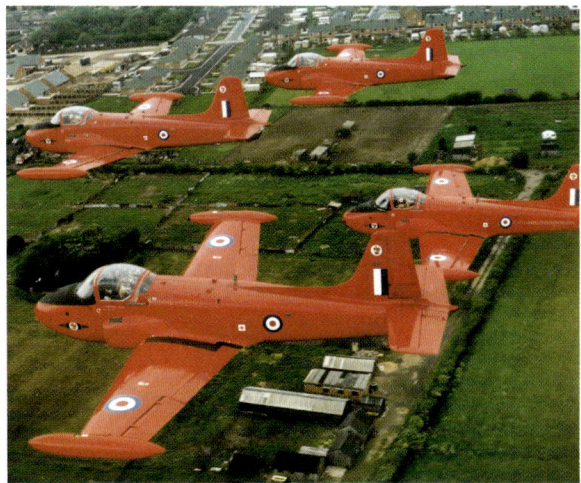

1957-60: No. 111 Squadron, "The Black Arrows", RAF North Weald, then Wattisham.

'Treble-One' provided the premier RAF team in 1957, and for the first time Hunters bore a special aerobatic colour scheme, having an all-black finish. This team started as a flight of four in 1956, led by Squadron Leader R. L. Topp and was the only Hunter team to be retained in 1957, when the formation was made up to seven, then to nine Hunter F.6s under the same leader. In this form, the team appeared in the 1957 SBAC display at Farnborough. Something of a sensation was caused by a formation loop and roll by nine aircraft, which had not been seen since the old biplane days. New manoeuvres and formations were added each year and in 1958 came the 'bomb-burst', the aircraft breaking formation at the end of a loop, trailing smoke, and pulling out in different directions.

Above: All dayglo-red Jet Provost T.4s of the C.F.S. *Red Pelicans* come in for a formation landing with smoke at Farnborough in September 1964. (Rolls-Royce)

Above left: Jet Provost T.4s of the C.F.S. *Red Pelicans* in the later postbox-red scheme, applied during the 1966-69 period. (British Aerospace)

Top: 5 Jet Provost T.4s of the C.F.S. *Pelicans* in formation over Farnborough, September, 1962. (D. W. J. Cross)

In 1958, the team was increased to sixteen aircraft, but the most noteworthy performance by *The Black Arrows* was the celebrated 22-Hunter loop seen during the 1958 Farnborough display week in September of that year. Still led by Squadron Leader Topp, the display began with the 22 Hunters being looped twice. After the six outside aircraft peeled off, the remaining sixteen were rolled. Following a nine-aircraft loop, they performed a bomb-burst, then five aircraft reformed to carry out several close formation passes. For the 22-Hunter loop, eight Hunters were borrowed from other squadrons, which retained their camouflage colours. This feat was quite remarkable, in view of the perfect timing and positioning of the Hunters, flying at about 400 mph and only 4 feet apart at times. This is the maximum number of aircraft ever looped together to date, the previous record being held by the Pakistan Air Force with 16 F-86F Sabres.

The Squadron was stationed at North Weald, Essex, but moved to Wattisham towards the end of 1958. It was at this time that Squadron Leader P. A. Latham, took over command of No. 111 Squadron and the team held the premier position until the end of 1960. The team then disbanded and No. 111 Squadron re-equipped with the Lightning F.1.

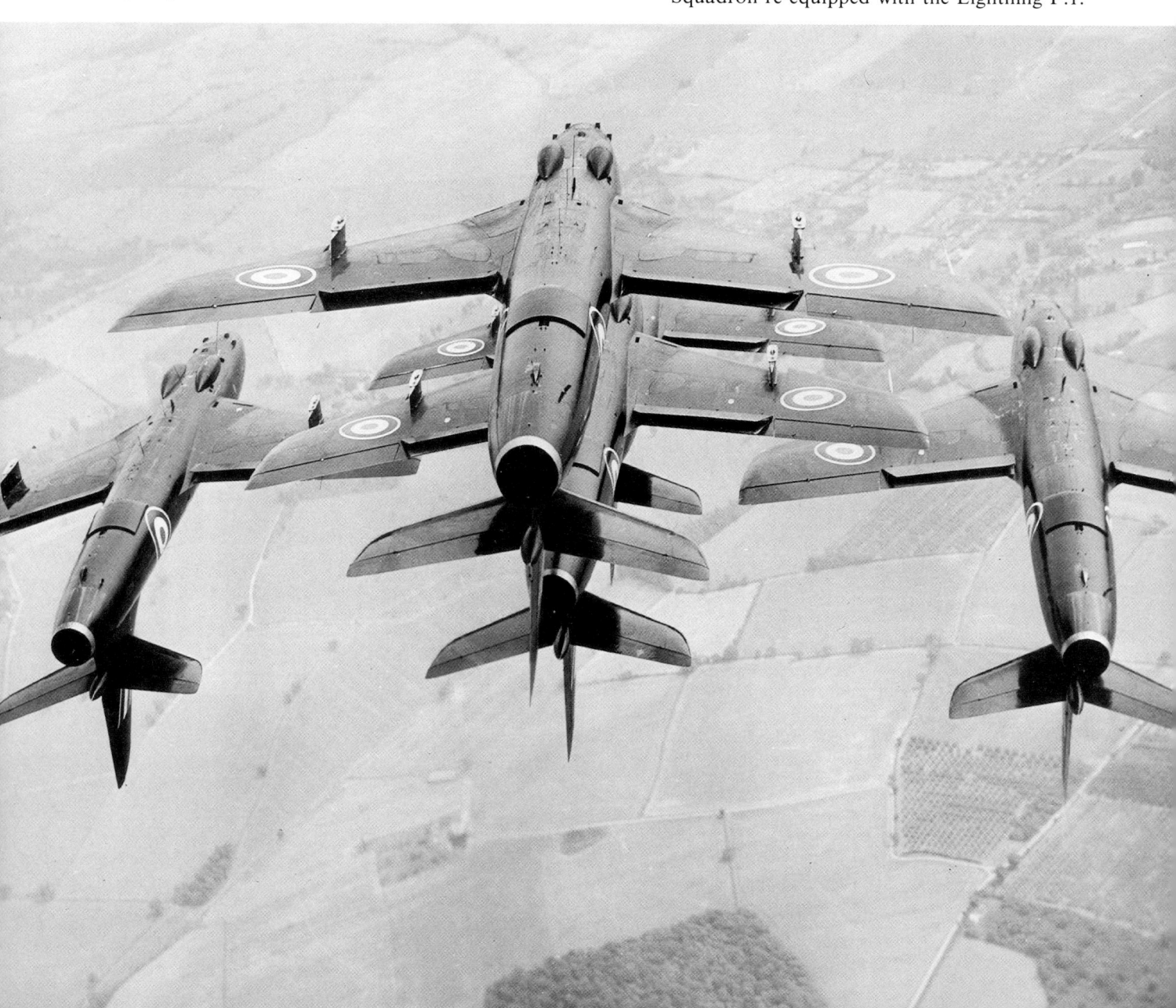

Below: Hunter F.6s of the *Black Arrows* at the top of a loop early in 1960. (via W. T. Larkins)

The overall gloss black colour scheme was derived from several little-known paint scheme experiments, which were tried out on the Hunters. Firstly, there were trials with a huge arrow-like cheat line the entire length of the fuselage, initially red then yellow. Another scheme tried was the painting of the wings and tailplane all-yellow, the trials aircraft also wearing a striking yellow arrow insignia for a time. Next, a Hunter was painted red overall with huge white letters 'RAF' painted on its underside — we nearly had the *Red Arrows* eight years early! Another less exciting scheme was a black Hunter with a white arrow painted on the underside of its fuselage from the tip of the nose to the end of the jet pipe. But, in the end, the more sober overall black finish prevailed. From 1958 onwards, the roundels and fin flash were outlined in white. The serial numbers were applied to the rear fuselage only, in minuscule 4" high red characters. A small red letter code appeared above the fin flash and on the nose-wheel door. On the port side of the nose was a small traditional squadron crest, flanked by gold bars in outline style. On the starboard side of the nose was a small Union Jack. The team leader's aircraft was a Hunter T.7 two-seater, which bore the inscription "Treble-One Squadron" in gold script on the nose. The aircraft flown by *The Black Arrows* over the 1958-60 period were: XE584, XE592, XE616, XE653:S, XE656, XF416:T, XF430:V, XF437:A, XF446:R, XF506:X, XF511:P, XF515, XG129:F, XG160:U, XG170:G, XG171:E, XG189:D, XG190:C, XG191, XG193:A, XG194:N, XG200:Q, XG201:B, XG205, XG266, XJ687, XJ715:H and XL610:Z (T.7).

It is interesting to note that, of these, XF511 and XG194 were still flying in 1984 with the TWU at RAF Brawdy.

During the 'reign' of *The Black Arrows,* other aerobatic teams were formed with Meteors and Hunters. The RAF Flying College provided a team of Meteor T.7s in 1957, 1960 and 1962, and quartets of the same type were supplied by the RAF College of Air Warfare in 1963 and 1964 with Mk.8 Meteors. The CAW team usually comprised silver and dayglo Meteor F.8s WH301, WK655, WL181 and WL190.

Vampire trainers were also used in 1960. Five teams of four aircraft each were provided by the RAF College, Cranwell, and Nos. 1, 5, 7 and 8 FTSs. In 1960, the RAF had no less than fifteen display teams!

Apart from *The Black Arrows,* there were five other official teams using Hunters, usually with four or five aircraft. These were from Nos. 56, 74, 92 and 208 Squadrons and 229 Operational Conversion Unit. Of those teams, it was No. 92 Squadron that continued as the RAF's premier team in 1961.

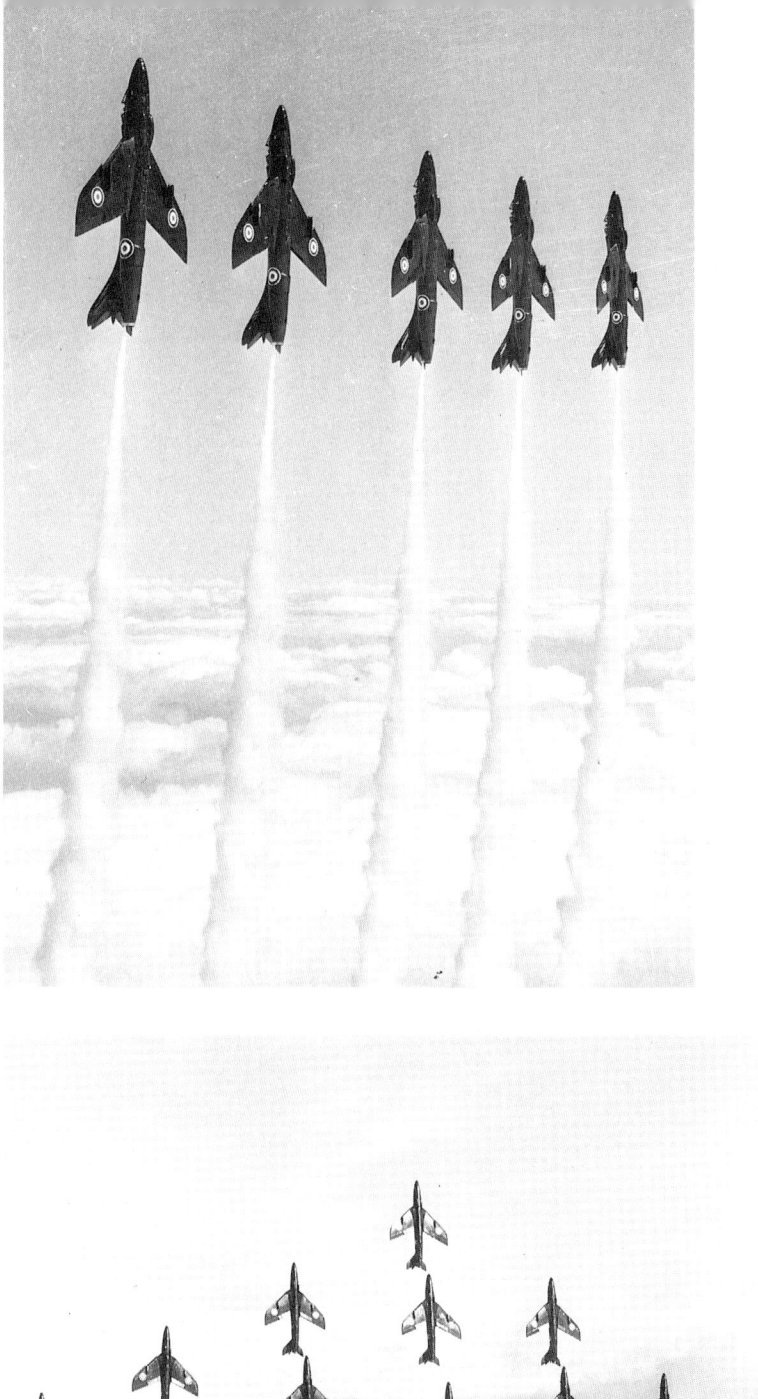

Above right: Five Hunter F.6s of No.111 Squadron *The Black Arrows* looping in May 1958. (MoD)

Right: The famous 22-Hunter loop by No.111 Squadron *The Black Arrows*, seen during Farnborough week, September 1958. Eight Hunters were borrowed from No.56 Squadron for this feat, which were not painted black. (MoD)

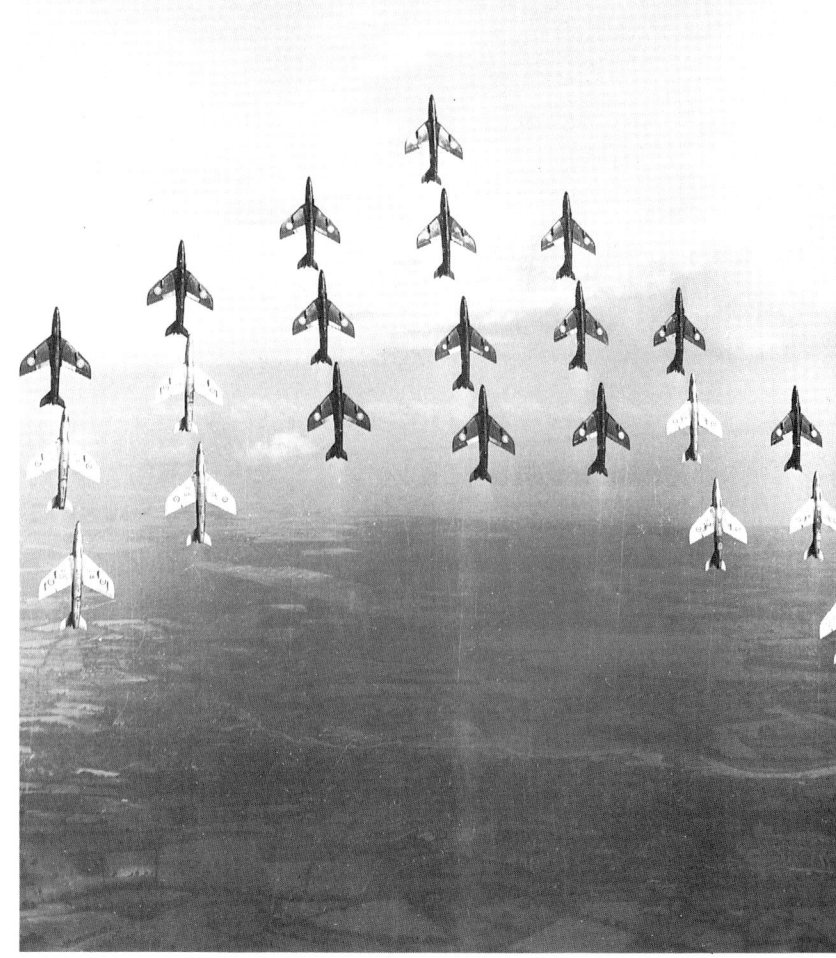

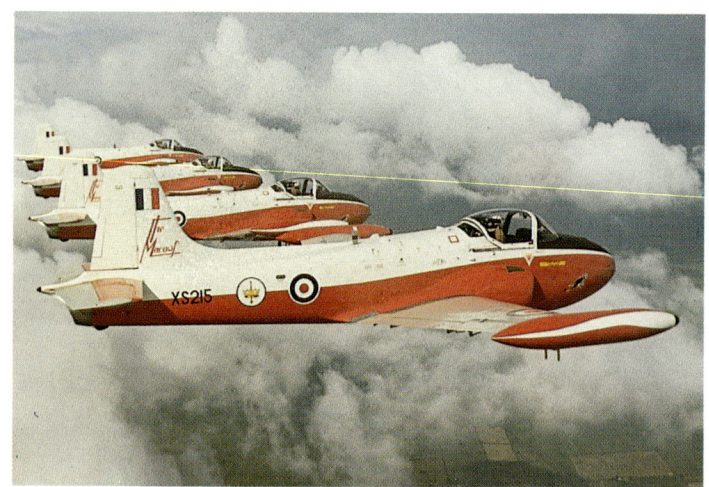

1959: Central Flying School, "The Redskins", RAF Little Rissington, Gloucestershire.

The Sparrows disbanded at the end of 1958 season, with their Jet Provost T.1s, and a pair of these aircraft continued during the 1959 season called *The Redskins*.

The CFS were supported by a nameless quartet of Jet Provost T.3s from 2 FTS in 1960 and well as the other un-named teams from the Central Navigation Control School and 6 FTS. At the end of the 1959 season, *The Redskins* disbanded and in the following year *The Pelicans* were born, flying four Jet Provost T.3s (See *The Sparrows* for serial numbers of team).

Left: Jet Provost T.4s of the College of Air Warfare *Macaws* team in their 1969 markings after the standard red and white training colour scheme had been adopted. (via J. F. Merry)

Below: XP629 heads a line of Jet Provost T.4s from the RAF College of Air Warfare *Macaws* team in their 1968 colour scheme at RAF Colerne, Wilts, on 6 July 1968. (Adrian M. Balch)

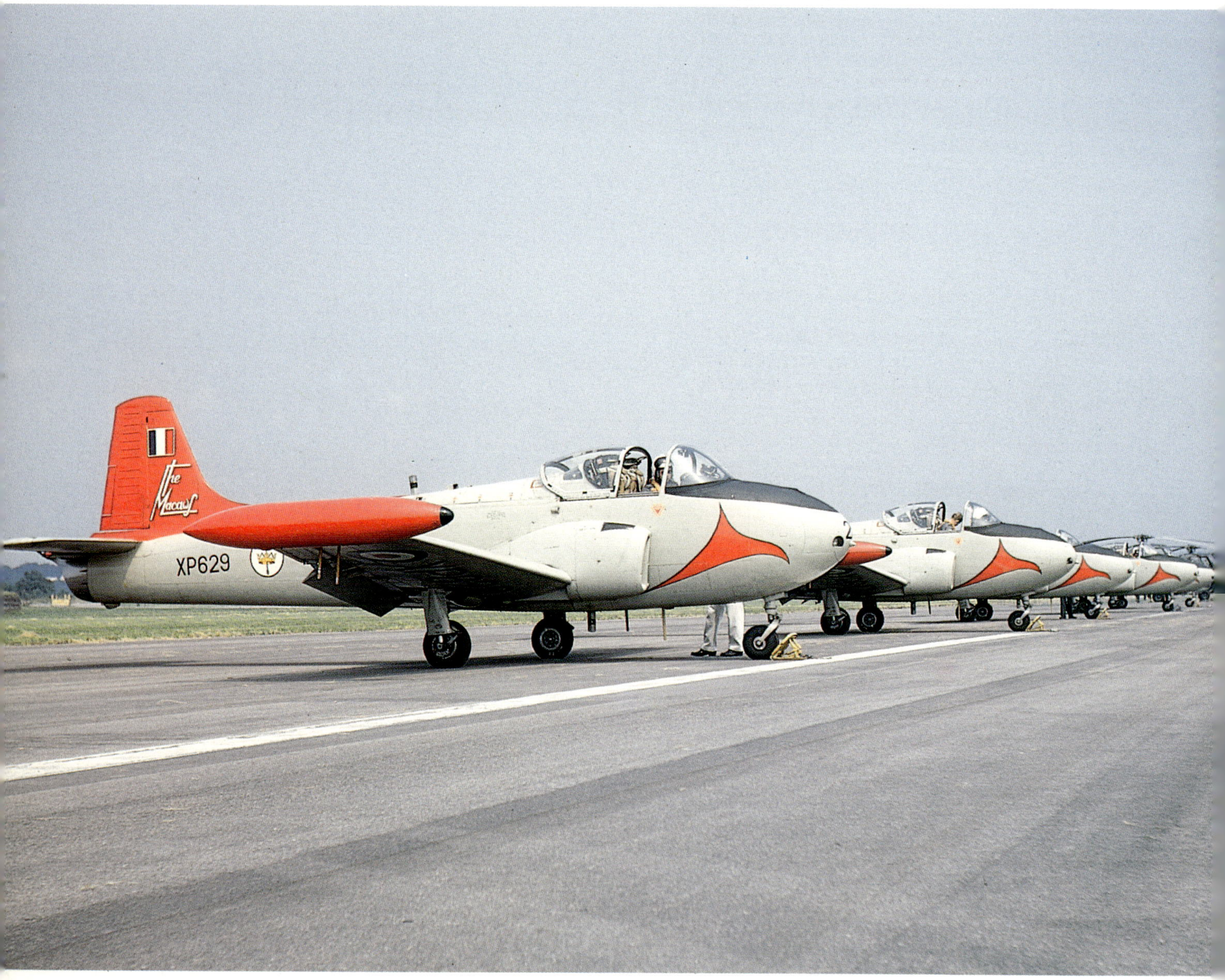

1961-62: No. 92 Squadron, "The Blue Diamonds", RAF Leconfield, Lincolnshire.

In 1961, No. 92 Squadron, under Squadron Leader B. W. P. Mercer, formed *The Blue Diamonds* and carried on the remarkable tradition of *The Black Arrows,* introducing some new formations and flying 16 blue-painted Hunters. The 16-aircraft formations were, at times, split into seven and nine so that one or the other of the formations was always in front of the audience. The team was initially named *The Falcons,* but quickly changed to the *The Blue Diamonds* in May 1961. Starting with twelve Hunters, the team was up to eighteen by the time it disbanded at the end of 1962, including two Hunter T.7s. They participated in shows all over Europe, including Farnborough and Paris. Colour scheme was roundel-blue overall with a thin white lightning flash down the fuselage sides and white wingtips. The national markings were outlined in white and the squadron markings of red/yellow checks were carried on the nose. Serial numbers were once again minuscule and carried on the rear fuselage in black. The team was drawn from: XG211:A, XE656:B, XG228:C, XF522:D, XG137:E, XG232:G, XG231:H, XG186:J, XF520:K, XE532:L, XG189:M, XG190:N, XG194:P, XG201:R, XG225:S, XL605:T (T.7), XL571:V (T.7), XG159:W, XF521:X, XG185:Z.

Of these, it is interesting to record that XE656, XG189, XG190, XG194 and XG201 were used by both *The Black Arrows* and *The Blue Diamonds*.

1961-62: No. 74 Squadron, "The Tigers", RAF Coltishall, Norfolk.

The largest and fastest RAF fighters to participate as official aerobatic team aircraft were the supersonic English Electric Lightnings, first appearing in 1960, when a quartet appeared at Farnborough in September of that year. In 1961, No. 74 Squadron increased the number to nine, under the leadership of Squadron Leader J. F. G. Howe, and became known as *The Tigers*. The team performed wing-overs and rolls in tight formation and in the following year they were led by Squadron Leader P. G. Botherhill, giving a co-ordinated display with *The Blue Diamonds* during Farnborough week, September 1962. During the 1961 season, the Lightning F.1As were natural metal overall, apart from the roundels and squadron markings. During 1962, the aircraft had their fins and spines painted black. For both seasons, nine aircraft were drawn from: XM143:A, XM142:B, XM139:C, XM141:D, XM165F, XM166:G, XM167:H, XM144:J, XM164:K, XM146:L, XM140:M, XM147:P and XM163:Q.

Top right: Five Hunters of No.92 Squadron *The Blue Diamonds* making smoke as they enter a loop in 1961. (MoD)

Above right: Hunter F.6s of No.92 Squadron's *Blue Diamonds* team with F-100Cs of the USAF's *Skyblazers* in 1961. The location is thought to be Wheelus Field, Libya. (RAF Museum)

Right: Squadron Ldr., B. W. P. Mercer and team of No.92 Squadron *The Blue Diamonds* at Leconfield in June 1961. The Hunter F.6 on the left is XE532:L with XG232:G on the right. (MoD)

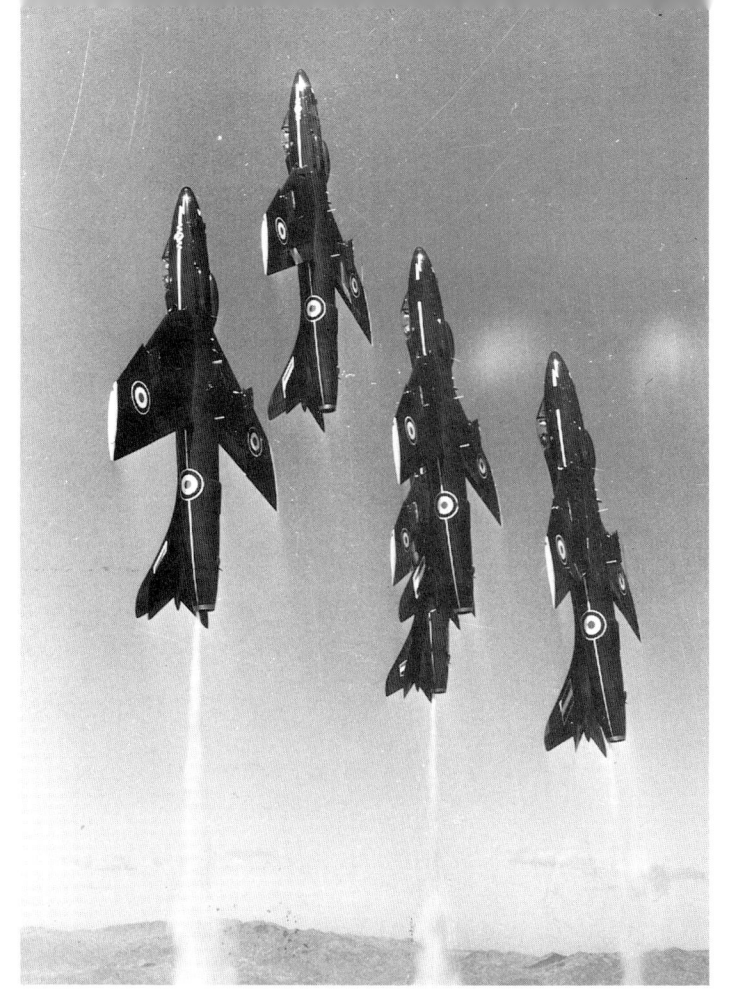

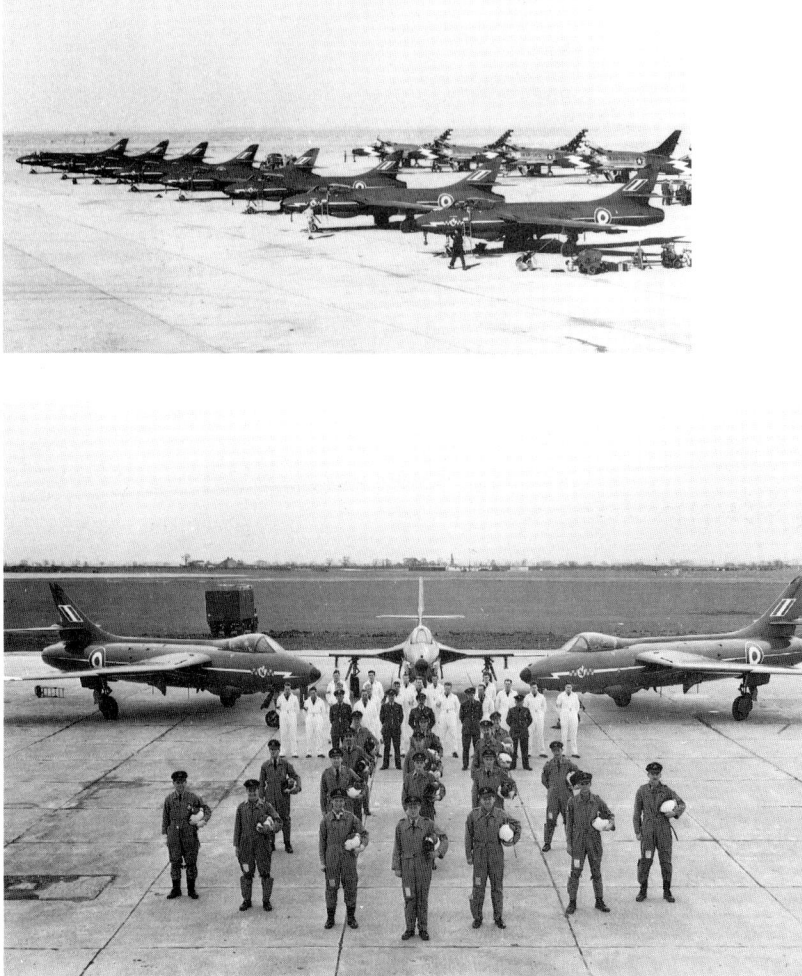

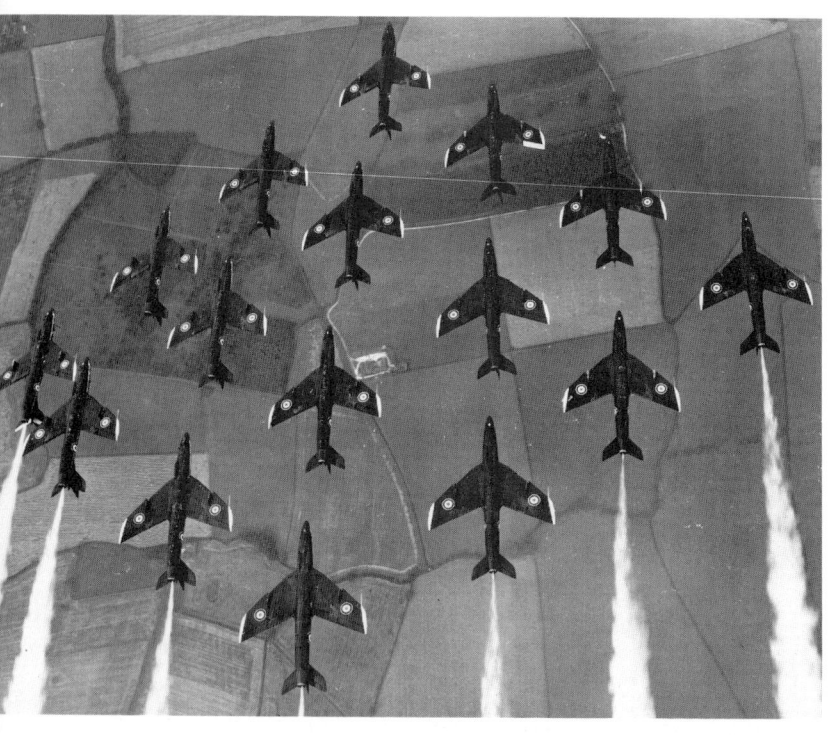

1963: No. 56 Squadron, "The Firebirds", RAF Wattisham, Suffolk.

The mighty Lightning held the position of the RAF's premier aerobatic team aircraft in 1963, when No. 56 Squadron formed *The Firebirds* — the name coming from the squadron's Phoenix badge. Led by Squadron Leader D. J. Seward, the team formed in March 1963 and was stationed at Wattisham, Suffolk, flying nine red-and-silver Lightning F.1As. They appeared at displays all over Europe, including shows at Paris and Farnborough. The aircraft were natural metal overall, with red fins, spines and leading edges to the wings and tailplanes, which tapered at the tips of each. Nine aircraft were drawn from: XM171:A, XM172:B, XM173:C, XM174:D, XM175:E, XM176:F, XM177:G, XM178:H, XM179:J, XM182:M, XM183:N, XM180:K, XM181:L and T.4 XM989:X. XM179:J was written off 6/6/63 in collison with XM174/D.

Left: Impeccable diamond formation at the top of a loop by 16 Hunters of No.92 Squadron *The Blue Diamonds* over Leconfield in September 1961. (MoD)

Below: 'Diamond-Nine' formation by Lightning F.1s from No.74 Squadron RAF in 1961, led by Squadron Ldr., J. F. G. Howe. (British Aerospace)

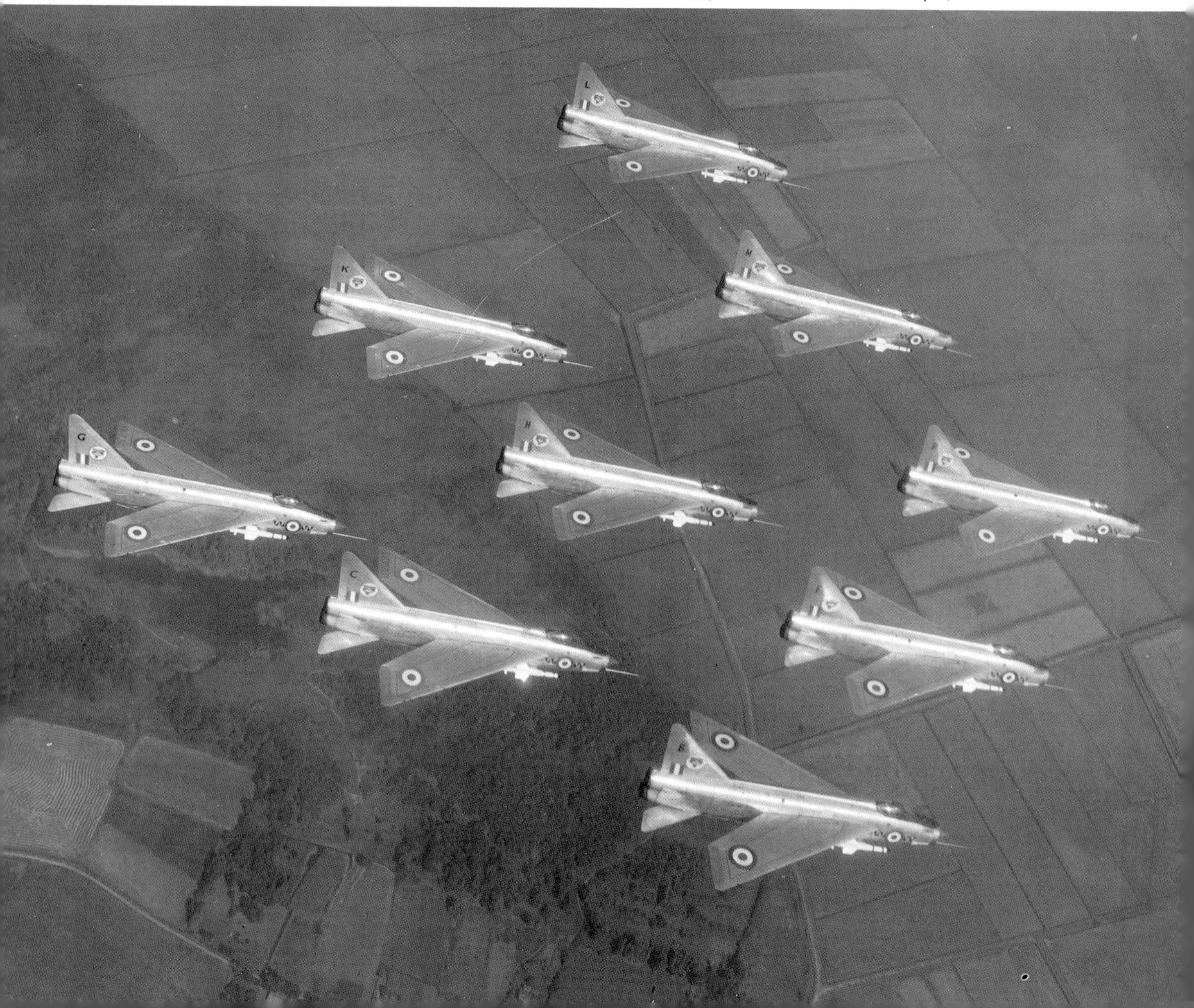

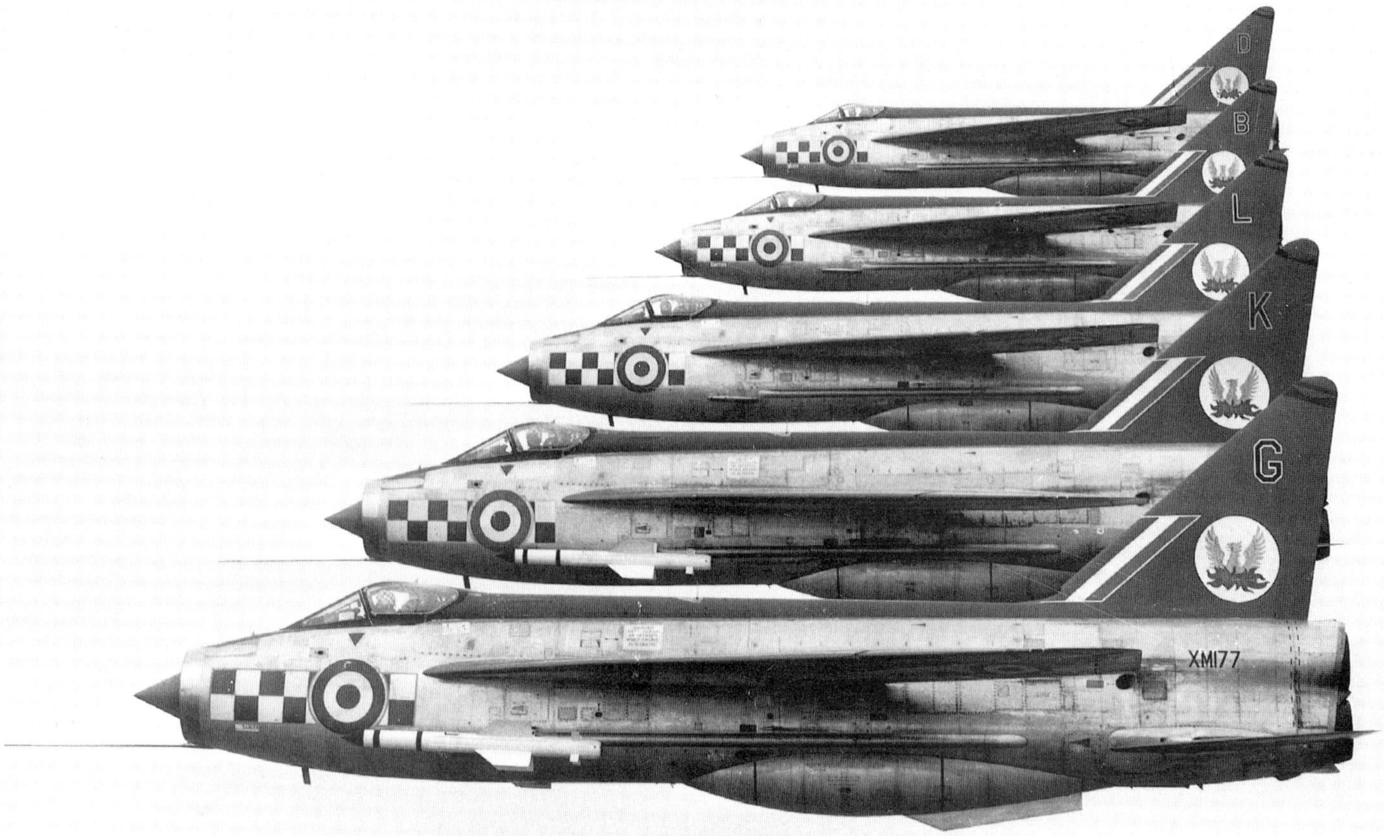

Above: A superb formation by No.56 Squadron *The Firebirds* with their Lightning F.1As in 1963. (MoD)

Below: Lightning F.1As of No.74 Squadron *Tigers* team performing at the 1962 Farnborough Air Show. Note black fins and spines. (British Aerospace)

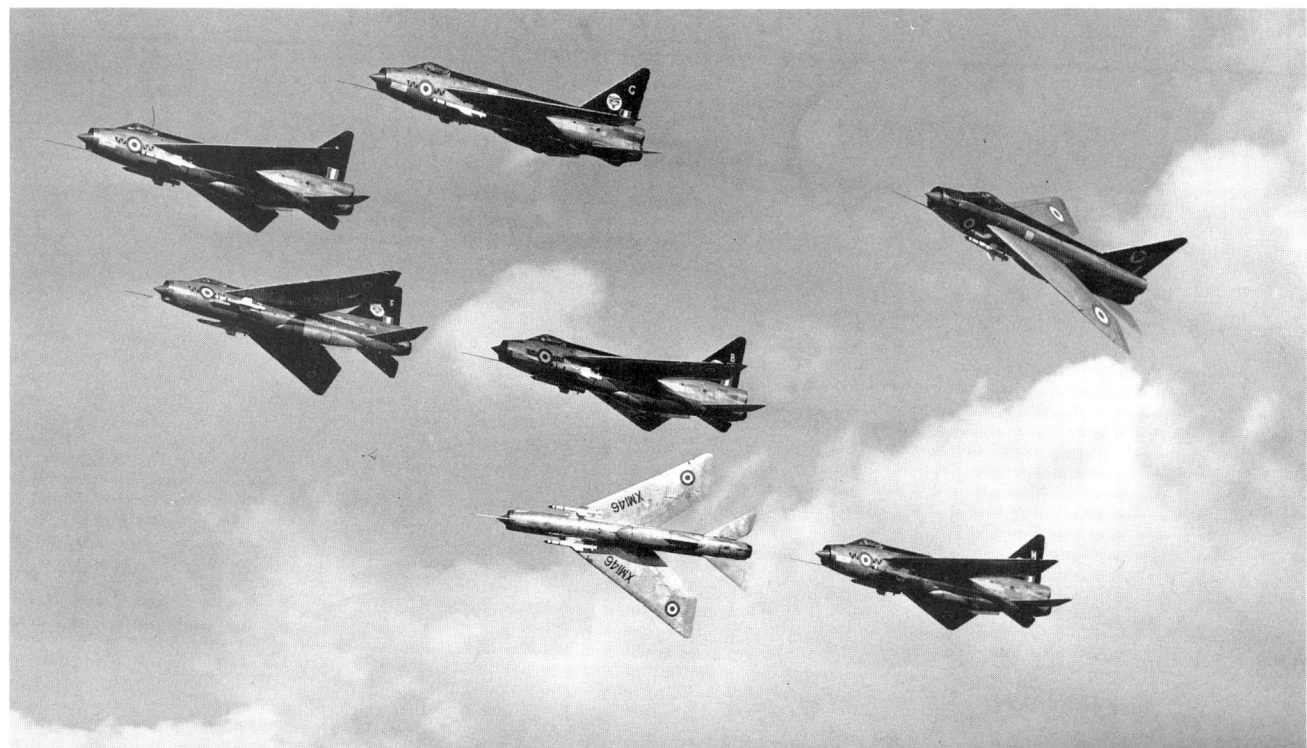

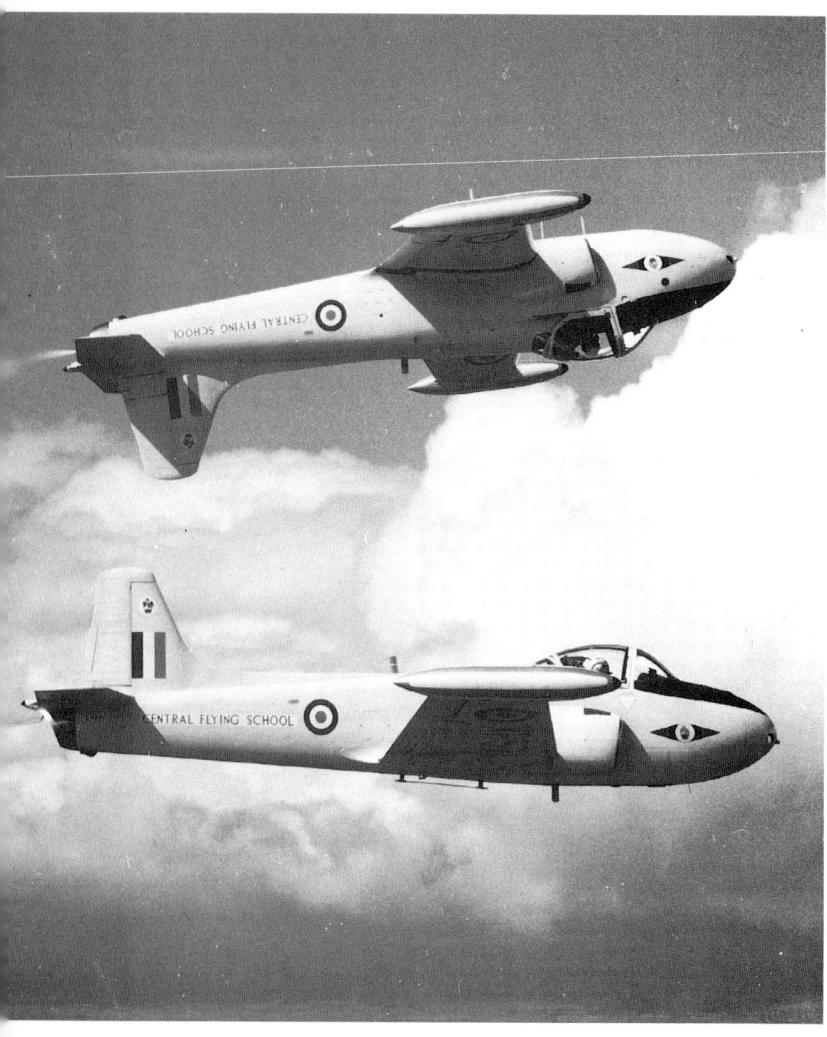

1960-73: Central Flying School, "The Red Pelicans", RAF Little Rissington, Gloucestershire.

Although the limelight was stolen by the Hunter and Lightning teams during the 1960-63 period, *The Pelicans* were formed in 1960 to represent the CFS. Flying four silver and dayglo-red Jet Provost T.3s, the machines were usually drawn from XM411:R-G, XM413:R-H, XM423:R-J, XM424:R-K and XM428:R-M. The 1961 team used slightly newer aircraft being drawn from: XN550:S-A, XN549:R-W, XN511:R-W, XN554:S-E, XN572:S-G and XN557:S-F. For the 1962 season, the team re-equipped with the Jet Provost T.4 and increased the number to five aircraft. The CFS changed from letter codes to numbers on its aircraft and the 1962 team were drawn from: XP549:40, XP550:41, XP551:42, XP552:43, XP553:44, XP554:45, XP571:47, XP572:48 and XP573:49.

These nine aircraft remained allocated to the team throughout the 1962, '63 and '64 seasons. In 1963, they were painted dayglo-red overall and became *The Red Pelicans,* being led by Flight Lieutenant I. Bashall. The 1963 team comprised six aircraft, which participated in displays in France, Belgium and events at home. By the end of 1963, the expense of front-line requirements were such that modern fighter aircraft could no longer be spared for display purposes and the honour of representing the RAF returned, after 44 years, to the Central Flying School. *The Red Pelicans* became the RAF Aerobatic Team for 1964. Led by Flight Lieutenant T. E. L. Lloyd, the team displayed in Belgium, France, the Netherlands and Norway, as well as in varied shows and events in England. During the latter half of the season and at the 1964 Farnborough Air Show, *The Red Pelicans* gave co-ordinated displays with *The Yellowjacks* Gnats. In 1965, *The Red Pelicans* took a step down as the RAF's premier aerobatic team, as *The Red Arrows* were formed in that year. The six dayglo-red, smoke-equipped Jet Provosts were relinquished and replaced by four postbox-red aircraft without the smoke facility. The team, in this form, continued to fly for five years using XN468:41, XS212:40, XS222:43, XS217:50 and XS225:47. The 1970 season saw a change of aircraft once again, when *The Red Pelicans* changed to the Jet Provost T.5, led by Squadron Leader E. D. Evers. As the aircraft were not full-time aerobatic team machines, they wore the standard training colour scheme of red, white and grey. The only additions were *The Red Pelicans* badge on the fin and the team's titling down the rear fuselage. The 1972 and '73 seasons saw the titling and Pelican badge take on a new improved style and the team continued until the end of 1973, when they disbanded. The T.5s used by *The Red Pelicans* were drawn from: XW288:81, XW289:82, XW290:83, XW291:84, XW292:85, XW293:86, XW294:87, and XW295:88. (See Page 41 for colour photographs).

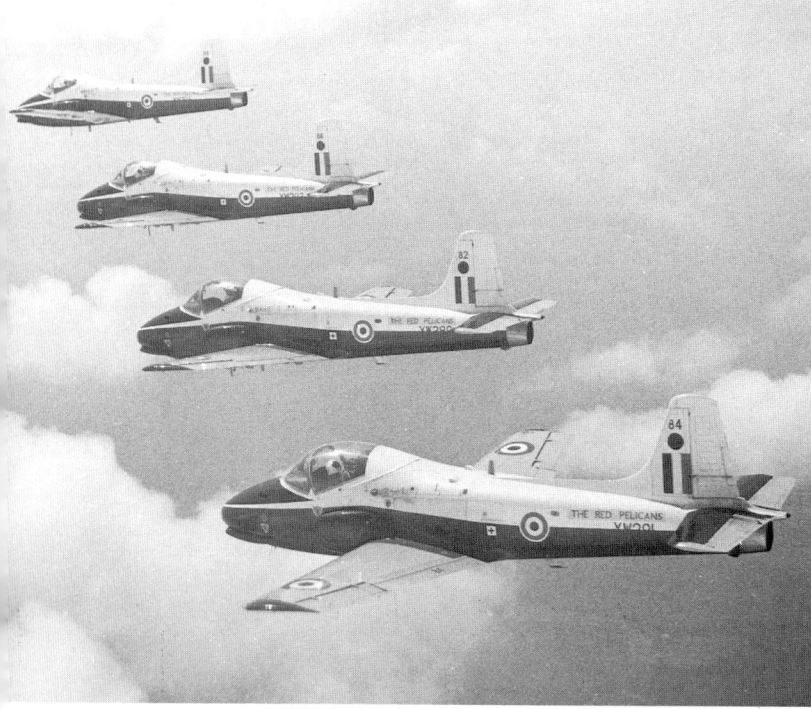

Top left: Two all-dayglo red Jet Provost T.4s of the C.F.S. *Red Pelicans* in 'mirror' formation during 1964. Lower aircraft is XP571. (MoD)

Left: The 1970 *Red Pelicans* with Jet Provost T.5s. Nearest aircraft is XW291. (MoD via S. Wolf)

1964: No. 4 Flying Training School, "The Yellowjacks", RAF Valley, Anglesey.

In 1964, it was decided to form a Gnat team from instructors at No. 4 FTS at Valley, on the Isle of Anglesey, to display the RAF's new trainer. The name *Yellowjacks* was derived from a radio callsign and the aircraft were painted bright lemon yellow overall. The team was led by Flight Lieutenant Lee Jones, an ex-*Black Arrows* pilot who had joined the RAF in 1946 and become a very experienced fighter pilot. The first public appearance of *The Yellowjacks* was at RNAS Culdrose Naval Air Day on 25th July 1964, followed by Open Days at Kemble and Little Rissington, among others. Although the team flew only five Gnats in their display, they had ten allocated to them, as the excellent serviceablility of the Gnat had yet to be proven. At the 1964 Farnborough Air Show, *The Yellowjacks* formated with *The Red Pelicans* Jet Provosts to begin their displays.

As an aerobatic team mount, the Gnat had proved itself and had brought back the sleek appearance the public had grown accustomed to in the formation displays of earlier years. It was an attractive aircraft and the ease of control and manoeuvrability resulted in the type being chosen as the RAF Aerobatic Team's mount for 1965 — *The Red Arrows*.

The aircraft were lemon yellow overall, with serials in roundel-blue. One little-known fact is that they all wore 'Moon-Eyes' decals on top of the nose, above the nose light. The five aircraft were drawn from XR991, XR992, XR993, XR994, XR995, XR996, XR986, XR987 and XR540.

1967-71: Central Flying School, "The Skylarks", RAF Little Rissington, Gloucestershire.

This team of four De Havilland (Canada) Chipmunks was formed in 1967 by Flight Lieutenant J. F. Merry. Although quite tame, compared with the smoke-making jet teams, they showed the Chipmunk off to its best with formation loops and rolls and synchronised manoeuvres in pairs. The team operated standard silver and dayglo-red Chipmunks from the CFS, which were repainted light grey overall with dayglo panels during the last two seasons. The aircraft had dark green spinners and a dark green lightning flash down the fuselage, upon which was the CFS crest. In 1970, a team badge was added above the fin-flash, comprising a black Skylark bird on a white disc. The team was drawn from: WB550:08, WB562:10, WB650:09, WB684:08, WD299:06, WD347, WG403:04, WK521:12, WK628:13, WP807:15, WP844, WZ847 and WZ877.

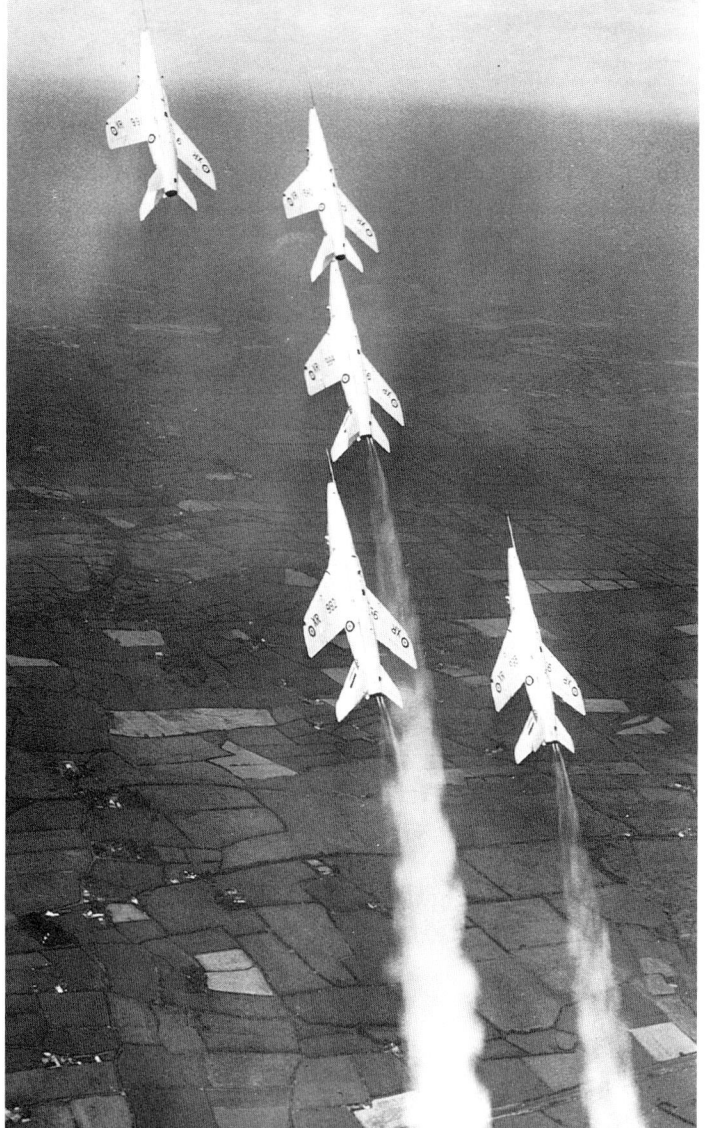

Top right: 'Card Five' formation by the *Yellowjacks* Gnats from No.4 F.T.S. at Valley, Anglesey. (British Aerospace)

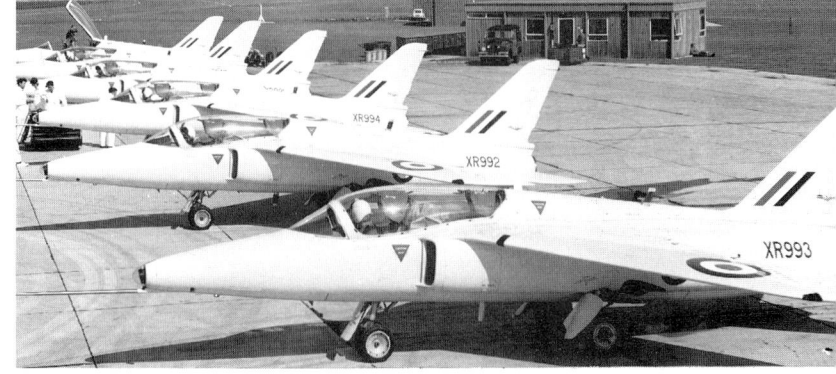

Above right: Gnat T.1s of No.4 F.T.S. the *Yellowjacks* lined up at Little Rissington in 1964. (via R. Ward)

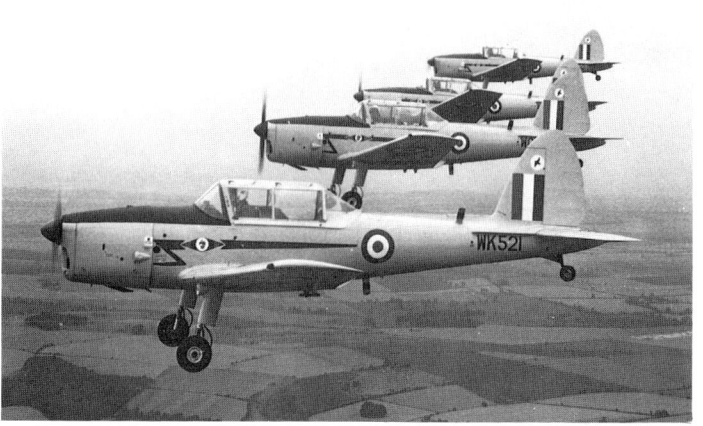

Right: Chipmunks of the C.F.S. *Skylarks* team photographed during a sortie from Little Rissington in 1970. (Peter R. March)

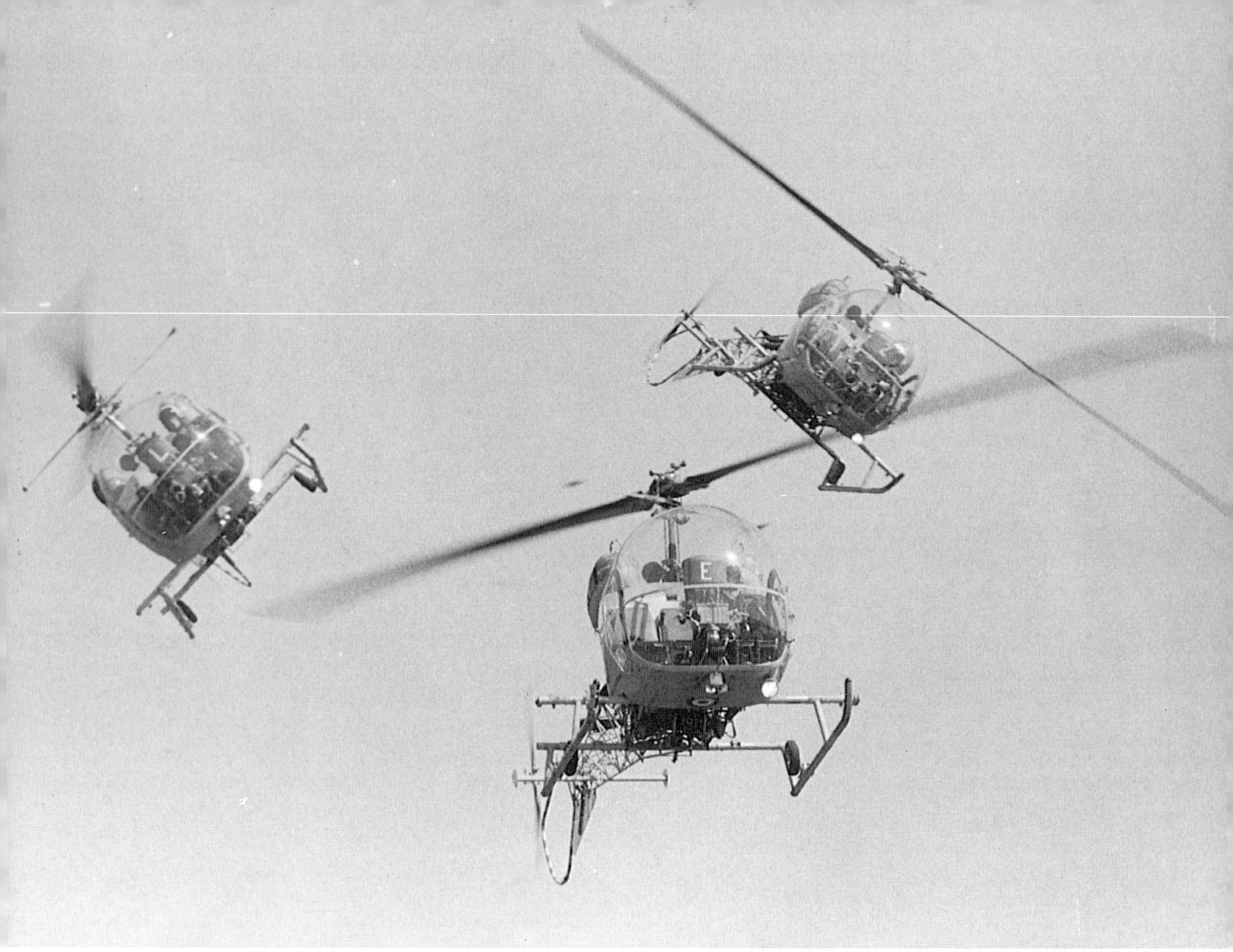

The Tomahawks — a trio of Westland-Bell 47G Sioux HT.2 helicopters from the C.F.S. Rotary Wing at Ternhill in 1968. (Peter R. March)

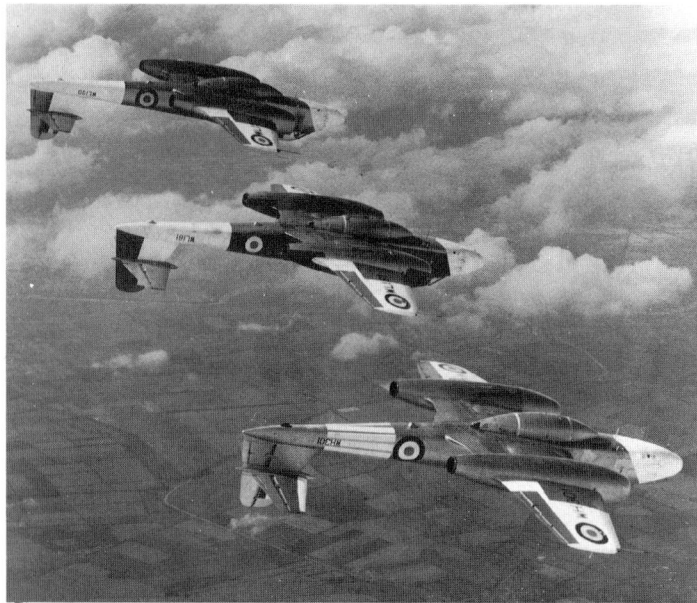

Above: Forerunner of the *Macaws*; three Meteor F.8s of the 1964 College of Air Warfare team at the top of a loop. Note different styles of dayglo application. WH301 (nearest) now resides in the RAF Museum, while WL181 (centre) is preserved at Lambton Park, Durham. (MoD via R. Ward)

1967-69: Central Flying School Helicopter Wing, "The Tomahawks", RAF Ternhill, Shropshire.

This was the first RAF helicopter team to be formed and comprised three Sioux HT.2s led by Flight Lieutenant J. Lloyd, an instructor at Ternhill. The team performed twice before Her Majesty The Queen, at the RAF's 50th Anniversary display at Abingdon in June 1968. Also at Little Rissington in June 1969 for the Royal Review of the CFS. The aircraft had dayglo-red fuselages with light grey boom and fins. *The Tomahawks* were drawn from: XV314:M, XV318:V, XV315:W, XV311:K, XV316:F, XV317:Z, XV319:N or XV323:L.

1967-72: College of Air Warfare, "The Macaws", RAF Manby, Lincolnshire.

This team was first called *The Magistrates,* when they formed in 1966 — the name deriving from the letters 'J.P.' However, this was changed early in 1967 and the team continued flying four silver and dayglo Jet Provost T.4s under the name *The Macaws*. This name was made from *M*anby *C*ollege of *A*ir *W*arfare and the team comprised instructors from the School of Refresher Flying, a component part of the College. In 1968, the team was given its own colour scheme, when the Jet Provosts adopted a smart light grey and red colour scheme. For the 1969-71 seasons, the aircraft adopted the new standard training colours of red, white and grey with the addition of the team's name in red on the fin and a Macaw in perched attitude on the nose during 1969.

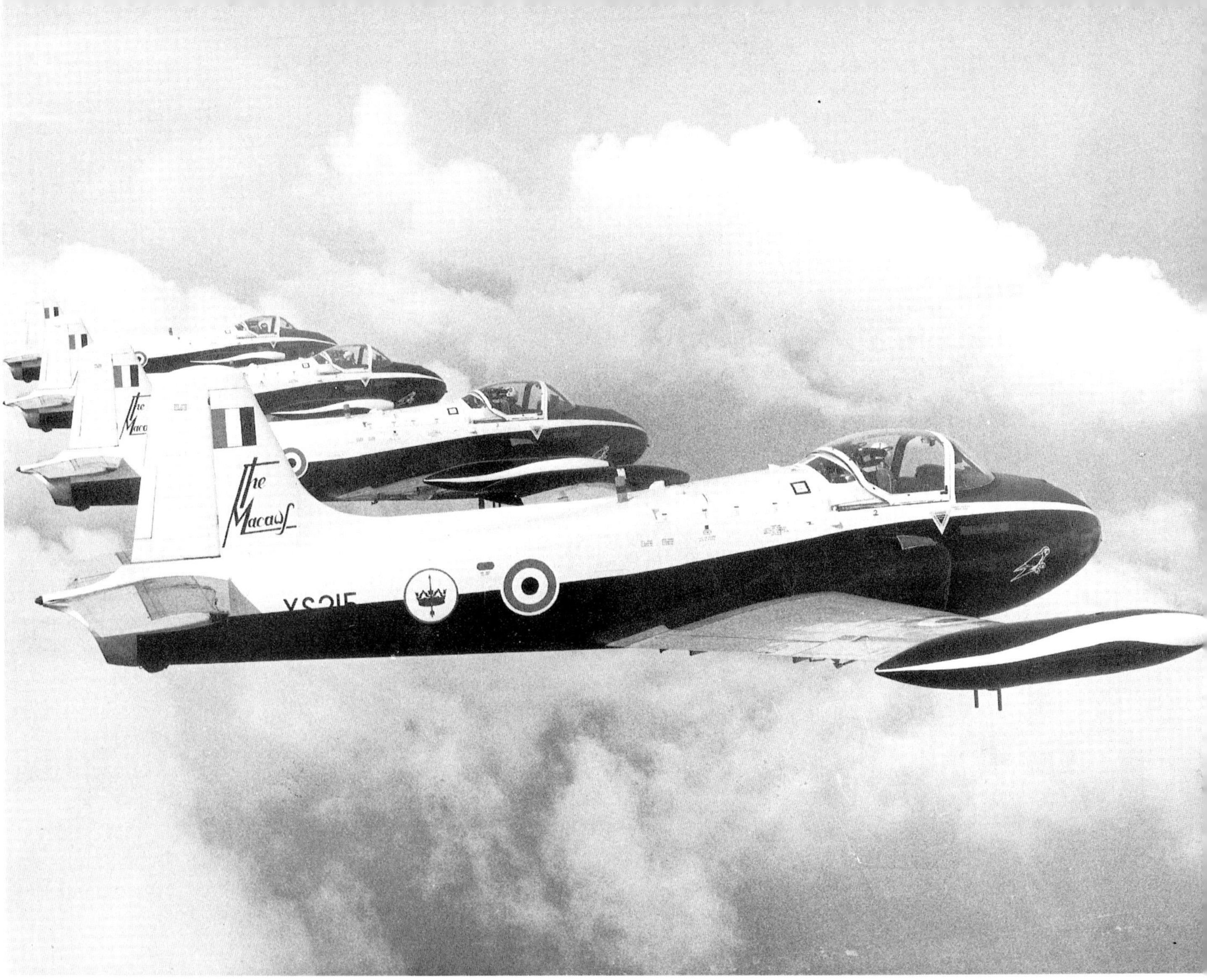

For their last three seasons, 1970-72, the Macaw on the nose was restyled 'in-flight' and the tail markings were slightly altered. Flight Lieutenant Brian Hoskins led the team during 1971 and later went on to lead *The Red Arrows*. The team flew six basic formations and their display culminated in a 'Petal Break', or flat bomb-burst towards the crowd.

The Macaws 1968 team operated XP629, XP686, XR704 and XS179. For the 1969-72 seasons, four aircraft were drawn from: XP680, XR654, XR660, XS180, XS210, XS211, XS215, XS216.

1968-69: No. 2 Flying Training School, "The Vipers", RAF Syerston, Nottinghamshire.

Another team flying the Jet Provost T.4 was *The Vipers*, which operated four aircraft from Syerston, near Nottingham. They flew a similar show to *The Macaws* and their aircraft were in standard silver and dayglo training colours with the addition of *The Vipers* in small black letters on the wingtip tanks. For the 1969 season, the fin, rudder and wingtip tanks were painted white. The team's titling moved on to the fin and a snake in a triangle formed the figure '2' on the fin — obviously a Viper! The team's name came from the engine that powered the Jet Provost T.4, the Bristol Siddeley Viper. The team's aircraft were: XP617:49, XP619:40, XR644:36, XR707:45 and XP641:34.

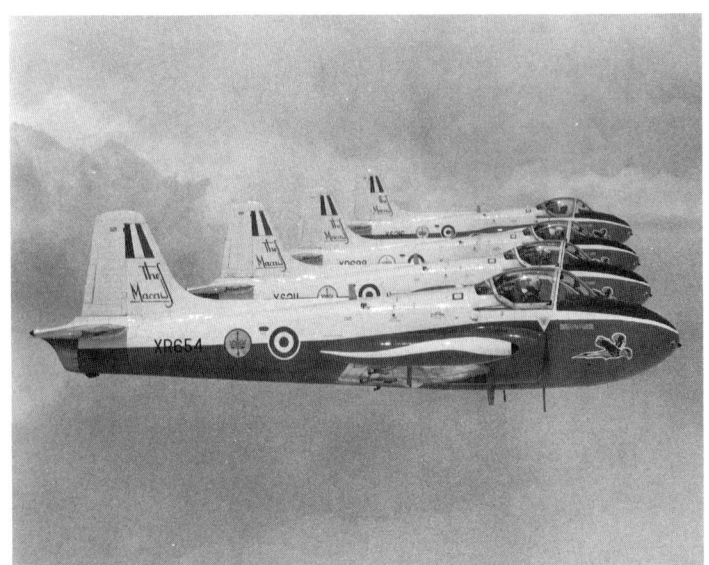

Above: During the 1970-71 seasons, the *Macaws* scheme was slightly modified to incorporate a flying Macaw on the nose and swept-back lettering and fin flash. Nearest aircraft is XR654 (MoD via S. Wolf)

Top: Jet Provost T.4s of *The Macaws* from the College of Air Warfare at Manby. They are shown in their 1969 markings with a Macaw in perched attitude on the nose, short vertical style fin flash and tail lettering angled forward. Nearest aircraft is XS215 (MoD)

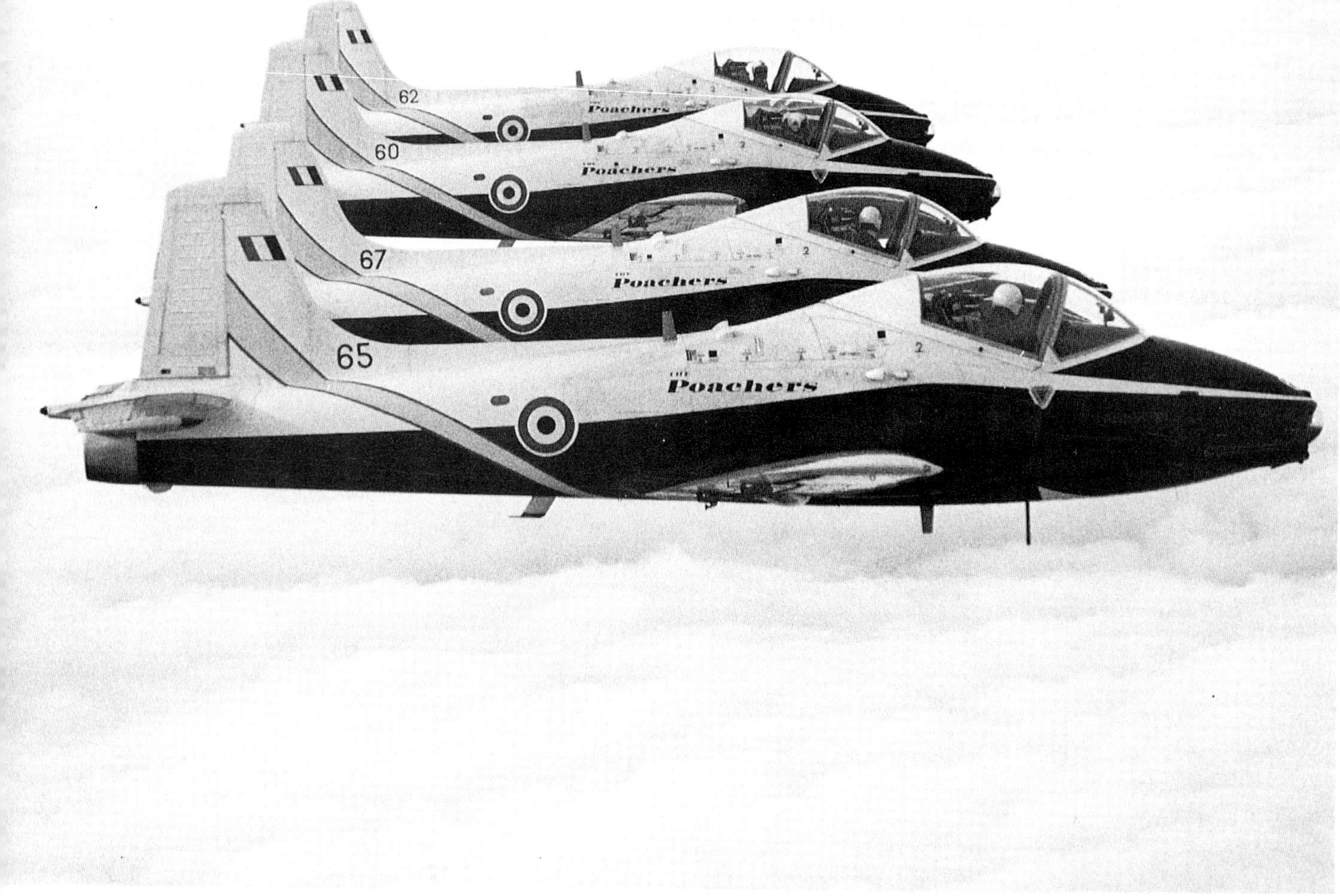

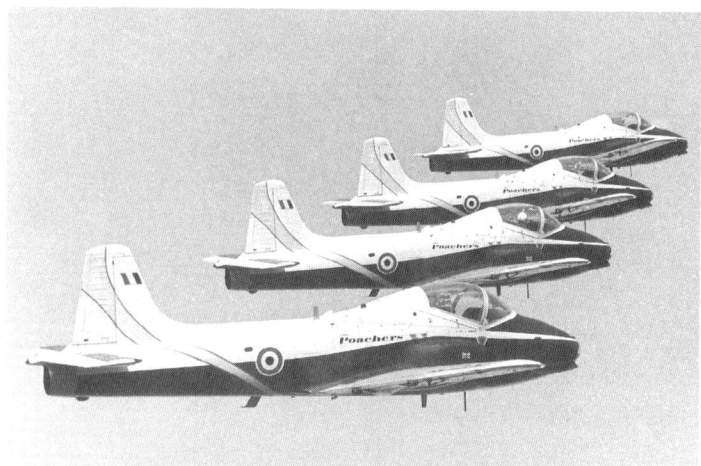

Above: The Poachers flying Jet Provost T.5s from the RAF College, Cranwell in 'echelon' formation during October 1972. Note the light blue sash now continues across the rudder and each aircraft has a white tail number code. Nearest aircraft is XW358 coded '4' (MoD)

Top: The Poachers Jet Provost T.5s, from the RAF College at Cranwell, in 1971 scheme. Nearest aircraft is XW354 coded '65' (MoD)

1969-76: RAF College, "The Poachers", Cranwell, Lincolnshire.

This team flew its Jet Provost T.4s in the later standard red, white and grey colour scheme with the addition of the RAF College pale blue band round the rear fuselage. Another team of four, the aircraft had a stylised 'CP' added to their fins during 1970, standing for "Cranwell Poachers". Before that, they had displayed 'Cranwell Poachers' in bold white letters along the wingtip tanks. Four aircraft were drawn from: XP555:70, XP556:71, XP563:78, XP583:87, XP584:88 and XR662:98.

In 1971, *The Poachers* re-equipped with the Jet Provost Mk.5 and continued with four-aircraft displays for five years on this type, until they disbanded at the end of the 1976 season. The aircraft wore the standard red, white and grey training scheme. Under the nose was a white triangle within which were three small red triangles representing aircraft. From these, three pale blue strips extended, one along the centre of the fuselage and the others round the fuselage and up the fin, becoming thicker as they went, representing smoke trails. For the 1976 season, the wings were painted white with a red sunburst scheme over them. Four aircraft were drawn from XW352, '353, '354, '356, '357, '358, '359, '360, '363, '420 and '438.

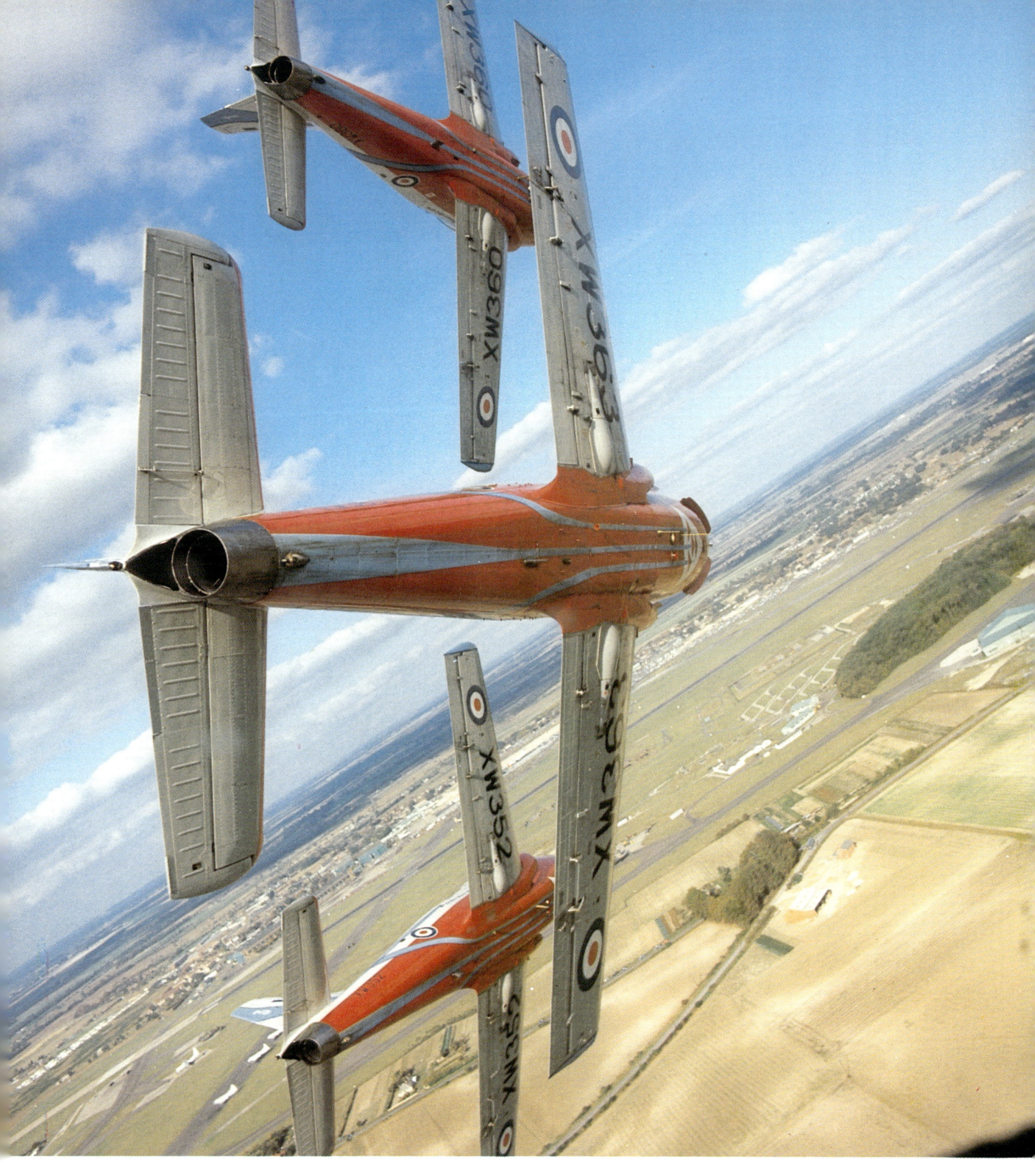

1967-69: No. 1 Flying Training School, "Linton Gin", RAF Linton-on-Ouse, Yorkshire.
Yet another team of Jet Provost T.4s, this team were first known as *The Gin Four*, when they formed in 1967. Colour scheme was standard silver and dayglo and no special aircraft were used. By 1969, the later red, white and grey training scheme was adopted and a stylised 'Linton GIN' was painted on the wingtip tanks. The aircraft used included: XP634:49, XR670:54 and XR672:43. The team disbanded at the end of 1969.

Above: Flying with an aerobatic team — Jet Provost T.5s of the RAF College's *The Poachers* performing at Mildenhall, Suffolk in 1975. XW363 is flanked by XW352 and XW360, showing the underside paint scheme to advantage. (MoD)

1970-73: No. 1 Flying Training School, "The Blades", RAF Linton-on-Ouse, Yorkshire.

Unlike the other Jet Provost teams mentioned previously, *The Blades* never operated the Jet Provost T.4 under their name, but started off in 1970 with the Mark 5. Again, they were a four-aircraft team, which performed a similar display to all the other Jet Provost teams, but mainly confined their displays to the north of England, being stationed at Linton-on-Ouse. The colour scheme was the standard red, white and grey training colour with the addition of a team badge on the engine intake and at the top of the fin. This comprised a large white Rose of York mounted on two crossed swords. By 1972, the badge was replaced by a single large yellow sword painted vertically up the rudder. The 1973 scheme retained the standard training colours, but with the top of the fuselage and fin painted dark blue. Unfortunately, this smart colour scheme didn't last long, as *The Blades* gave their last display in June 1973, when they disbanded. The aircraft used included: XW301:60, XW307:66, XW302:61 and XW409:78.

Above: Jet Provost T.5s of 1 F.T.S., *Linton Blades* over snow-covered Linton-on-Ouse in February 1973. Standard red, white and grey scheme with roundel-blue upper fuselage and fin. Nearest aircraft is XW310. (MoD)

1970-73: No. 3 Flying Training School, "Gemini Pair", RAF Leeming, Yorkshire.

Unlike the other Jet Provost teams, Gemini comprised only two Jet Provost T.5s, which gave synchronised displays all over the country. The highlight of their display was the 'mirror', where the two aircraft flew back-to-back at very close quarters and rolled together in this configuration. The *Gemini Pair* were stationed at RAF Leeming, Yorkshire and the leader during the 1973 season was Flight Lieutenant Clive (Bob) Thompson, with No. 2 being Flying Officer Graham Miller. Both were Qualified Flying Instructors at No. 3 FTS. The usual training scheme of red, white and grey was retained, with the addition of 'GEMINI' lettering on the fin. The 1973 scheme included a dark blue cheat line down the fuselage. Although there were only two aircraft in the team, at least seven Jet Provosts wore the team's markings. These were: XW319:35, XW325:37, XW331:46, XW332:45, XW406:48, XW407:50 and XW410:51. *Gemini Pair* disbanded at the end of the 1973 season.

1970-72: No. 2 Flying Training School, "The Blue Chips", RAF Church Fenton, Yorkshire.

Like the *Gemini* team, *The Blue Chips* were only a pair of aircraft, but this time two Chipmunks, which carried out formation and synchronised aerobatics. Stationed at Church Fenton, Yorkshire, the aircraft wore the newly-adopted red, white and grey training scheme, with the addition of a pale blue rectangle on the fuselage sides, below the cockpit. Upon this was mounted the crest of No. 2 FTS. Chipmunks used included: WG470:32 and WG348:28.

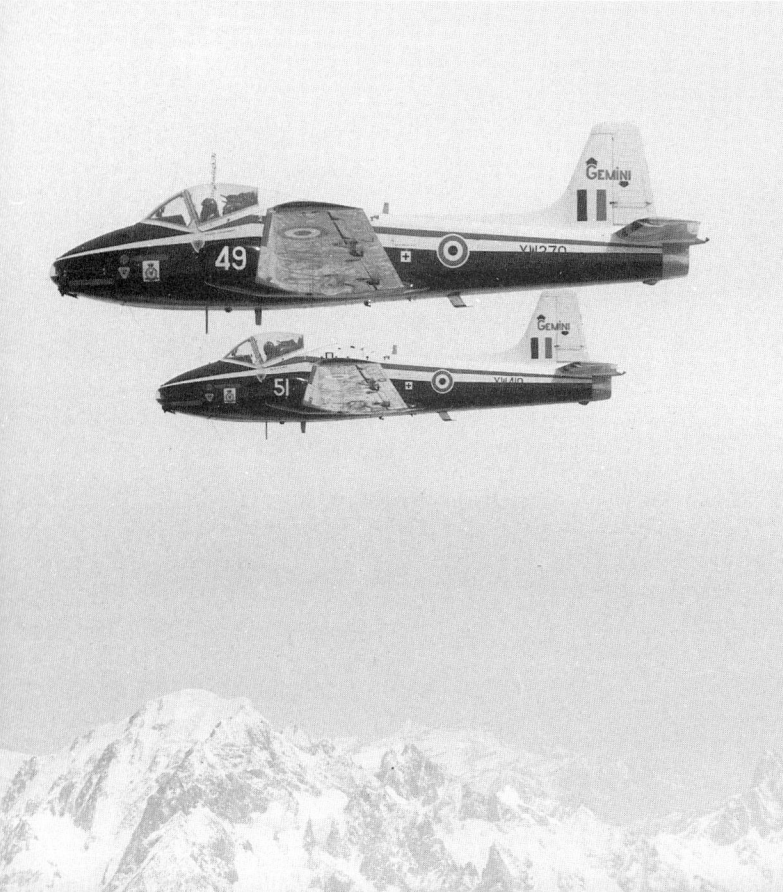

Left: Jet Provost T.5s, XW370:49 and XW410:51 of *Gemini Pair* from 3 F.T.S., at Leeming in 1973 scheme. (MoD)

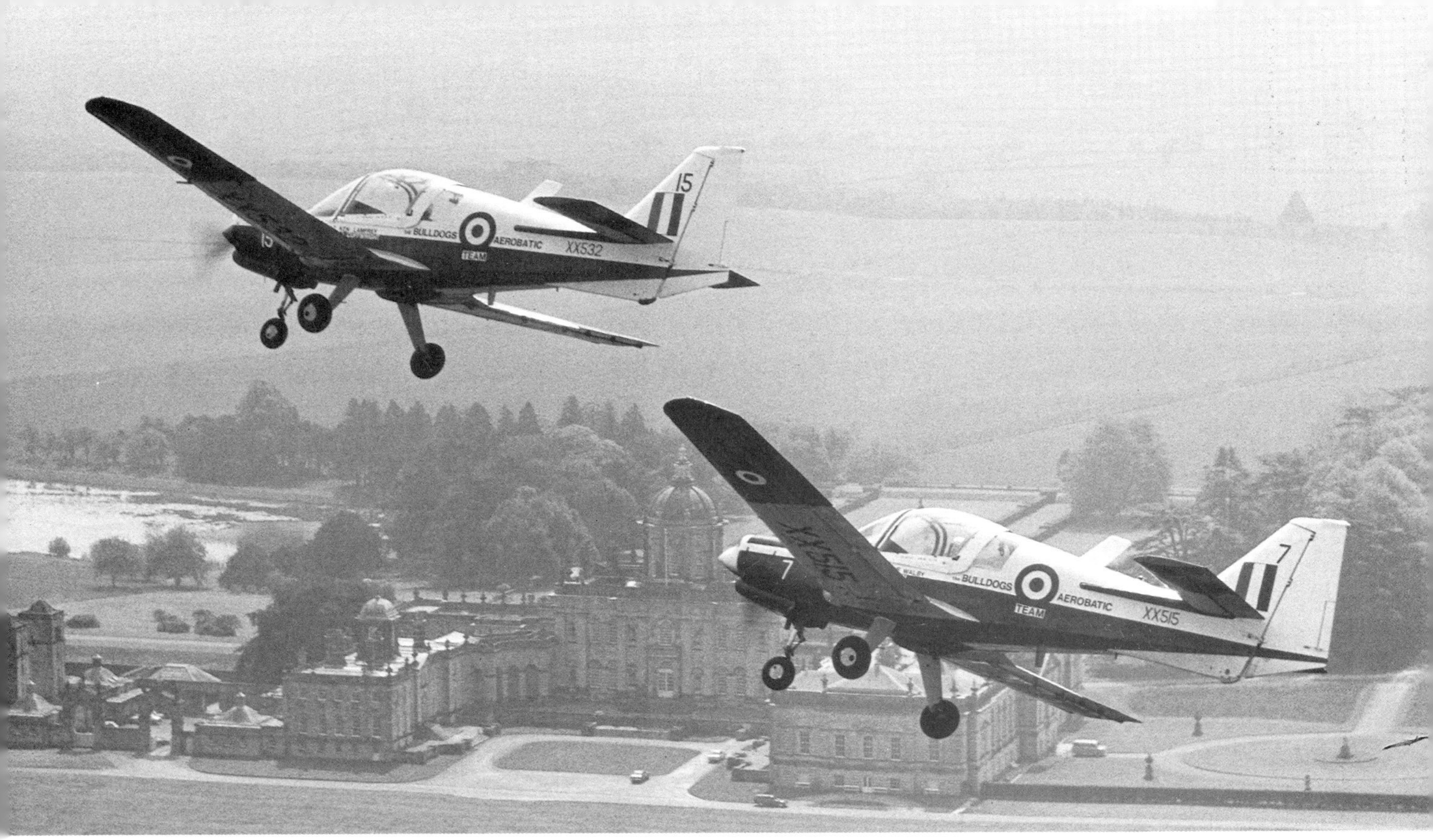

The Bulldogs aerobatic team — a pair of Scottish Aviation Bulldogs from 2 F.T.S. during 1973. (MoD)

1973-74: No. 2 Flying Training School, "The Bulldogs", RAF Church Fenton, Yorkshire.

The Bulldogs succeeded *The Blue Chips,* when No. 2 FTS re-equipped with Scottish Aviation Bulldogs at Church Fenton and relinquished its Chipmunks. The team was led by Squadron Leader P. J. Drummer, with Flight Lieutenant M. W. Watkins or Lieutenant A. J. Griffiths, RN, taking up the second position. The team continued the fine performance of *The Blue Chips* using two Bulldogs painted in the standard red, white and grey training colours. The legend, "Bulldogs Aerobatic Team" appeared on the rear fuselage sides and a badge appeared on the fin, comprising a white rose on a pale blue disc. The team disbanded at the end of 1974 and the aircraft used were drawn from: XX515:7, XX519:1, XX520:2, XX523:5, XX526:8, XX529:11, XX528:10 and XX532:15.

1974: No. 3 Flying Training School, "The Swords", RAF Leeming, Yorkshire.

The Swords only operated for the one season, flying four Jet Provost T.5s. The team took its name from RAF Leeming's station crest — a sword.

Flight Lieutenant Clive 'Bob' Thompson led the team after being a member of the 1973 *Gemini Pair* team. *The Swords* took part in several displays up and down the country, including Greenham Common and Weston-Super-Mare. Colour scheme was the standard red, white and grey training scheme with the addition of a dark blue cheat line down the white fuselage top and a large yellow sword up the fin. The whole rudder was painted red, white and blue and *The Swords* appeared on the engine intake in gold script. The Jet Provost T.5s flown by *The Swords* were drawn from: XW406, XW407:50, XW370:49, XW428:54, XW426:53, XW326 and XW424:52. The team's publicity material was promoted by the Wilkinson Sword Company.

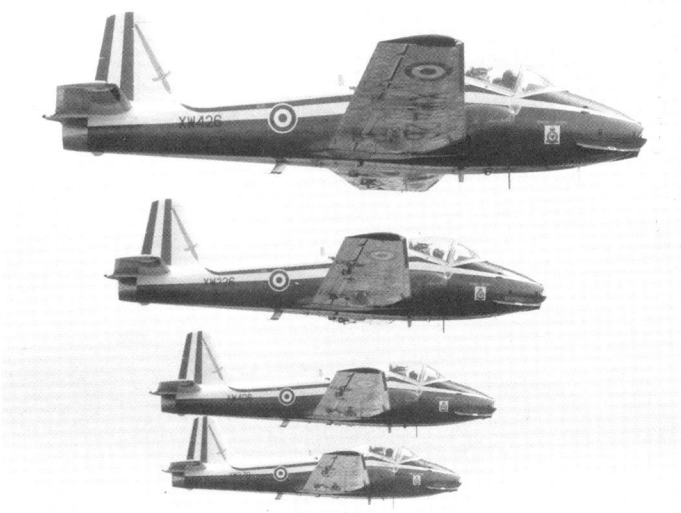

Above: Perfect line-abreast formation by Jet Provost T.5s of *The Swords* team from No.3 F.T.S., RAF Leeming during 1974. (MoD)

Below: The *Gazelles* flying Gazelle HT.2s from the C.F.S. at Ternhill in 1975. (MoD)

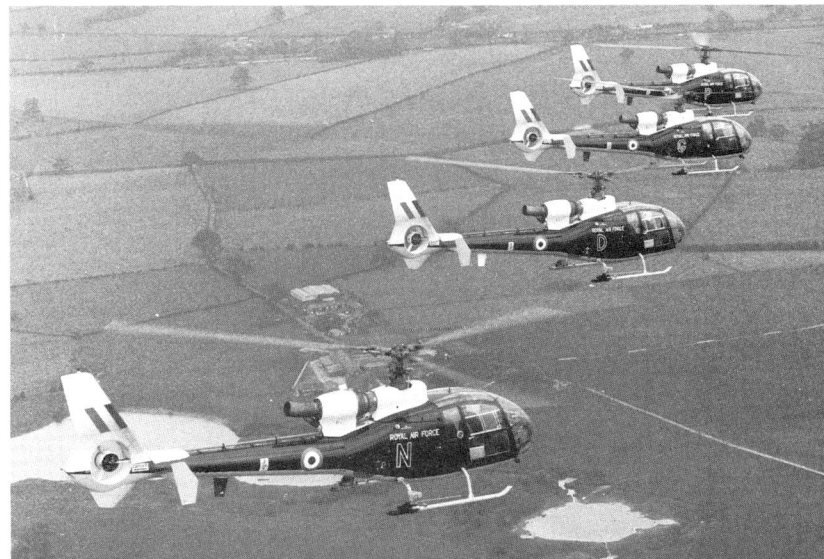

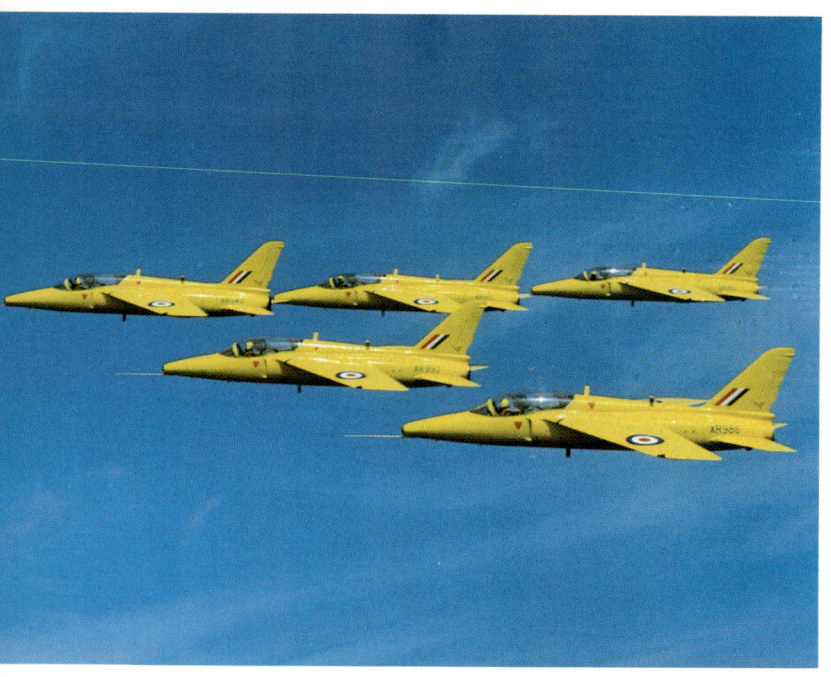

Above: Gnats of the 1964 *Yellowjacks* from No.4 F.T.S., Valley. (Rolls-Royce)

Below: The C.F.S. *Red Arrows* Gnat T.1s performing the 'undercarriage roll-back' at RAF Abingdon, September 1978. (Adrian M. Balch)

1974-76: Central Flying School Helicopter Wing, "The Gazelles", RAF Ternhill, Shropshire.

When the Sioux was replaced by the Gazelle with the CFS at Ternhill at the end of 1973, it was decided to form a display team with the type. The team formed at the end of June 1974, with their first display at RAF Little Rissington in July 1974 before HM The Queen Mother. *The Gazelles* flew four Gazelle helicopters in standard red, white and grey training colours with the addition of smoke-making containers attached to the skis. They performed at ten displays throughout the 1974 season culminating in film-making for the BBC at Ternhill in October.

Led by Flight Lieutenant D. F. Southern, the team formed up again in May 1975 to participate in another ten displays including the Paris Air Show in June. The last season was 1976, when *The Gazelles* flew to a dozen venues from May to September, now led by Flight Lieutenant B. Howley. These included the International Air Tattoo at Greenham Common, the final show being at Waterbeach in September. The team disbanded at the end of the 1976 season. The team's Gazelle HT.3s were usually drawn from: XW852/A, XW862/D, XW898/G, XX396/N and XX406/P.

1965-to date: Central Flying School, "The Red Arrows", RAF Fairford, RAF Kemble, Gloucestershire, then RAF Scampton, Lincolnshire.

Following the success of *The Yellowjacks,* it was decided to establish a permanent team of Gnats for the 1965 season. Flight Lieutenant Lee Jones, who led *The Yellowjacks,* formed *The Red Arrows* at Fairford in March 1965. The team was on permanent detachment to Fairford, which was a short distance from the CFS Headquarters at Little Rissington. The aircraft used by *The Yellowjacks* were repainted red and the team increased its number from five to seven.

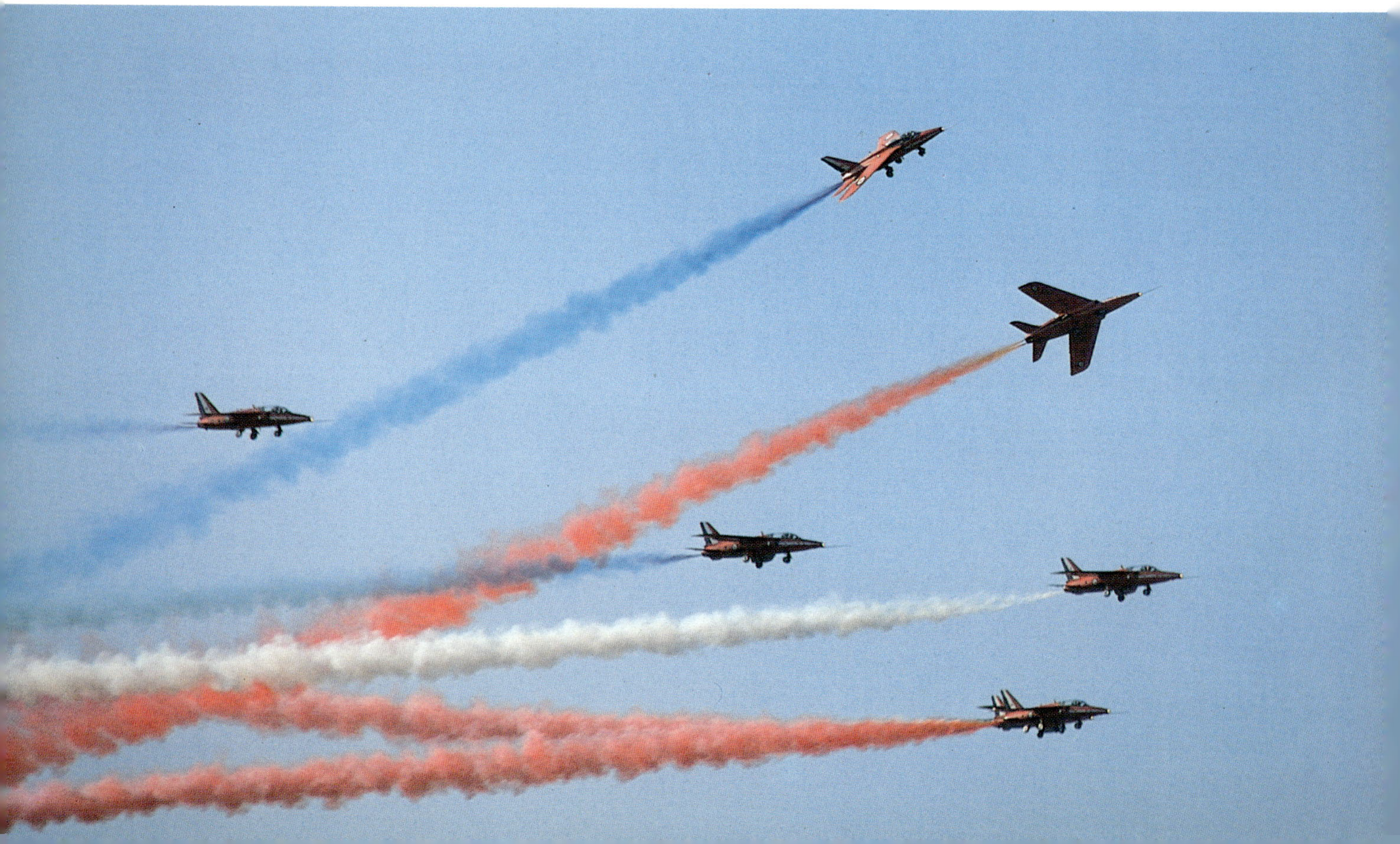

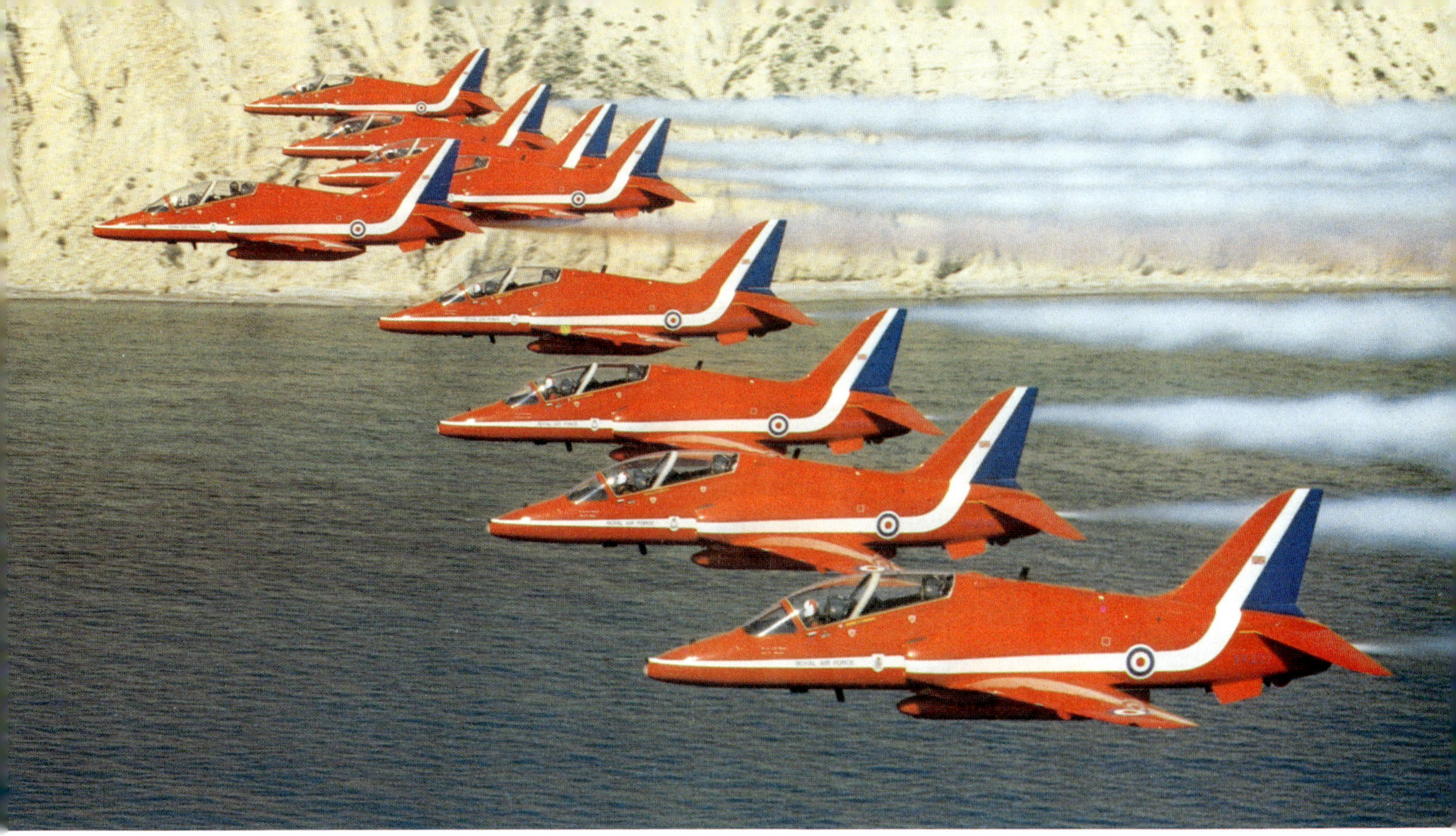

Above: Early in 1981, the *Red Arrows* deployed their Hawks to Cyprus for rehearsals in fine weather. (British Aerospace)

The unit came under the command of Squadron Leader Dick Storer, who was appointed Team Manager and the team's first public performance was at the Biggin Hill Air Fair in May 1965. The 1965 team could be identified by the Gnat's fin markings, which sported a raked fin flash and a CFS crest on a white disc. In 1966, the CFS crest was moved to the nose and the fin had a Union Jack above the fin flash. Squadron Leader Ray Hanna took over the leadership in 1966 and the team had flown nearly 100 shows by the end of that year. They performed all over Europe, including Norway, Germany, Belgium, France and Italy. From July until the end of the season, the team increased in number from seven to nine. Towards the end of the 1966 season, the team made a tour of the Mediterranean, which included Cyprus, Malta and Jordan.

In 1967, *The Red Arrows* were once again reduced to seven aircraft, the Gnats now sporting red, white and blue fins.

1968 was the 50th Anniversary of the RAF and *The Red Arrows* flew nearly 100 shows again. The serviceability of the Gnats was so good that they never failed to provide a full complement of aircraft. The team was back to nine aircraft in 1968 and all nine participated at every show. To do this out of a total ten was no mean achievement on the part of the maintenance personnel. For the 1968 season, the white lightning flash was added to the fuselage of the Gnats.

Squadron Leader Denis Hazell took over as leader in 1970 and it was hoped that he would retain the lead for the following season but, unfortunately, he suffered a broken leg when ejecting from an aircraft early in the between-season training period in November. That was the first of a series of setbacks to befall the team in the winter of 1970-71.

In early January 1971 another member left for medical reasons and a few days later in a tragic accident, two aircraft were lost and four pilots killed.

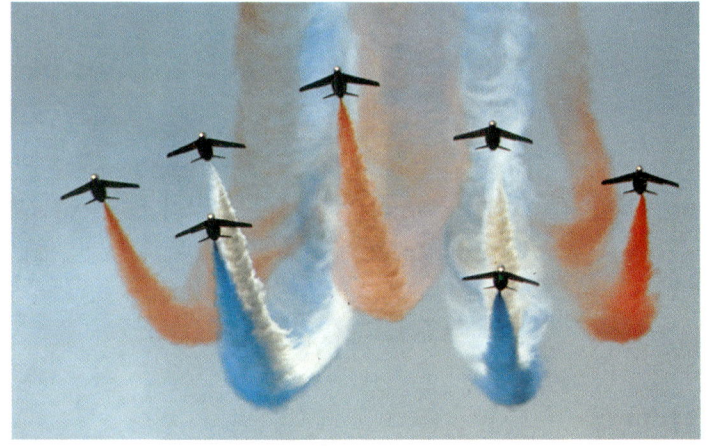

Above: Thick red, white and blue smoke being trailed by the Gnats of the *Red Arrows* in 1972 during their U.S.A. tour. (U.S. Air Force)

Below: The daring 'roulette' crossover by two *Red Arrows* Hawks is perfectly captured here during a display in 1981. (British Aerospace)

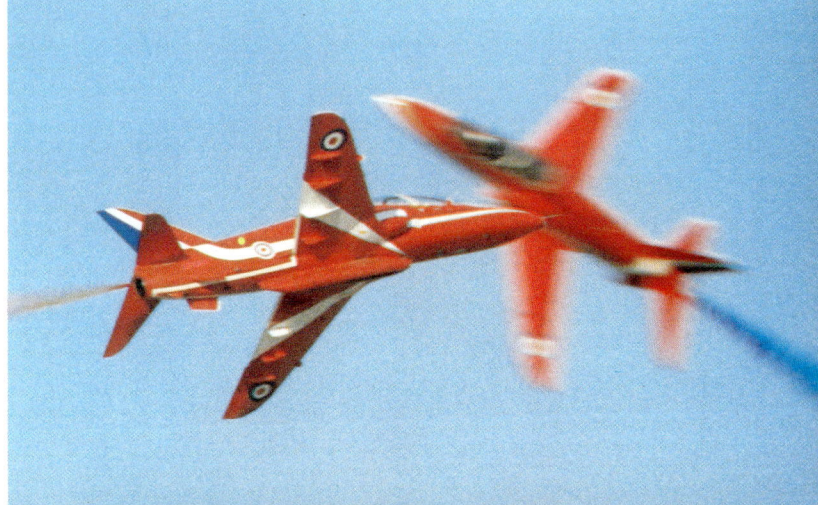

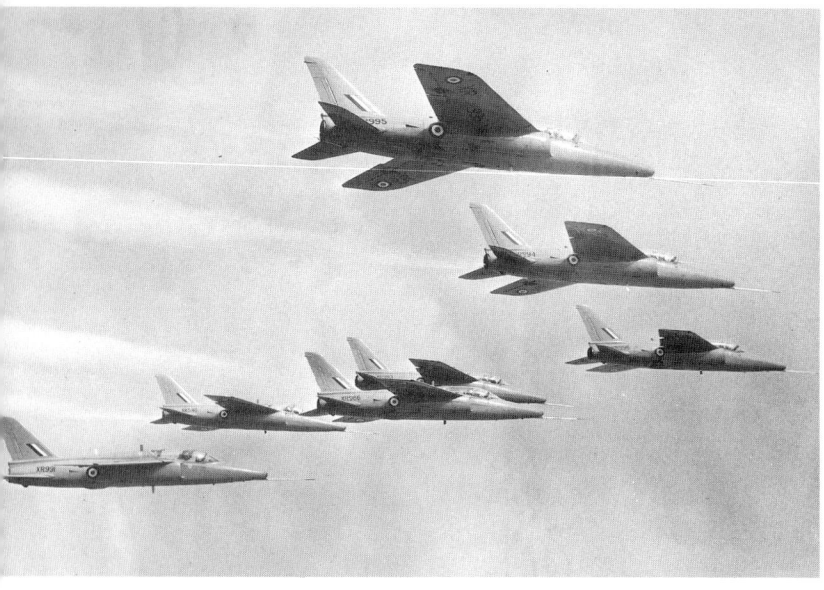

The *Red Arrows* Gnats photographed early in 1965, just after they were repainted from their *Yellowjacks* scheme. (Hawker Siddeley Aviation)

Below: The *Red Arrows* Gnats in their 1965 scheme, lined up at Little Rissington. Note C.F.S. badge above raked fin flash (MoD)

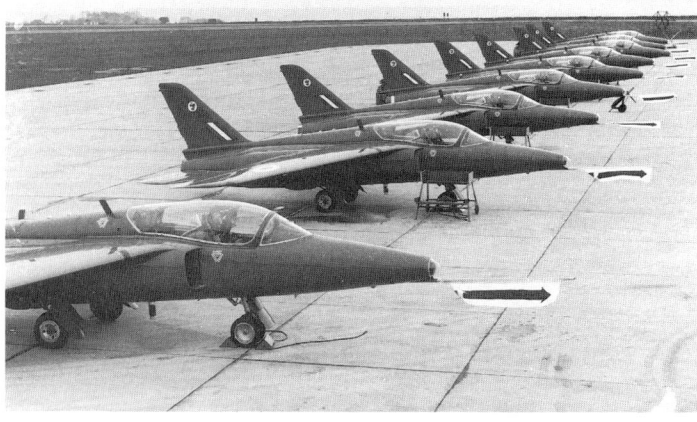

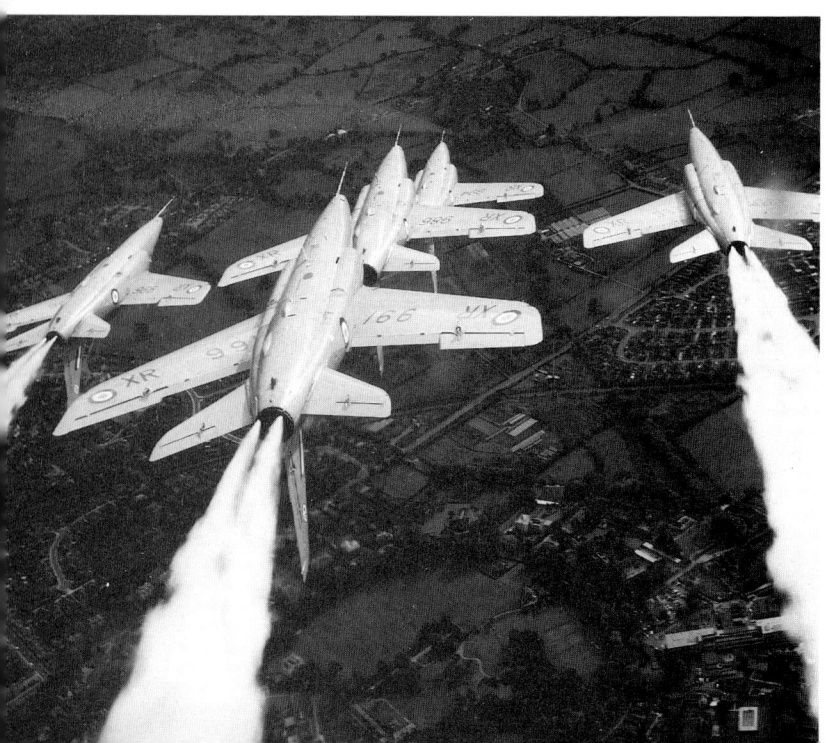

Squadron Leader Bill Loverseed was appointed leader for the 1971 season, but due to the loss of aircraft, only seven were displayed that year. In 1972, Squadron Leader Ian Dick became *The Red Arrows* leader and remained so for three seasons. In 1974, *The Red Arrows* display season was postponed until July due to the "energy crisis". Squadron Leader Dickie Duckett returned as leader for the 1975 season, after flying with the 1968, '69 and '70 teams. He led the team during the following year and then it was the turn of another *Red Arrows* member to return as leader in the form of Squadron Leader Frank Hoare. He had flown with the 1966, '67 and '68 teams, so had plenty of experience with the team. 1977 was the Silver Jubilee of Her Majesty The Queen and a new manoeuvre called "Jubilee Break" was devised in her honour. Jubilee Celebrations included the Royal Review of the RAF at Finningley on 29 July. This was preceded by a flypast over Buckingham Palace on 11 June. At the end of the 1977 season, the team had chalked-up 109 displays.

In 1978, *The Red Arrows* flew a record 123 displays, closing this very busy display season with a deployment to Malta. During the year, all the European teams met at Salon to celebrate the 25th anniversary of *La Patrouille de France* and there was a joint dinner with Italy's *Frecce Tricolori* after a display in Florence.

For the final season with the Gnats, 1979, Squadron Leader Brian Hoskins took over as leader. He was an ex-member of *The Macaws* Jet Provost team and led *The Red Arrows* through the conversion from the Gnat to the Hawk. By the end of the 1979 season, the Gnats had flown 1,292 displays and had shown the flag in Belgium, Canada, Cyprus, Denmark, Finland, France, Germany, Greenland, Ireland, Italy, Jordan, Malta, Netherlands, Norway, Portugal, Sweden and USA. For the last two seasons, the Gnats had "ROYAL AIR FORCE" in white on the nose. Rumour has it that some people thought they were a privately-owned aerobatic team! The leader's aircraft had "RAF" in large white letters under the wings, to make sure everyone knew whose team it was.

Apart from one Gnat operated by the Royal Aircraft Establishment, *The Red Arrows* were the last unit to use the type in the RAF. Unfortunately, just before the type was withdrawn from the team, they could only muster eight aircraft for the last few displays. The final displays were on Battle of Britain Day in September 1979 at Abingdon and St. Athan.

The 1965 *Red Arrows* Gnats at the top of a loop over Little Rissington. (MoD)

The Red Arrows converted to the Hawk during the winter and flew to Cyprus to complete their training in better weather conditions, in time for the show season. Squadron Leader Brian Hoskins led the team of nine Hawks throught the 1980 and '81 seasons, followed by Squadron Leader John Blackwell, who took over leadership from 1982 for three years. After a four-year absence from the team, Squadron Leader Richard Thomas returned as leader in 1985 after being a member of the team during the last three years with the Gnat and during the first year with Hawks.

A change of base came in April 1983, when *The Red Arrows* moved from Kemble, Gloucestershire, which had been their home since 1966. Kemble became a USAFE maintenance base and the team moved to RAF Scampton, Lincolnshire. The original *Red Arrows* Gnats during the 1965-67 seasons were: XR991, XR992, XR993, XR994, XR995, XR996, XR986, XR987, XR540 and XS111, of which the latter was the last Gnat built. Due to attrition and accidents, the following have also served with the team since then: XP501, XP505, XP514, XP515, XP531, XP533, XP535, XP538, XP539, XP541, XR537, XR545, XR571, XR572, XR574, XR955, XR977, XR981, XS101, and XS107, making a grand total of 30 Gnats that have flown in *Red Arrows* colours! Hawks used by the team from 1980 to date are: XX227, XX243, XX251, XX252, XX253, XX257, XX258, XX259, XX260, XX262, XX264, XX266, XX304, XX306 and XX308. Of these, XX262 was written-off on 17 May 1980, when it hit a yacht's mast during a display off the coast at Brighton; Squadron Leader S. Johnson ejected safely. XX257 was also ditched in the sea off Sidmouth on 31 August 1984, when engine problems developed and the pilot once again ejected safely. XX251 crashed at Akrotiri, Cyprus on 21 March 1984 during winter training.

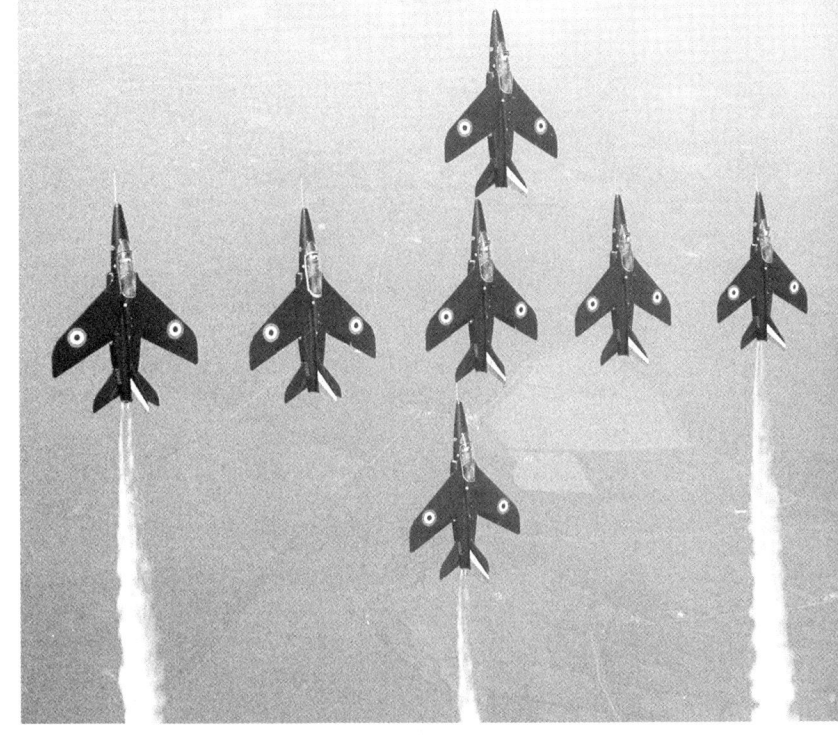

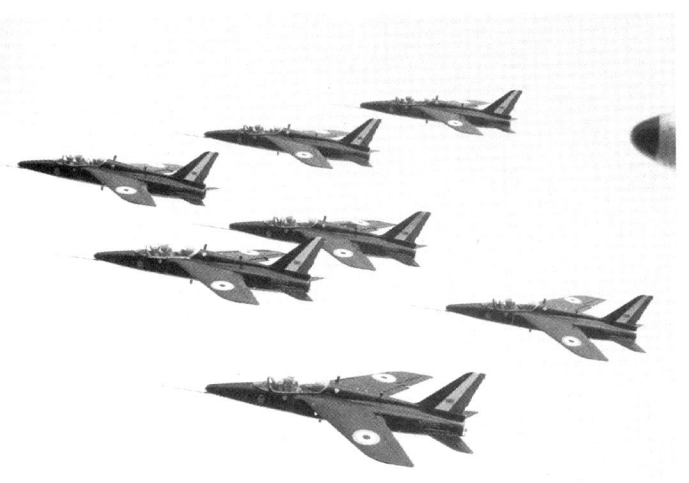

Top: Gnats of the 1967 *Red Arrows* in 'Kings Cross' formation. Due to fuel economy, the team only operated seven aircraft that year. (MoD)

Centre: The 1967 *Red Arrows* again, seen in 'Arrow' formation. 1967 was the first year that the tri-coloured fin was introduced. (MoD)

Bottom: In 1968, the *Red Arrows* reverted to nine Gnats and introduced a white lightning flash on the nose, which was retained until the end of the 1977 season. Nearest aircraft is XS111, which was the last Gnat to be built. (MoD)

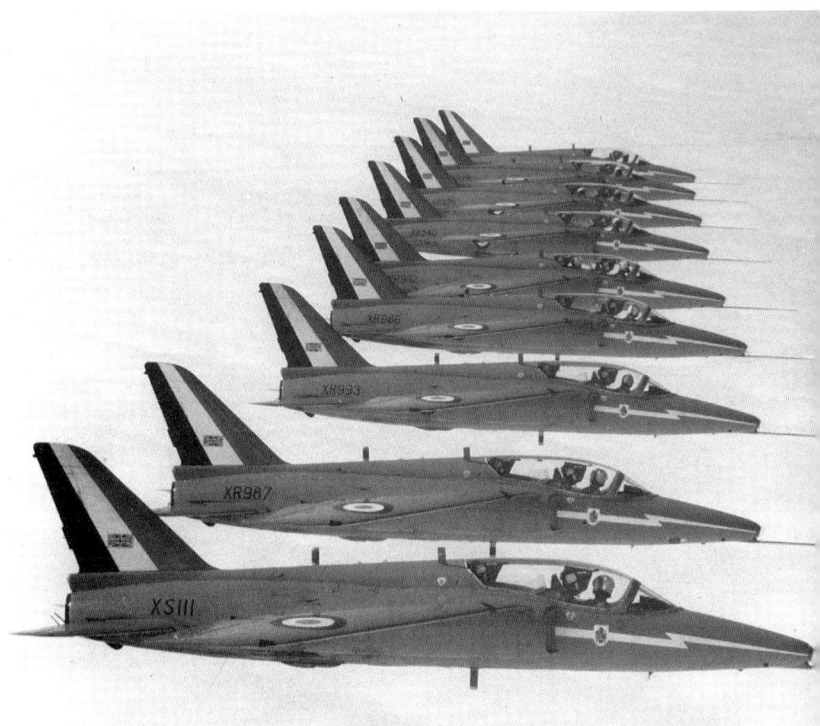

GREAT BRITAIN
The Royal Navy, Fleet Air Arm

The Fleet Air Arm flew several formations during the 1930s, but nothing that could be called an aerobatic team until after the Second World War. It was in the 1950s that squadron teams began forming, as they found the Sea Hawk was an ideal aerobatic mount. Nos. 800 and 898 Squadrons formed teams of Sea Hawks during the mid-'50s. During 1954-56, No.898 Squadron flew a team of six Sea Hawk F.1s, which included WF182:101, WF184:102, WF213:103, WF185:104 and WF170:109.

The current FAA display team, *The Sharks* from No. 705 Squadron. From 1980 onwards, *The Sharks* adopted the RAF colour scheme for their Gazelles of red, white and grey. (Royal Navy)

1957: 738 Squadron, "The Red Devils", RNAS Lossiemouth, Morayshire.
This was the first named Fleet Air Arm team and formed just for the one season. *The Red Devils* flew five Sea Hawk F.B.3s and were based at Lossiemouth in Scotland. They participated in several displays all over the country, with their all-red, smoke-equipped Sea Hawks, which wore large white 'ROYAL NAVY' titles under the wings. *The Red Devils* were best known for their participation in the 1957 S.B.A.C. display at Farnborough. The aircraft used by the team were: WM934, WM975, WM999, WN105 and WV831, the leader being Lieutenant Commander A. J. Leahy, D.S.C.

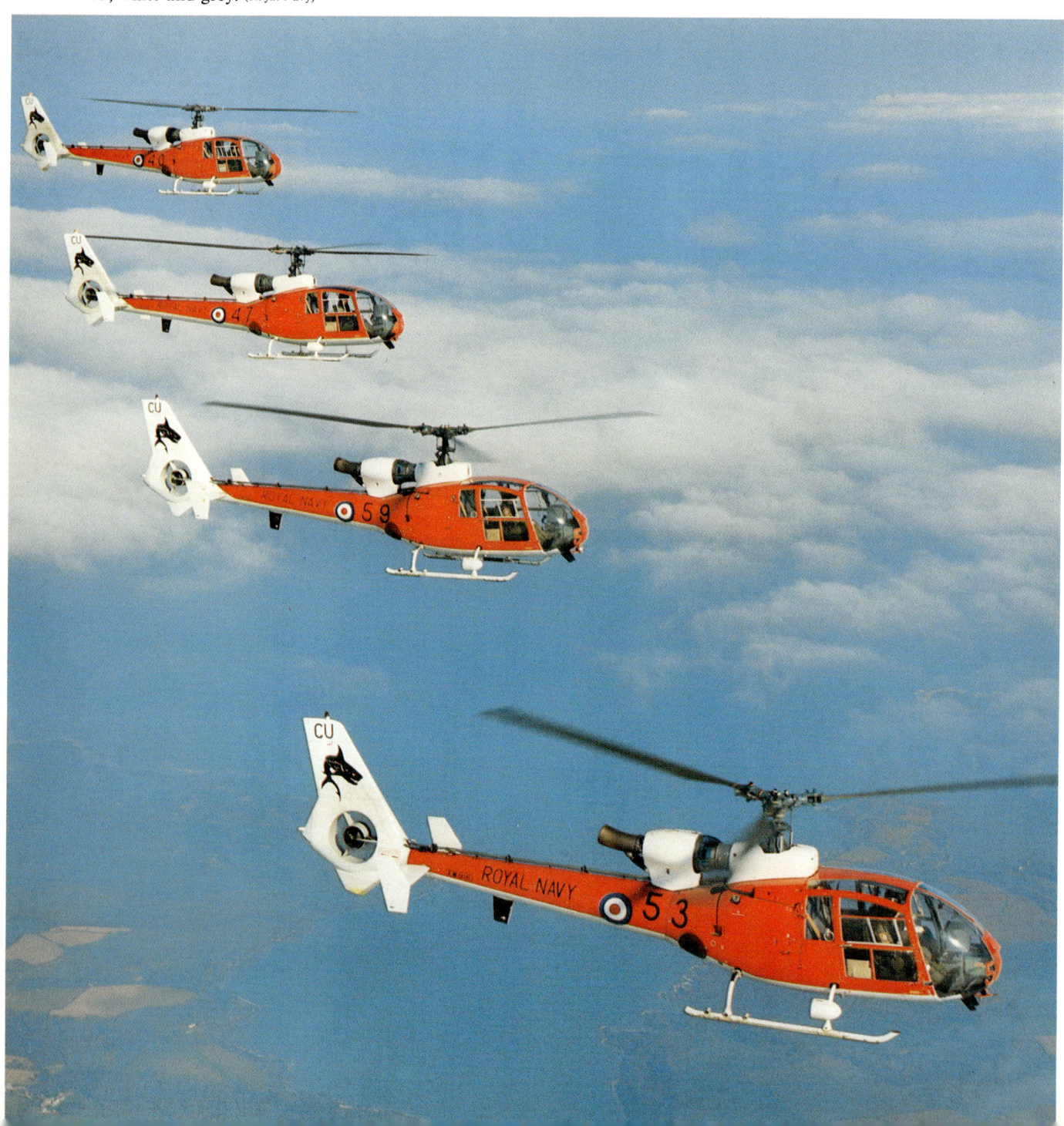

When *The Red Devils* disbanded, No. 800 Squadron formed a team of Sea Hawks and took part in the 1958 Farnborough display. This team comprised seven aircraft, which retained their standard colour scheme of dark sea grey and pale green undersides. Operating from HMS *Ark Royal*, the team's aircraft were drawn from: XE342, XE462, XE406, XE385, XE386, XE438, WV844, WV907, WV805 and WV912. The team participated daily at Farnborough, but XE462 crashed at Blackbushe on 1st September 1958.

Scimitar teams.

Those squadrons equipped with Scimitars were starting to try the type out with aerobatic manoeuvres in the late 1950s. Although a much bigger and heavier aircraft than the Sea Hawk, it was found to be a very stable and graceful aerobatic mount and could also be easily adapted to make smoke. The first Scimitar team to appear at the annual Farnborough Air Show was provided by No. 803 Squadron, who flew a team of four at the 1958 display and shared the limelight with No. 800 Squadron's Sea Hawks. The aircraft used were drawn from XD234, XD235, XD237, XD238, XD239 and XD240. No. 803 Squadron continued to provide formation displays right up until 1964, when the squadron disbanded. The 1964 Farnborough display was the team's last public performance.

1959 saw the formation of another Scimitar team, this time coming from No. 807 Squadron, which provided a display with seven aircraft led by Lieutenant Commander K. A. Leppard. Based at Lossiemouth, the team's main formation comprised four aircraft, whose aerobatics were interspersed with solo demonstrations by two other aircraft. One of them carried a full load of underwing stores and demonstrated an 'over-the-shoulder' bombing technique. The other, in addition to solo aerobatics, used its hook to snatch a high-speed towed target, of the kind used for live air-to-air firing practice. This display was given at the Farnborough Air Show in September 1959 and introduced a new manoeuvre to Farnborough, in which each aircraft did an individual and very quick roll whilst in formation. They concluded their act with a remarkable landing drill, in which the solo pair landed together from one end of the runway, folded their wings whilst still in motion to permit a third Scimitar coming from the opposite direction to land between them! It was hoped that it frightened the pilots less than it did some of the spectators! The aircraft wore the standard dark grey and white colour scheme worn by all Scimitars, with the addition of the squadron's Scimitar insignia on the fin, which was white with a yellow handle. The seven aircraft in the team were usually: XD244:191/R, XD245:192/R, XD248:195/R, XD249:196/R, XD250:197/R, XD267:193/R and XD268:194/R. The 'R' in the codes indicated that the aircraft were based on *HMS Ark Royal*, but were detached to Lossiemouth.

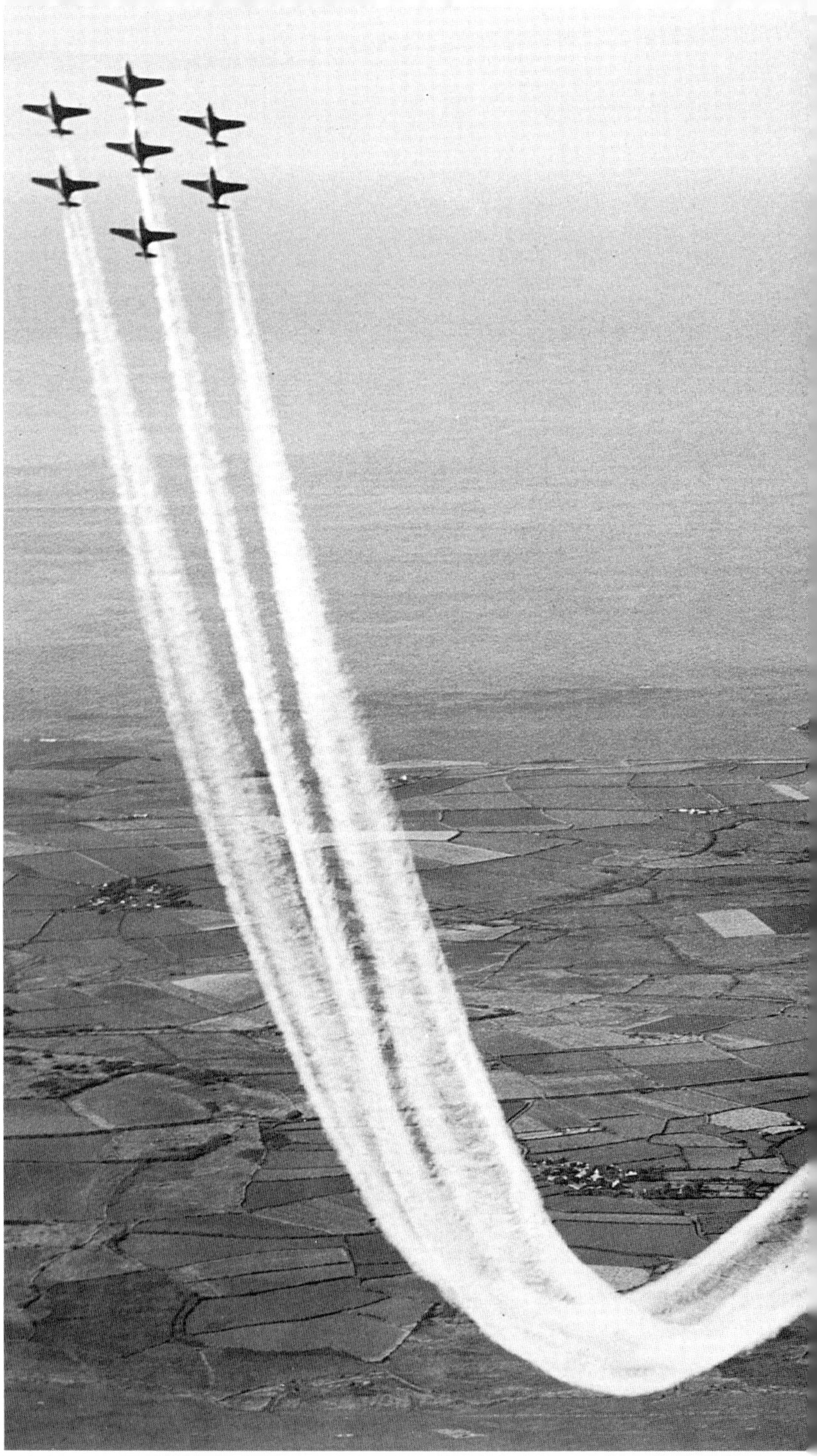

All-red Sea Hawks of No.738 Squadron's *Red Devils* team during rehearsals in 1957 near Lossiemouth.
(Flight International via R. Ward)

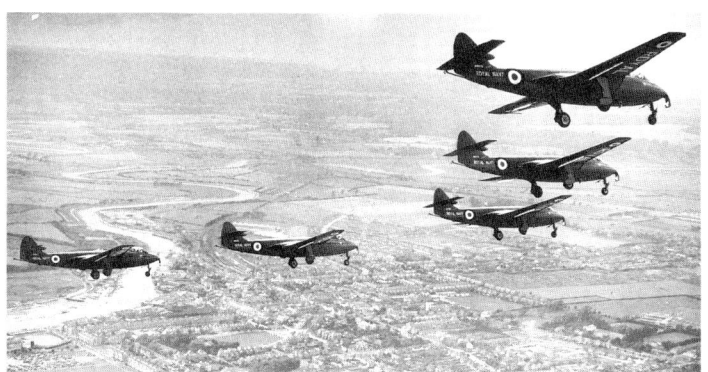

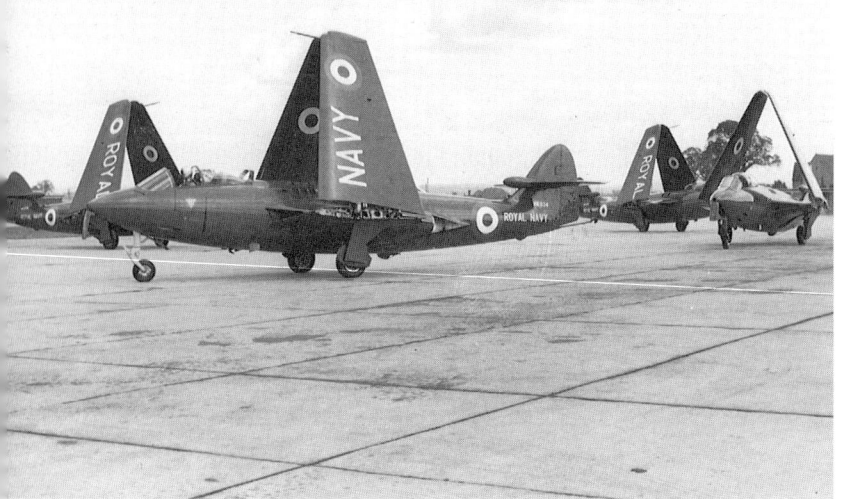

Above: The Sea Hawks of 738 Squadron's *Red Devils* taxy out for a display at Lossiemouth in 1957. Note the white 'ROYAL NAVY' lettering under the wings, on overall red aircraft. (Fleet Air Arm Museum)

Below: Sea Vixen FAW.1s of the 1962 F.A.A. aerobatic team, *Fred's Five*. Nearest aircraft is XJ565. (MoD via R. Ward)

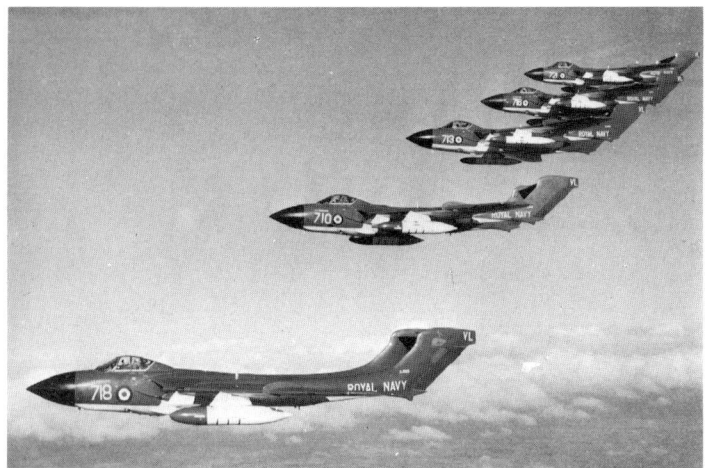

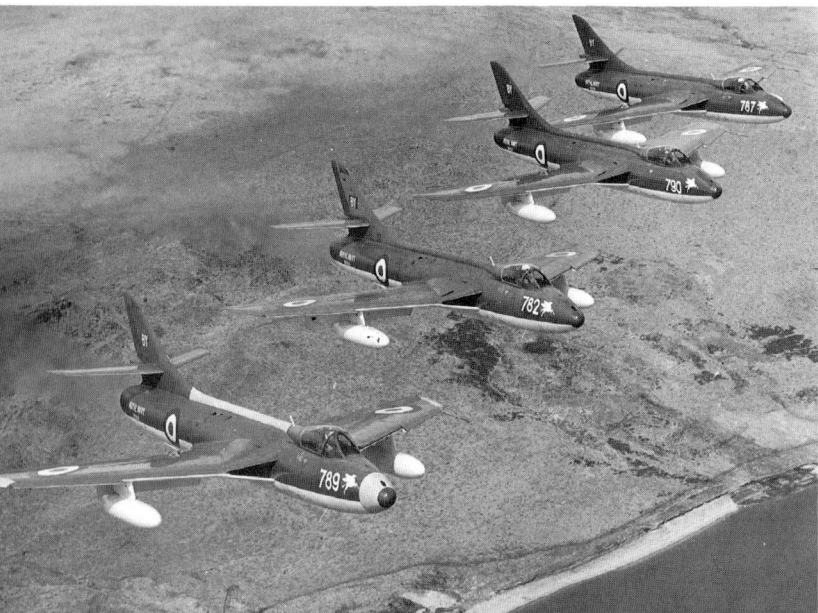

Above: Hunter GA.11s of No. 738 Squadron's *Rough Diamonds* flying near Brawdy in 1967. Note the dayglo-red nose, spine and wingtips of the leader's aircraft, which is XE680 coded 789/BY. (Royal Navy)

1961 saw a team of Scimitars from No. 800 Squadron, also detached to Lossiemouth from *HMS Ark Royal*. Also equipped to make smoke, No. 800 Squadron had a nine-aircraft team led by Lieutenant Commander D. P. Norman A.F.C., which participated in the Paris Air Show in May and in the 1961 Farnborough display. One of the highlights of their display was a 'Diamond-9' formation flypast with everything down, including arrestor hooks. The aircraft wore the standard grey and white colour scheme, with the addition of a red fin panel with 'R' in white, denoting *HMS Ark Royal*. The aircraft in the team were drawn from: XD276:100, XD277:101, XD278:102, XD279:103, XD246:104, XD265:105, XD322:106, XD250:107, XD231:108, XD239:109 and XD267:110.

Formation flypasts were also made by Scimitars from Nos. 736 and 804 Squadrons in 1961 and '62, but these were not regarded as aerobatic teams.

1962: No. 766 Squadron, "Fred's Five", RNAS Yeovilton, Somerset.

It was not until 1962 that another named Fleet Air Arm aerobatic team came into being. This was *Fred's Five*, comprising five Sea Vixen FAW.1s from No. 766 Squadron at RNAS Yeovilton. This was the first team to use the Sea Vixen, which despite being a heavy aircraft, proved very manoeuvrable in displays and was equipped with smoke-making apparatus. Led by Lieutenant Commander P. B. Reynolds, they participated in the 50th Anniversary of Military Aviation display at Upavon on 16 June 1962 and at Farnborough the following September. The aircraft were in the usual dark sea grey and white scheme with no special markings, although the front section of the underwing tanks was red. The aircraft in the team were drawn from: XJ513:710, XJ576:711, XJ524:712, XJ482:713, XN697:714, XJ480:715, XJ565:718, XN698:719 and XJ575:720. Apart from the 700 series nose codes, all aircraft carried a white 'VL' on top of the fins, denoting Yeovilton-based. *Fred's Five* disbanded at the end of the 1962 season.

1965-69: No. 738 Squadron, "The Rough Diamonds", RNAS Brawdy, South Wales

Although several squadrons provided formations for air displays, it was not until the summer of 1965 that an official aerobatic team was formed. This was *The Rough Diamonds*, flying four Hawker Hunter GA.11s, whose main display venues were events at Royal Naval establishments. Flying from Brawdy, in South Wales, the team did not get its name from a poor diamond formation, but from the shape of the Hunter! The team comprised a formation of four, with the spare aircraft often joining in for certain displays. Lieutenant Commander Christopher Comins was the team leader in 1967, who took the team through eight minutes of loops and rolls in various formations. The Hunters were not able to make smoke, as they were standard aircraft drawn from No. 738 Squadron. The aircraft wore the standard F.A.A.

Opposite: No. 800 Squadron's Scimitars rehearsing near Lossiemouth in 1961. (Fleet Air Arm Museum)

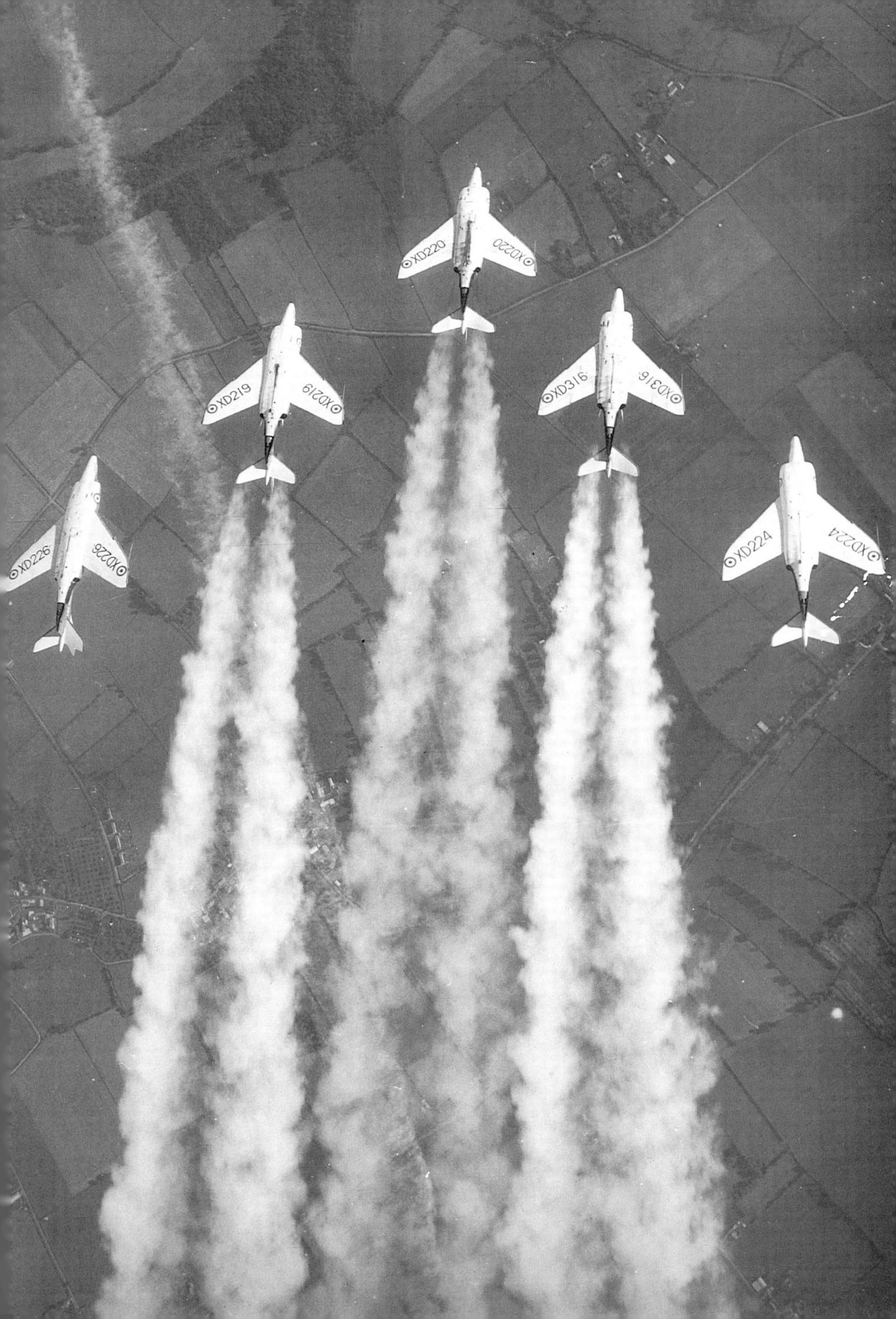

dark sea grey and white scheme, with white lettering and the squadron's Pegasus winged-horse on the nose. The team leader's aircraft had a dayglo-red nose, spine and wingtips. Three aircraft were known to have worn these markings — XF291:789, XF297:781 and XE680:789. The rest of the team were usually drawn from: WV380:794, WT711:783, WW659:793 WT713:787, XF301:791, WV374:795, WV256:794, XE674:788 and XE712:785. All aircraft wore the 'BY' tail code in white, denoting Brawdy-based.

1968: No. 892 Squadron, "Simon's Sircus", RNAS Yeovilton, Somerset.

In February 1968, No. 892 Squadron disembarked from *HMS Hermes* to RNAS Yeovilton. Three weeks later, *Simon's Sircus* was formed by Lieutenant Commander, Simon Idiens, flying six Sea Vixen FAW.2s. The aircraft were fitted out with smoke-making equipment and the team underwent intensive rehearsals for their first public display on 9 May at the Biggin Hill Air Fair. The team only operated for the one season, but gave many displays around the country including shows at Brawdy, Yeovilton and Farnborough. Towards the end of the season, they flew co-ordinated displays with *Phoenix Five* — the Buccaneer display team from 809 Squadron. *Simon's Sircus* aircraft wore the usual dark grey and white colour scheme, with a black and yellow wolf's head badge on their fins. The front of the underwing tanks was red. The six Sea Vixens used were drawn from: XN650:301, XN687:307, XJ609:306, XN690:304, XN694:305, XJ604:303 and XN705:302.

1968: No. 809 Squadron, "Phoenix Five", RNAS Lossiemouth, Morayshire.

This was the only team ever to be formed using Buccaneers. Operating from Lossiemouth, the team's name derived from 809 Squadron's Phoenix badge and, of course, there were five aircraft. They only flew during the one season and gave co-ordinated displays with the Sea Vixens of *Simon's Sircus*. Following Yeovilton's Naval Air Day in September 1968, *Phoenix Five* flew daily in the Farnborough Air Show, which was their last public performance. The Buccaneers were unable to make smoke and wore the standard colour scheme of extra dark sea grey overall with pale blue codes, serials and lettering. No. 809 Squadron's official crest appeared on the engine intake and the red, yellow and white Phoenix badge adorned the fin. The team was usually drawn from: XT277:320, XV334, XV340:321, XV344:325, XT280:323, XV868:327 and XT279:322. All the Buccaneers carried a small 'LM' code under the fin badge, denoting Lossiemouth as their base. The following year, 1969, 809 Squadron's Buccaneers embarked in *HMS Ark Royal*.

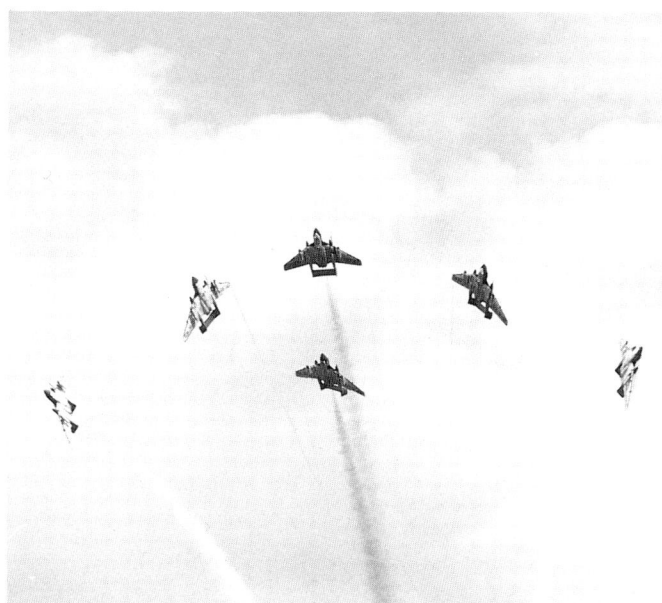

Above: Simon's Sircus Sea Vixen FAW.2s of No. 892 Squadron RNAS, Yeovilton in September 1968. (for colour photograph, see page 69). (Peter R. March)

Below: Simon's Sircus. Sea Vixen FAW.2s of No. 892 Squadron leading *Phoenix Five* Buccaneers from No. 809 Squadron in 1968 (Peter R. March)

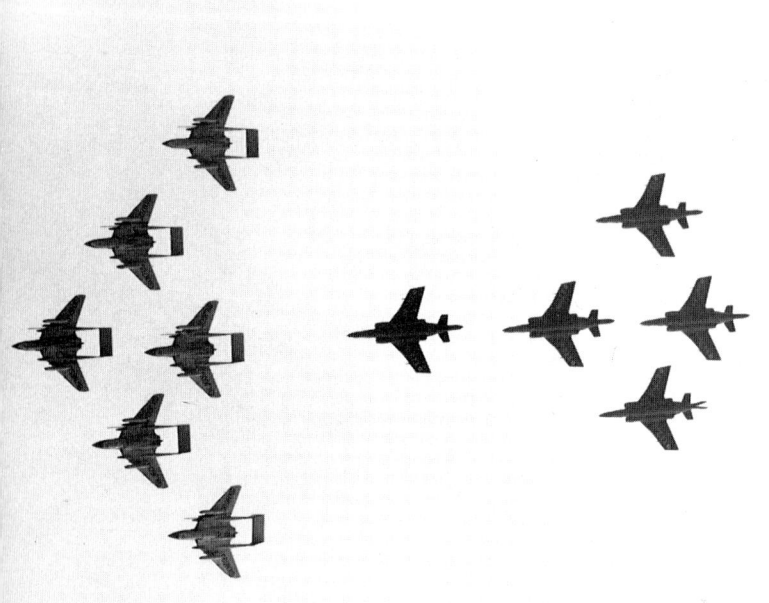

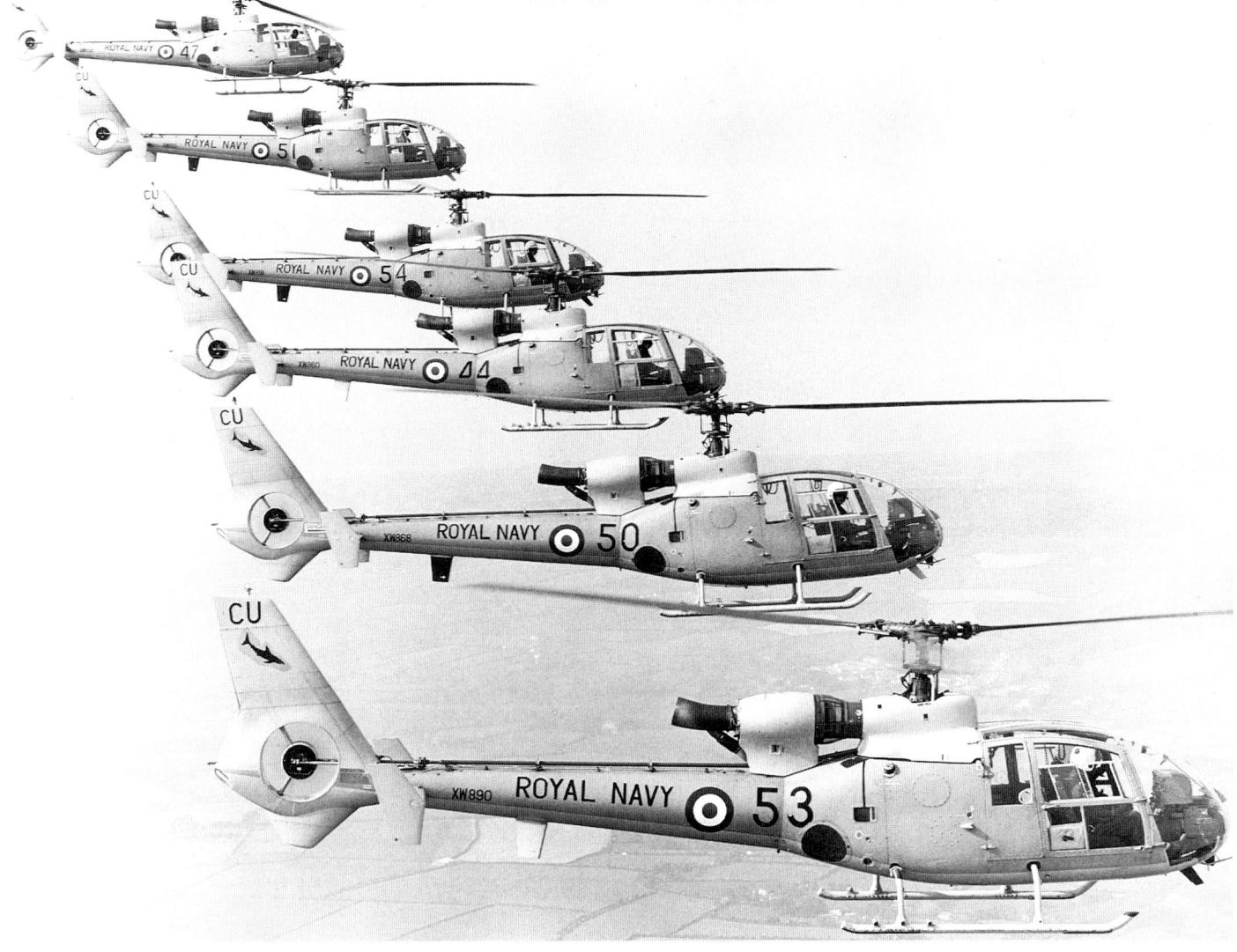

Above: The original *Sharks* livery in 1975-76 was dayglo orange, grey and white. Note traditional-style Shark insignia, which was black on a dayglo red background mounted on a grey fin. Compare with colour photograph on page 60. (Royal Navy)

1975—to date: No. 705 Squadron, "The Sharks", RNAS Culdrose, Cornwall.

Based at RNAS Culdrose, Cornwall, *The Sharks* were formed in 1975 with four Westland Gazelle HT.2 helicopters. The team pilots are all qualified helicopter instructors from 705 Squadron, which is the Royal Navy's basic flying training unit for helicopter pilots. Practices have to take place in the early morning or evening, as the team are required for normal instructional duties during the day. Using smoke cannisters attached to the skis, the team uses a colourful combination of orange and green smoke during its display. The standard Royal Navy Gazelle colour scheme was employed during the 1975-76 seasons, comprising orange-dayglo, grey and white. In addition, a black Shark emblem on a dayglo surround appeared on the fin. For the 1977-79 seasons, the fin and engine casing were painted gloss black and the Shark motif was modified to a rampant pose, which looked more aggressive. This appeared on the black fin in dayglo red. From 1980 to date, the Royal Navy changed the Gazelle colour scheme to that used by RAF aircraft, i.e. red, white and grey. The rampant Shark appears in black on a white fin and all lettering is in black. Lieutenant Commander John Beattie led *The Sharks* through the 1982 season, whose display venues were mainly at Royal Naval Establishments. From the time they were formed, the Gazelles of *The Sharks* have usually been drawn from: XW907:40, XW884:41, XW863:42, XX397:43 XW860:44, XW856:47 XW868:50, XW895:51, XW894:52, XW890:53 and XW891:54. All carry the 'CU' tail codes, indicating their base of RNAS Culdrose.

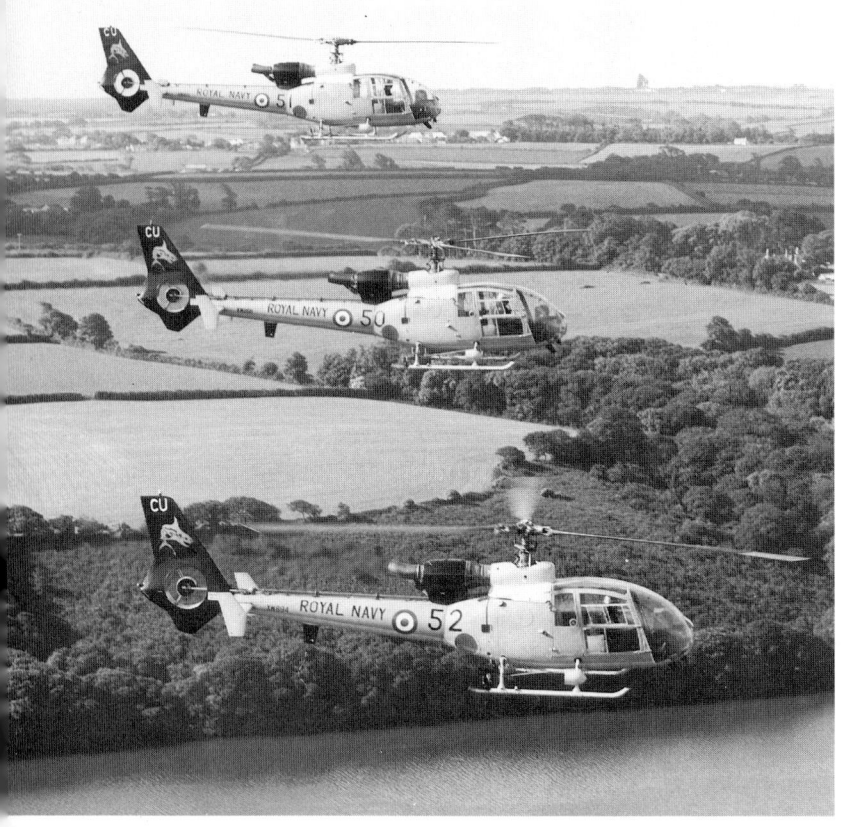

During 1977-79, *The Sharks* modified the original colour scheme on their Gazelle helicopters to incorporate a gloss black fin and engine surround. The Shark insignia was in rampant style and dayglo-red. This photo was taken in 1978. (Royal Navy)

Hunter GA.11s of the F.A.A. *Blue Herons* team at the top of a loop in 'Card Four' formation during 1977. (HMS Heron)

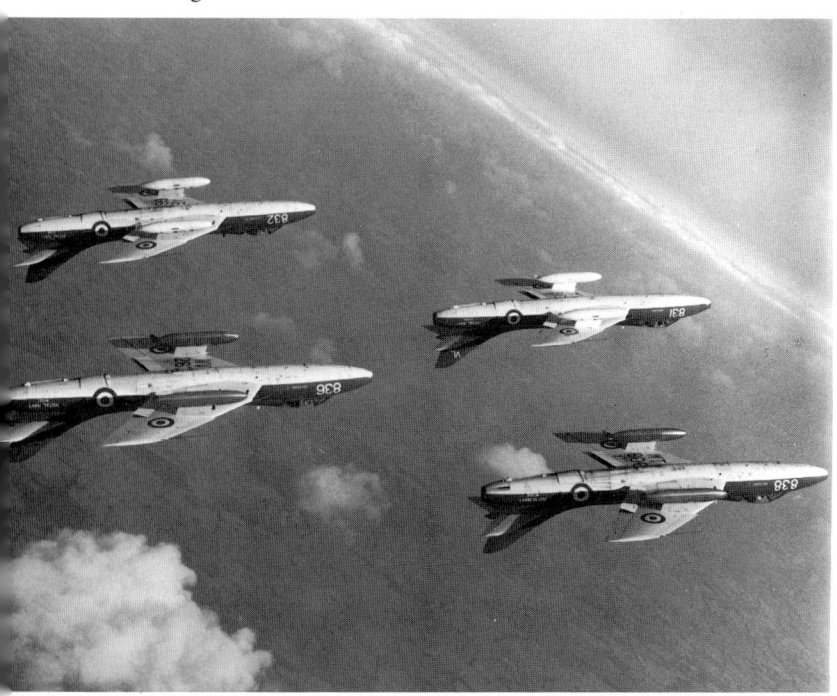

1975-80: FRADU, "The Blue Herons", RNAS Yeovilton, Somerset.

The Blue Herons aerobatic team was formed in July 1975 by pilots of the Fleet Requirements and Air Direction Unit (FRADU) at Royal Naval Air Station Yeovilton. It was formed originally to display only at RNAS Yeovilton Air Day 1975, but as the subsequent years proved, the team was soon in great demand at other shows.

It was the world's first civilian team to fly military jet aircraft and gave its first performance with the unit's Hawker Hunter GA.11s at RNAS Yeovilton in September; it's last at Battle of Britain Day, RAF Coltishall in September 1980.

The original team was founder/leader Derek Morter, No. 2 Godfrey Cornish-Underwood, No. 3 Jerram Gosnell and No. 4 Pierre Cadoret; Brian Grant replaced Jerram Gosnell in 1977 as No. 3, Mike Todd took over as No. 2 in 1979. These were the main members with Martin Holloway and Nigel Charles stepping in later as No. 4. No specific training periods were allocated to the team for practice; practices were gleaned at the end of normal unit tasks, in particular with the co-operation of the Air Direction Unit. Fortunately, the team members all had considerable Hunter experience; this showed in the routine demonstration by the team earning wide acclaim at the first public performance.

The Hunter GA.11s flown by the team were operated by Airwork Ltd. under contract to the Royal Navy. The civilian aircrew and the engineering personnel who maintain the aircraft were all employed by the firm. The Hunter GA.11s used by *The Blue Herons* were standard aircraft used for fleet requirements and fighter direction tasks and had a modified nose incorporating a powerful Harley light and an improved radio fit.

The Blue Herons name derived from the fact that the parent base was *HMS Heron* — RNAS Yeovilton and the pilots came from a RAF or Royal Navy background, being a mixture of the light and dark blues. Such was the achievement of the team, in the short time that it existed, in giving a public display of originality and quality, that it was awarded second prize in the Shell Trophy competition at the 1976 International Air Tattoo. At the Silver Jubilee International Air Tattoo held at Greenham Common in June 1977, with participants from all over the world, *The Blue Herons* won the Shell Trophy. It was awarded to their team by a panel of International judges for the best overall flying performance at the Tattoo on Sunday 26th June 1977. Unfortunately, due to the need for the Royal Navy to make substantial financial economies, the team was disbanded at the end of the 1980 display season.

The four Hunter GA.11s were painted in the standard Fleet Air Arm dark sea grey and white colour scheme with all lettering in white on the fuselage. For a short period, a *Blue Heron* badge was carried on the front of the underwing tanks. The aircraft used were usually drawn from: WW654:833, XE682:835, WT804:831, WT806:838, WV267:836, WT711:837, WV382:830.

GREAT BRITAIN
The Army Air Corps

Several fixed-wing and helicopter teams have been formed by the Army Air Corps during the 1960s, '70s and '80s, but mainly only for the biennial Army Air Days at Middle Wallop. The only team that has operated for a considerable time were *The Blue Eagles* with their Sioux AH.1s. No doubt a long-running Lynx team will form in the near future, if defence economies permit it.

1968-75: "The Blue Eagles", AAC Middle Wallop, Hants.

The Blue Eagles helicopter display team was formed by five instructors at the School of Army Aviation, Middle Wallop, in the Spring of 1968. Using training aircraft from the School, they gave displays in their spare time throughout the Summer, and the season culminated with the Farnborough Air Show.

The success of the first season's flying was such that the demand for a full-time team was met the following year. Their unique and spectacular routines were seen at over sixty public shows throughout the United Kingdom, at events ranging from Country Carnivals to Battle of Britain Anniversary air displays.

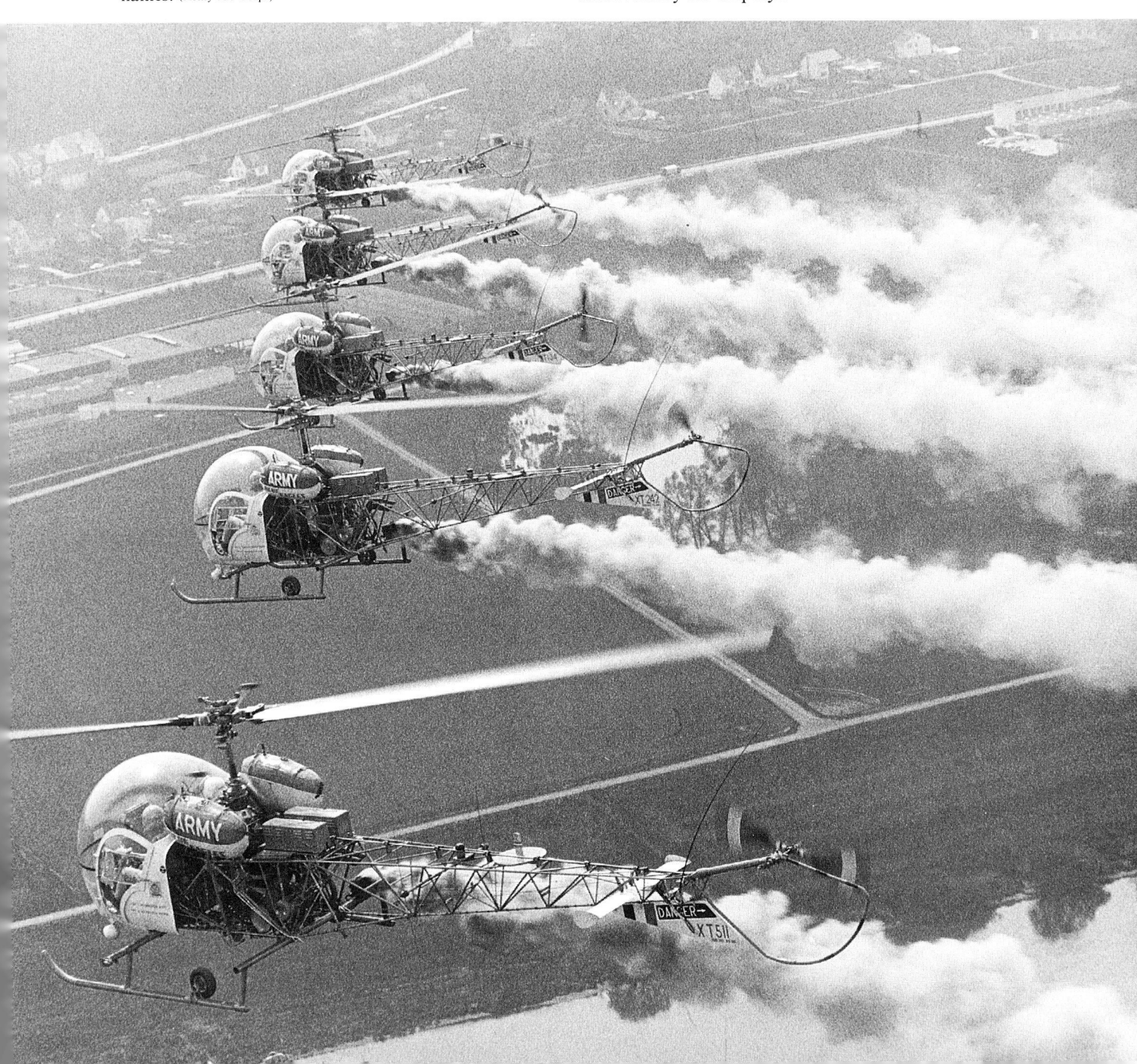

The *Blue Eagles* with Sioux AH.1s during their final year, 1975. Note fuselage roundels were replaced by crew names. (Army Air Corps)

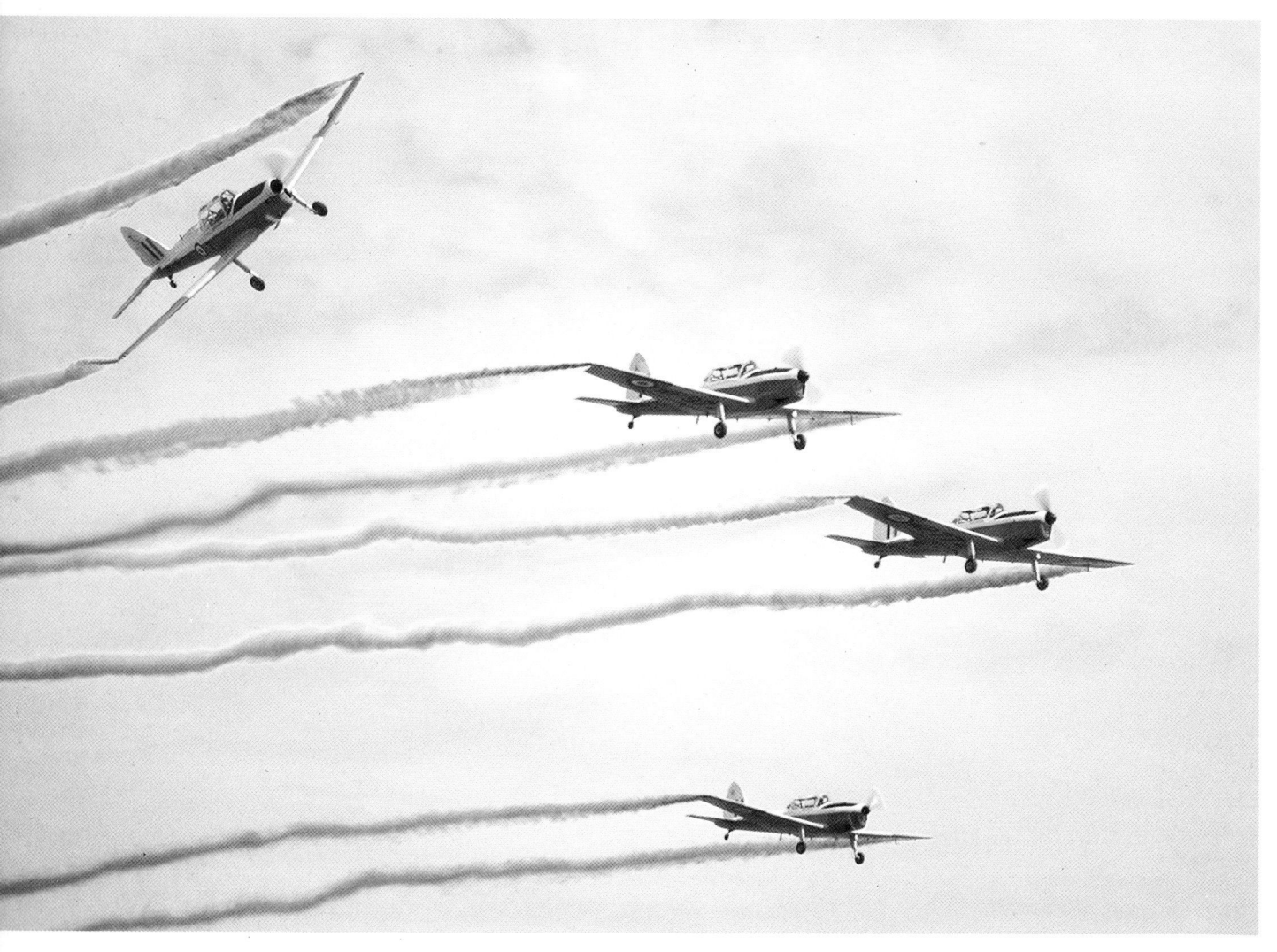

Above: Army Air Corps team of Chipmunks, the *Grey Owls* trailing red and green smoke at Middle Wallop in July 1975. (Adrian M. Balch)

The team flew five standard Sioux helicopters and the pilots, most of whom were NCOs, were selected from operational squadrons in the UK and overseas, to fly exclusively for *The Blue Eagles* from February to October. No formal instruction in formation flying techniques were included in the training and consequently all *Blue Eagles* pilots underwent eight weeks of intensive training and rehearsal before their first appearance in public. During their display, *The Blue Eagles* trailed red, yellow and blue smoke from canisters on the skis, which enhanced their display. The aircraft were painted in the standard Army green and brown camouflage for the 1968 and '69 seasons, but were given their own colour scheme of light and dark blue from 1970. However they reverted to camouflage for the 1971 season only, as the aircraft were required for other operational duties. The final season saw the fuselage roundels replaced by the crew names and the team's Westland-Bell 47G Sioux AH.1s were drawn from: XT511, XT242, XT134, XW192, XT193 and XT206. XW191 was used during the first two seasons, but was written-off in a display accident at Christchurch in August, 1969.

The author was privileged to fly with this team in June 1970 and take the colourful photograph opposite.

1975-79 "The Grey Owls", AAC Middle Wallop, Hants.

This was a part-time team of Army Air Corps Chipmunks, which participated in the 1975, '77 and '79 air displays at Middle Wallop. The team comprised eight Chipmunks, which split up into two formations of four, giving co-ordinated displays. They trailed red and green smoke from canisters on their wingtips, making the display quite spectacular for piston-engined aircraft. The aircraft were painted in the standard training colour scheme of red, white and grey, as used by the RAF. All lettering was in black and no special team markings were carried. *Grey Owls* Chipmunks often included: WB565, WB615/E, WB647/R, WB693/S, WB754/H, WD325/N, WG321/G, WG323/F or WG403/0.

1975-79: "The Sparrow Hawks", AAC Middle Wallop, Hants.

This was a team of six Gazelle helicopters from the Training Wing at the School of Army Aviation, Middle Wallop. They flew displays all over the country, giving similar performances to *The Blue Eagles*. The Gazelles trailed green and orange smoke during their display, but did not have a special colour scheme, being the standard green/black camouflage with orange-dayglo panels. *Sparrow Hawks* Gazelles included: XZ314:0, XW869:A, XW885:B, XW889:D, XW903:E and XZ290:J

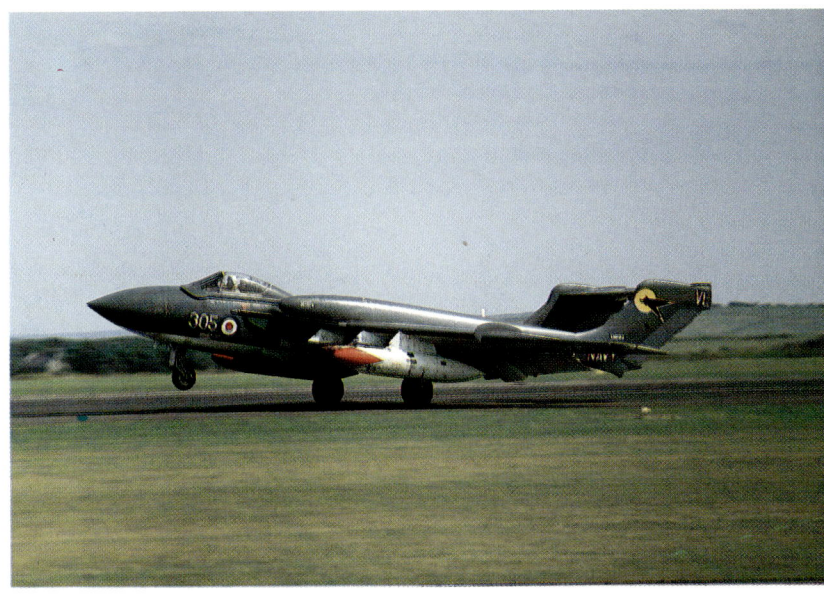

Fleet Air Arm Sea Vixen FAW.2, XN694, of No. 892 Squadron *Simon's Sircus* team landing at Brawdy in August 1968. See page 63 for team history. (J. W. Peck)

The Army Air Corps *Blue Eagles* team flying their Sioux AH. 1s near Middle Wallop on 18 June 1970. (Adrian M. Balch)

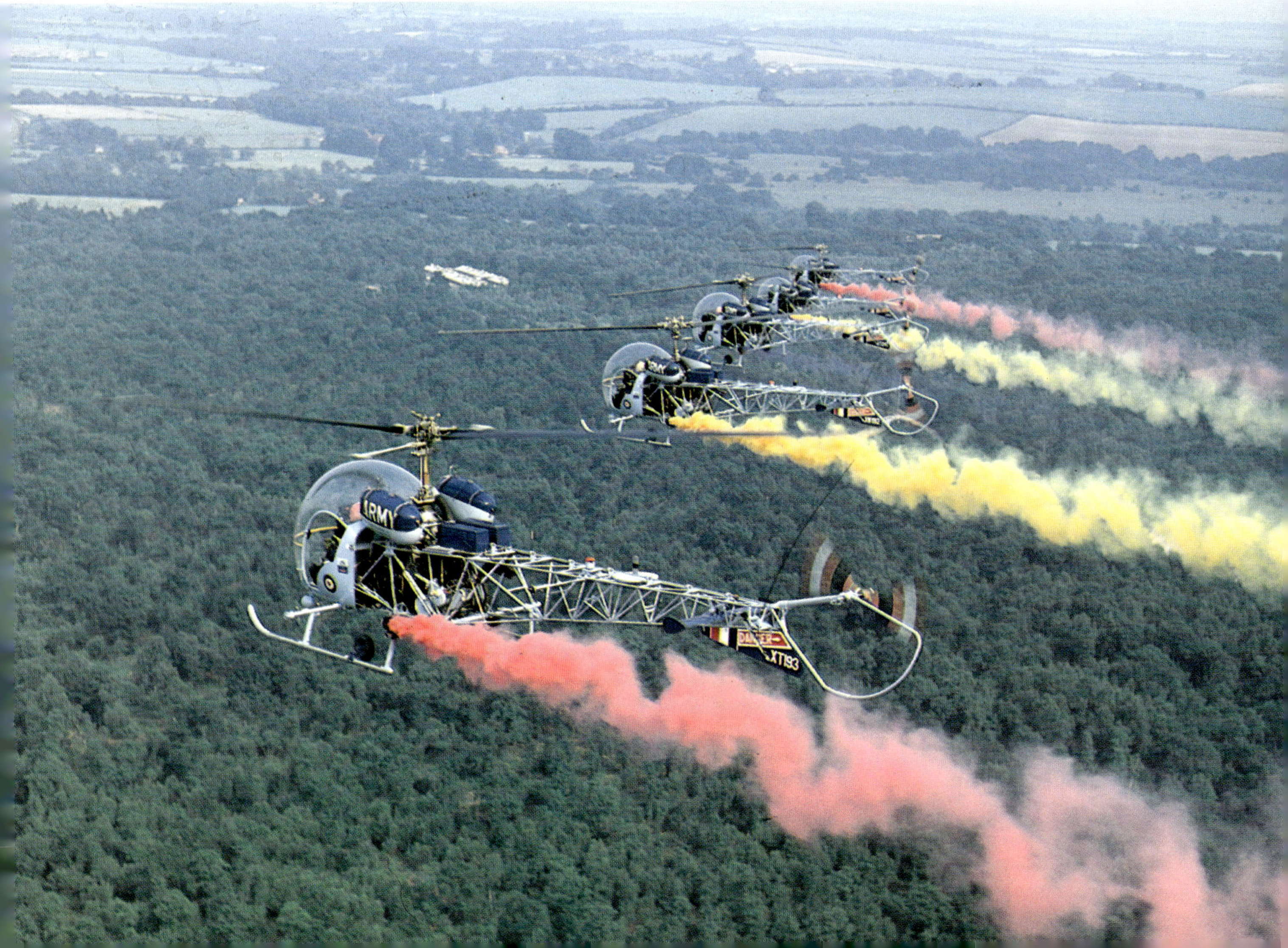

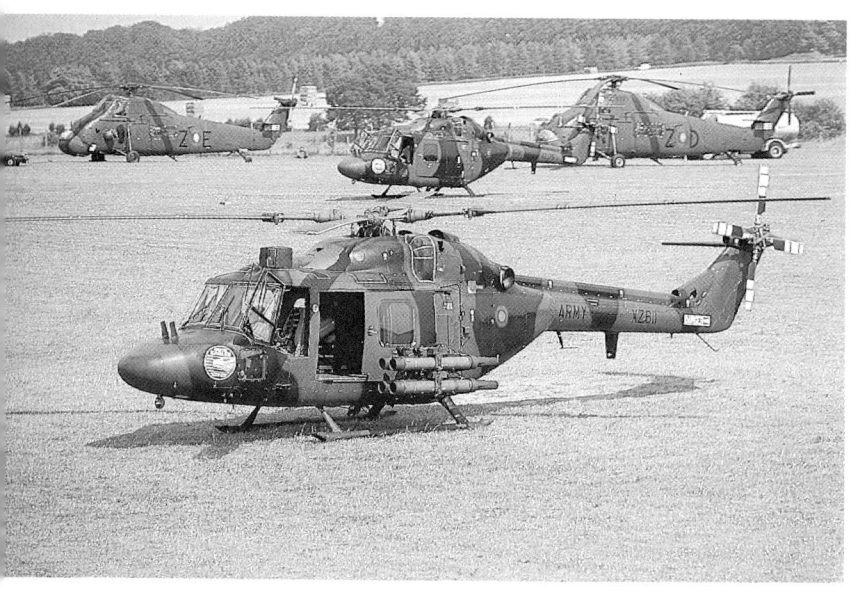

Westland TOW Lynx AH.1, XZ611, of the Army Air Corps *Silver Eagles* at Middle Wallop on 25th July 1982. (Adrian M. Balch).

Below: Scout AH.1s of the 1984 Army Air Corps *Eagles* team. Nearest Scout is XW797/T. (Army Air Corps)

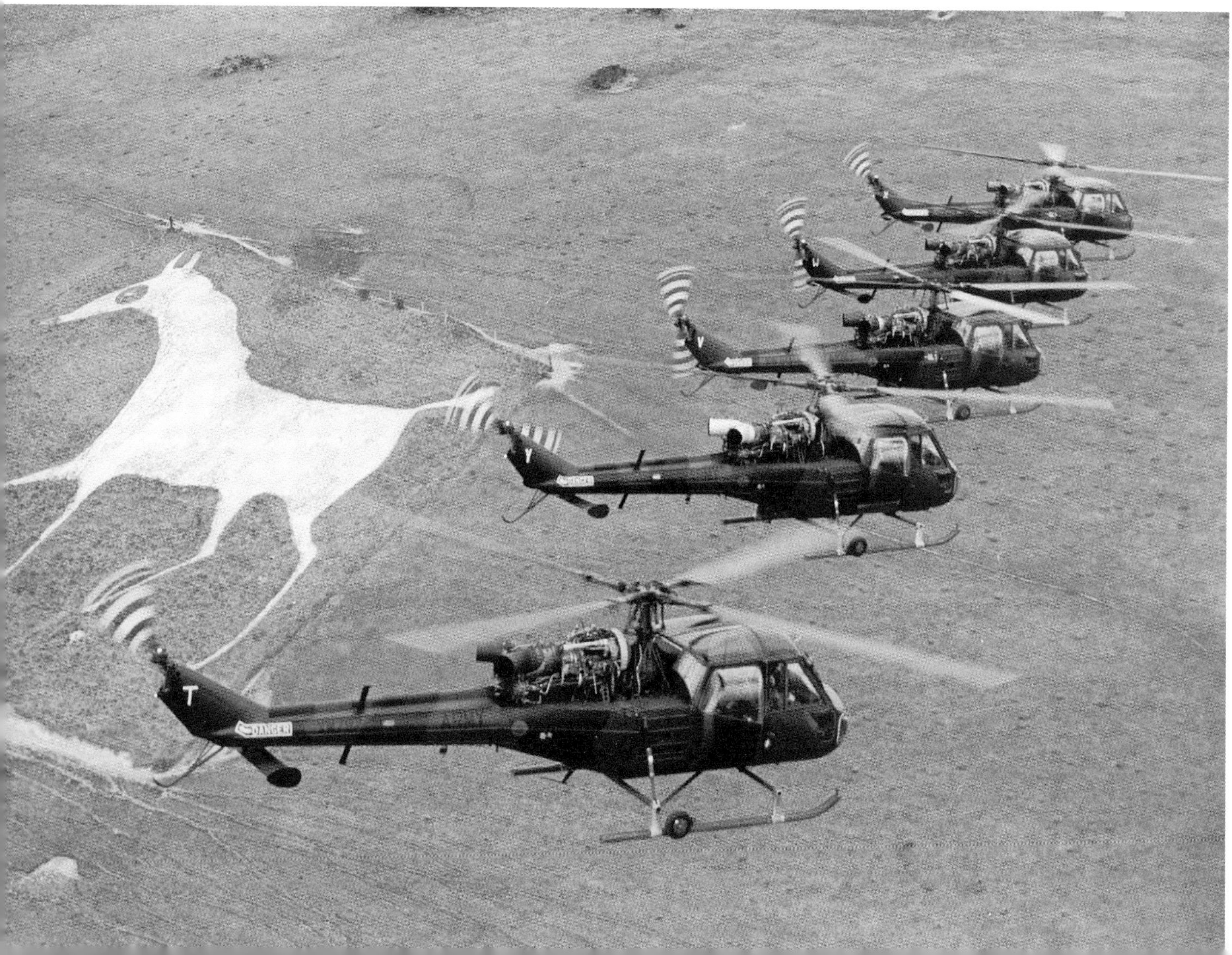

1982: "The Silver Eagles", AAC Middle Wallop, Hants.

This was a team of six Lynx helicopters, specially formed for the Army Air Corps Silver Jubilee. They were a part-time Army display team formed by instructors from the Lynx Conversion Flight at Middle Wallop, flying standard Army Lynx helicopters. Following the twenty-fifth Anniversary celebrations at Middle Wallop in July 1982, the team participated in displays at Odiham and Yeovilton, then disbanded. They flew a mixture of utility Lynx and TOW Lynx, the anti-tank missile-equipped version which is recognised by the sight on top of the roof, port side and the 4 round launchers each side of the centre of the aircraft. The standard green and black Army camouflage was retained, with the addition of a large team badge on either side of the nose in blue and silver. *The Silver Eagles* were led by Captain Rob. Wilsey and the Lynx AH.1s included: XZ172, XZ188, XZ222, XZ611 and XZ649.

1984: "The Eagles", AAC Middle Wallop, Hants.

Another annual helicopter team formed prior to the biennial Middle Wallop air display. This time, the team comprised five Scout helicopters led by Major Alan Wiles. The aircraft wore the standard Army Air Corps camouflage of olive green/black with *Eagles* stickers on the nose and fuselage sides. The team gave about a dozen shows before disbanding. Scouts used by the team included: XW797/T, XP885/Y, XW613/V, XT624/W and XT630/X.

GREECE
Hellenic Air Force

1953-58: "Skyblazers", Larissa then Elefsina

The first aerobatic team of the Hellenic Air Force was formed early in 1953 and was based at Larissa. After the Commander of 337 fighter-bomber Squadron had seen demonstrations by the USAF *Skyblazers* with F-84E Thunderjets at Elefsina Airport in 1952, he decided to form a team with the same name and using the same aircraft type. With four F-84G Thunderjets, the *HAF Skyblazers* underwent intensive training to participate in displays in Greece and abroad. The first appearance was in the Autumn of 1953 at Larissa Airport for the Chiefs of Staff to evaluate the team.

The first official appearance took place in May 1954 at Larissa and was attended by the Defence Minister. Initially, the Hellenic Air Force team copied the USAF *Skyblazers* from their 1952 demonstrations, but developed new manoeuvres once they had gained experience. In the autumn of 1956, 337 Squadron was relocated to 112 Combat Wing at Elefsina, which became the new base of the *Skyblazers*. In 1956, the team participated in international demonstrations abroad for the first time. They competed in Milan, Italy, against aerobatic teams from other NATO countries. In 1958, the *Skyblazers* participated in displays in Belgium and Holland. The aircraft originally wore a mainly natural metal finish, but by 1958 they were painted black overall with white-blue-white diagonal stripes on the fin and across the wings. Three of the HAF *Skyblazers* in the original finish were 51-10373, '746 and '697, while the only one known in the black colour scheme was 51-10047.

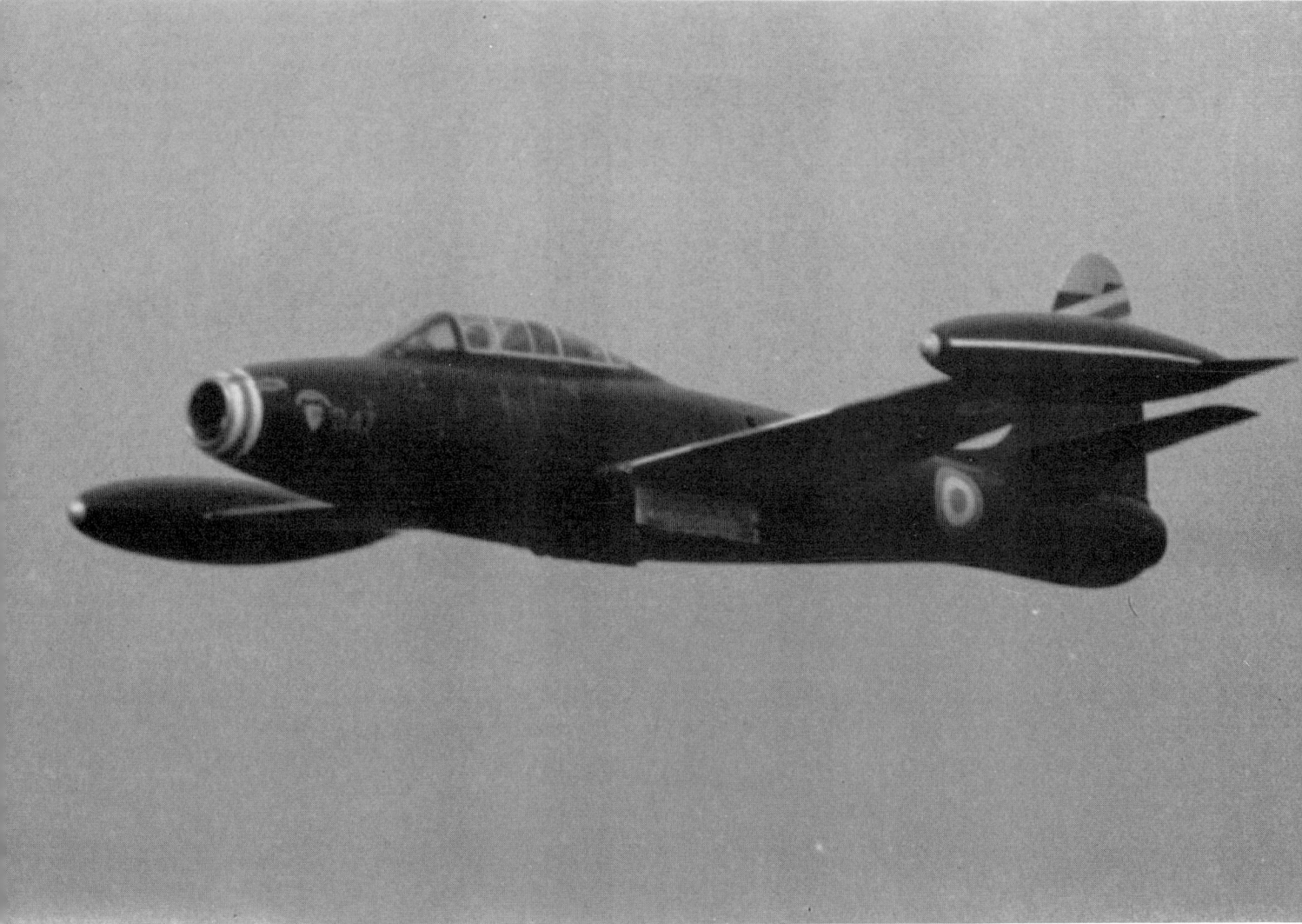

A rare shot of black-painted F-84G Thunderjet 51-10047 of the Greek Air Force team *Skyblazers* in 1958. (R. Neth A. F. via R. Ward)

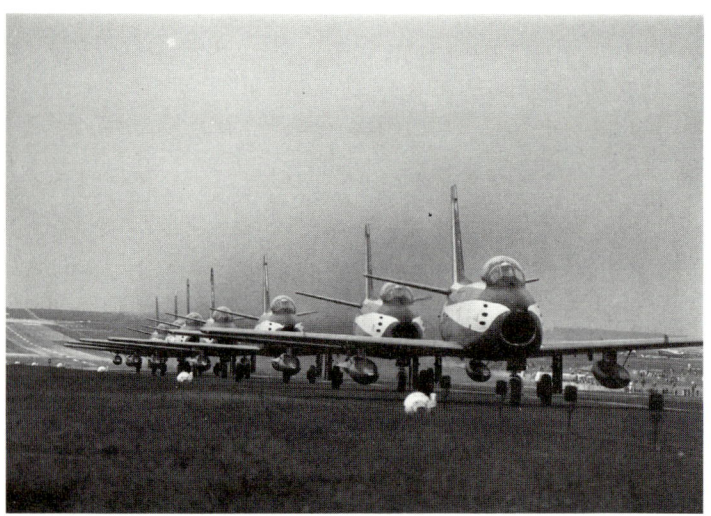

Above: Canadair Sabres of the Greek *Hellenic Flame* team taxying in line-astern at the 1963 Paris Air Show. (Werner Gysin)

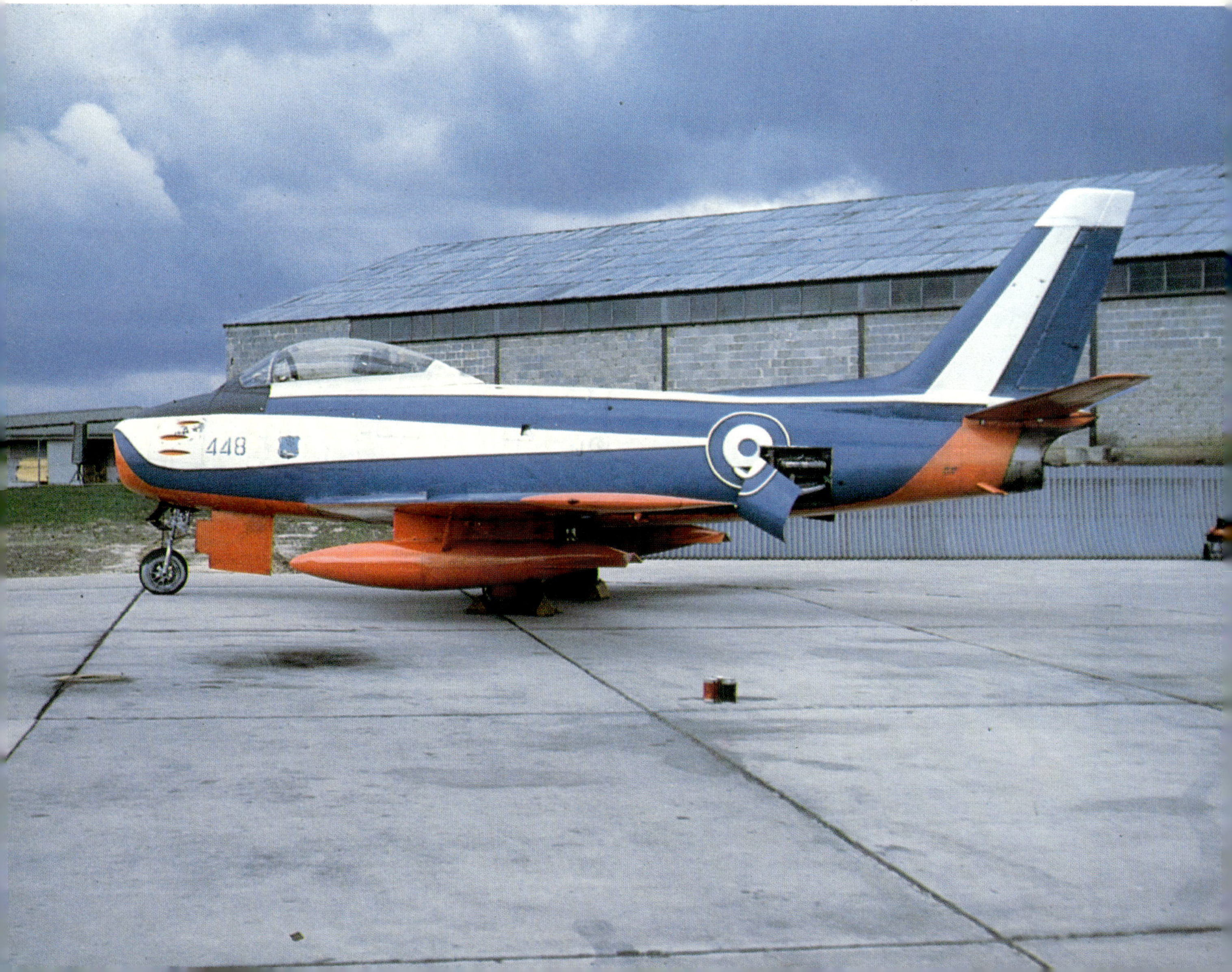

Below: Canadair CL-13A Sabre, 19448 of the Greek Air Force aerobatic team *Hellenic Flame* at Spangdahlem Air Base, Germany, in May 1962. The shield badge under the cockpit appeared port side only. (David W. Menard)

1958-64: "Hellenic Flame", Tanagra

In August 1958, after five years of action without incident despite the fact that there were no substitute pilots, the *Skyblazers* were dissolved and immediately replaced by another team — the *Hellenic Flame*. This team had already been training since September 1957 at Tanagra Air Base and was equipped with newer, more modern aircraft. It initially consisted of five Canadair-built F-86E Sabres, which was later increased to seven, the team belonging to 341 Interception Squadron which was part of 114 Combat Wing at Tanagra.

The first official appearance of the *Hellenic Flame* was in May 1958, when the *Skyblazers* were still in existence. A number of successful demonstrations followed in Greece as well as abroad. It performed in the honour of, among others, General de Gaulle, the President of Italy, the President of the U.A.R., Naser and Air Marshals Lindsay and Le May.

During the years 1959, '60 and '61, the *Hellenic Flame* participated in air shows held at Fürstenfeldbruck near Munich and Wiesbaden, West Germany, during the USAF Armed Forces Day. The Chief of Staff of the German Air Force was particularly impressed by the team. The *Hellenic Flame* also appeared in Naples, Italy, in July 1961, in Toul, France and again at Fürstenfeldbruck in the same year.

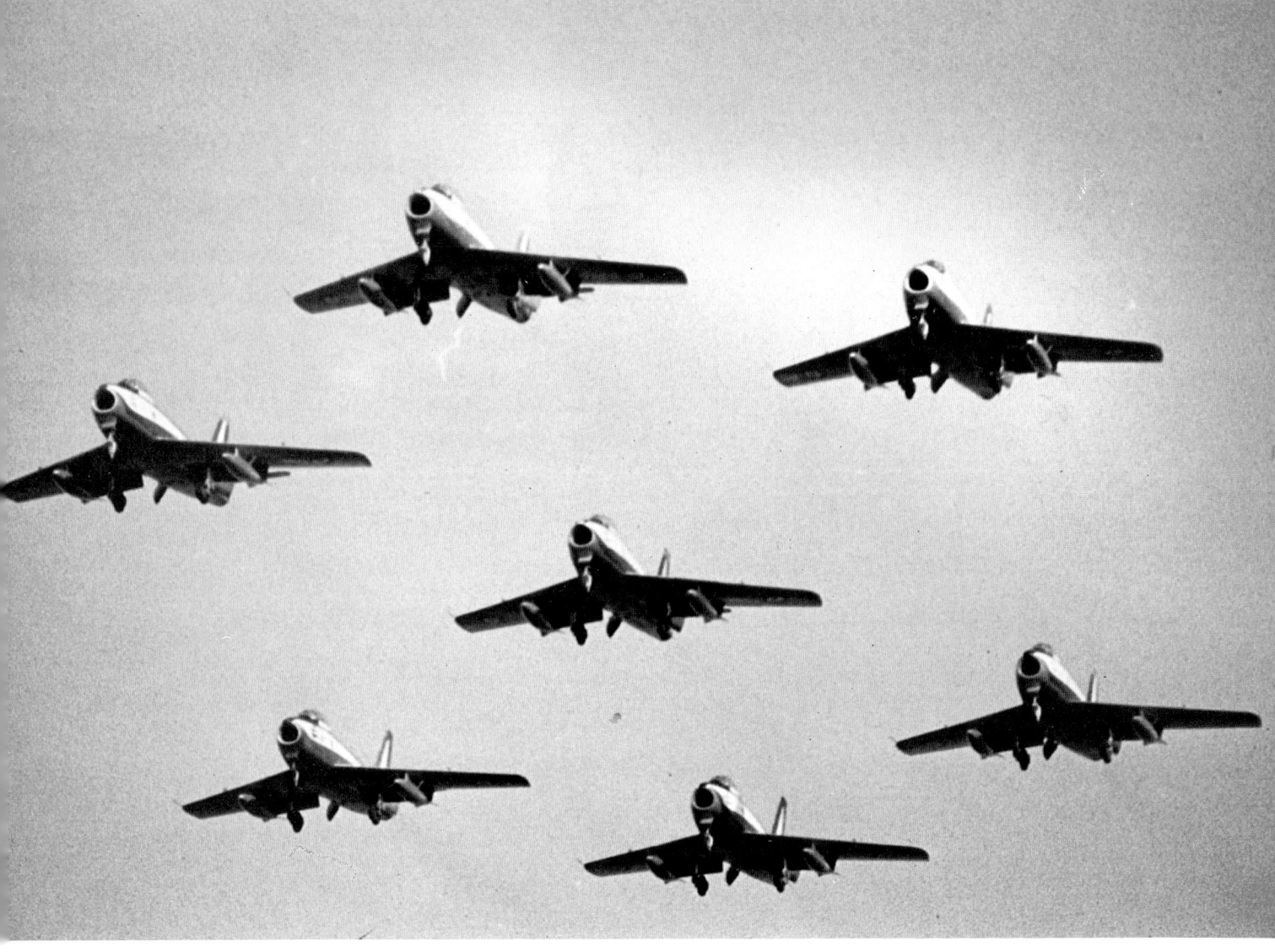

Above: Seven Canadair CL-13A Sabre Mk.2s of the Greek Air Force aerobatic team *Hellenic Flame,* seen performing at Fürstenfeldbruck in 1961. (Werner Gysin)

At the end of the 1961 season, the team was relocated to the airport of Anghialos. It took part in demonstrations in Aviano, Italy and Spangdahlem, West Germany, in May 1962. After the demonstration, the American Commander of Spangdahlem Air Base announced that the *Hellenic Flame* was one of the best aerobatic teams he had ever seen. 1963 took the team to the Paris Air Show, France, followed by displays in Italy and Turkey. 1964 was the final year for the team and once again, they displayed at Aviano, Italy. After six years of operation and several awards and decorations, *Hellenic Flame* disbanded in September 1964. The colour scheme applied to the team's Sabres was mainly blue and white with orange undersides. The upper surfaces of the wings were striped blue-white-blue and five of the team's aircraft were 19294, '377, '382, '392, and '448', all being ex-RCAF Canadair Sabre Mk.2s.

1967: "New Hellenic Flame", Anghialos
Three years after the *Hellenic Flame* disbanded, the Hellenic Air Force Command decided to form a new aerobatic team with the Northrop F-5A, since the F-86E had become antiquated. The new team, under the name *New Hellenic Flame*, started its training in July 1967 and made its first official appearance on 20th October 1967 at Anghialos, where it was based. It consisted of five F-5As and appeared only once more before it finally terminated its activities in late 1967.

INDIA
Indian Air Force

Like most other air forces, the Indian Air Force has employed aerobatics as part of their pilot training, but no official team was formed until recently. In 1970, a team of 4 MiG-21s was formed by No. 47 Squadron, called the *Red Archers*. These aircraft were silver with dayglo red nose, wings, upper fuselage and fin . . . quite spectacular! However, they only performed on squadron occasions and are not known to have appeared in public. There have been other squadron teams of Hunters, MiG-21s, HF-24 Maruts and HAL Kirans, but not until 1982 did the Indian Air Force have an official team.

1982-to date: No. 20 Squadron, "The Thunderbolts", Hashimara

This team was formed on the occasion of the IAF's Golden Jubilee and comprises nine Hunter F.56As painted in an an attractive dark blue colour with white lightning flashes over the wings and fuselage. Wing Commander P. S. "Ben" Brar, was selected as leader with Squadron Leader J. S. Thakur as his deputy. The selection of the aircraft was not so easy. Although most types of aircraft are capable of putting on some form of solo flying display, formation flying and aerobatics require an aircraft to have well defined qualities of manoeuvrability and an aesthetically pleasing appearance. A good power/weight ratio and responsive engine controls are essential, bearing in mind that the leader of the formation would have to manoeuvre using less than full power in order that his team members can keep up with him. The Indian Air Force narrowed its choice down to three types — the Kiran jet trainer, the Hunter and the MiG-21. The former had been used in a three-aircraft team in 1981, but the effect was very tame. The latter had excellent power/weight ratio, but a formation flying MiG 21s would need extensive areas of sky in carrying out the enormous repositioning manoeuvres. The Hunter was selected unanimously and accordingly No. 20 (Lightning) Squadron flying the F.56A variant at Hashimara was chosen to form *The Thunderbolts*.

The team uses some of the RAF *Red Arrows'* formations and manoeuvres and made their first public appearance during the Republic Day week in January 1982. The team initially comprised six Hunters, but this was subsequently increased to nine. With the added attraction of smoke, *The Thunderbolts* present loops and rolls in different formations before climaxing with a spectacular bomb-burst. The display lasts 18 minutes and encompassess 20 manoeuvres and six changes of formation.

The serial numbers of the team's aircraft are unknown, but modellers should note that the white lightning flashes appear on the fuselage and upper surfaces of the wings and tailplanes. All undersides are plain dark blue with roundels in six positions.

Below: The *Thunderbolts* — Indian Air Force Hunter F.56As of No.20 Squadron in 1982. In the centre is Wg. Cdr. P.S. 'Ben' Brar (now Group Capt.) who is the leader. (Pushpindar S. Chopra)

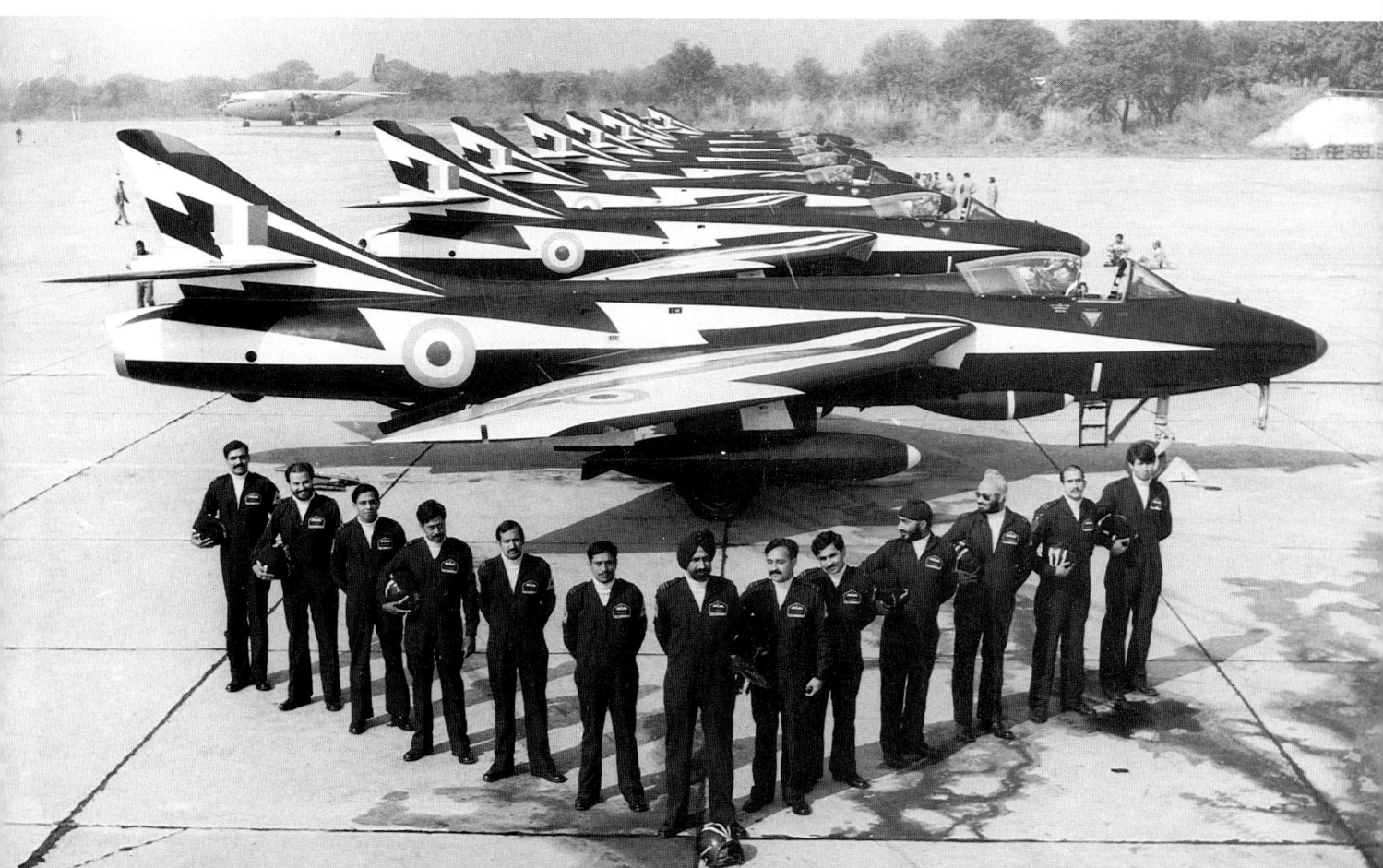

IRAN
Imperial Iranian Air Force

1958-79: IIAF "Golden Crown" Team, Shiraz

The IIAF *Golden Crown* team consisted of four F-84G Thunderjets, when established in 1958 and demonstrated their first official air show on 8th April in the same year, in the presence of His Imperial Majesty the Shahanshah Aryamehr. (See Page 98 for colour photograph).

F-5E Tigers of the Imperial Iranian Air Force aerobatic team *Golden Crown* lined up at Shiraz in November 1977. (Author's collection)

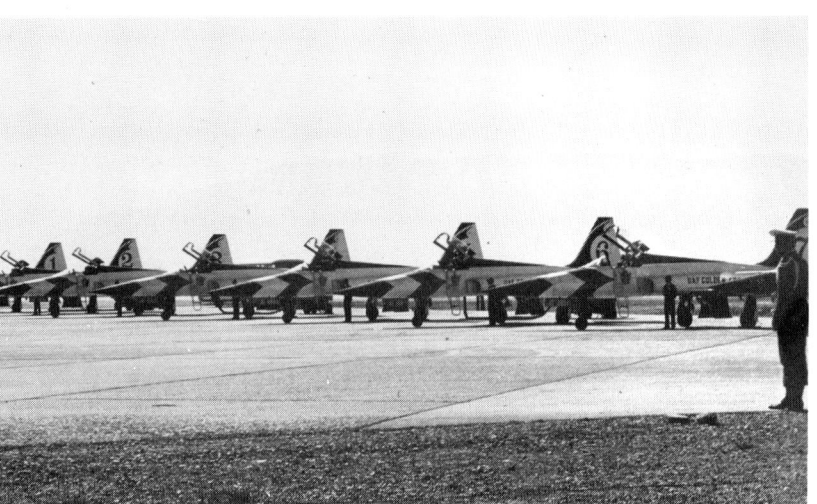

Below: Not the USAF *Thunderbirds* but F-5Es of the Imperial Iranian Air Force aerobatic team *Golden Crown* performing at Shiraz in November 1977.
(Author's collection)

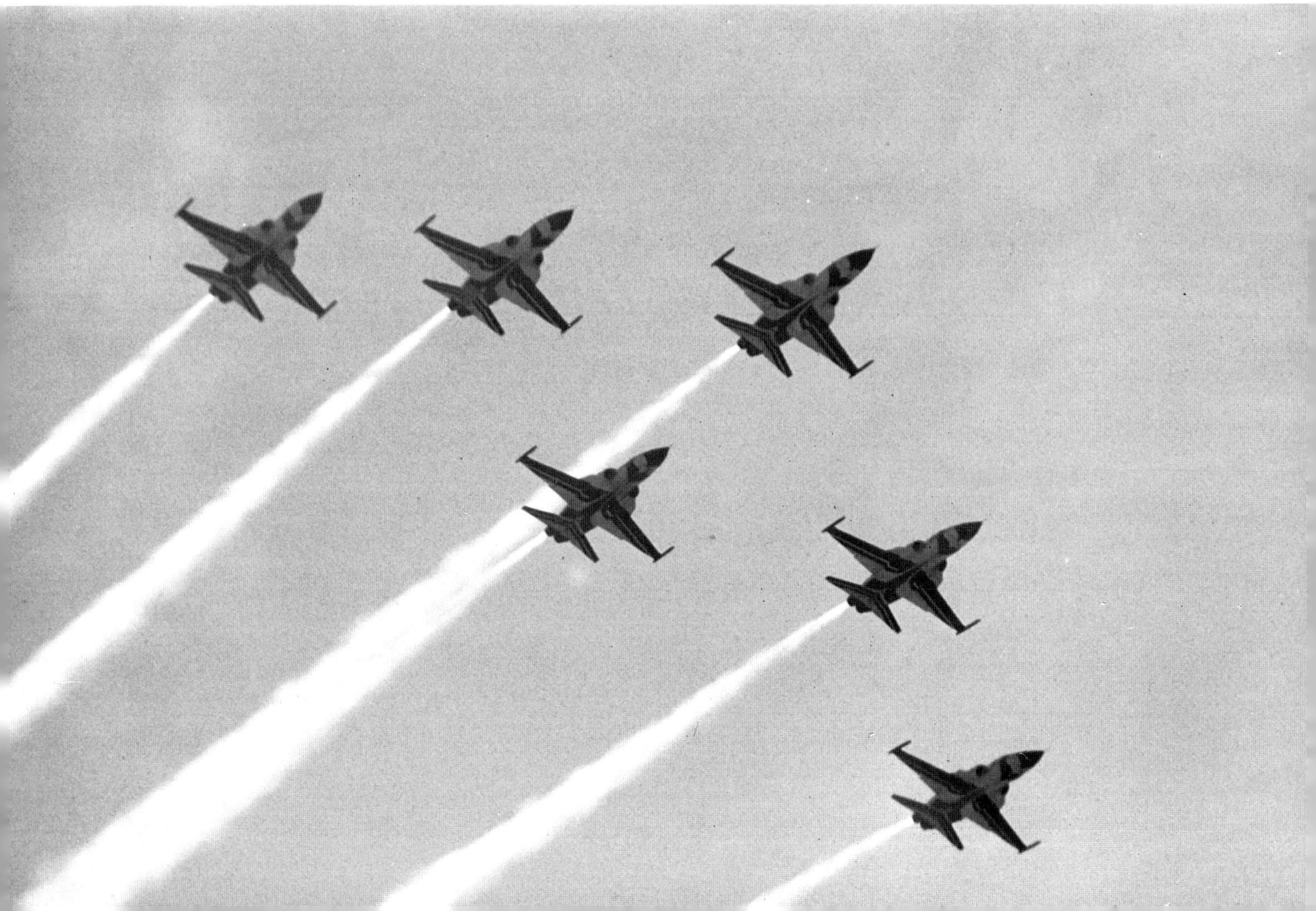

In 1960 the F-84Gs were replaced by F-86F Sabres and the team started practising with the new aircraft. In a very short time, they were prepared for their demonstrations. The team continued with F-86F Sabres until the type was withdrawn from service in 1970. Although the F-5A had been in IIAF service since 1966, the *Golden Crown* Sabres were not replaced until 1971, when they received six F-5A Freedom Fighters. These were replaced by the more powerful F-5E Tigers around 1975, when the F-5As were sold. The team flew six smoke-equipped F-5Es at official engagements in Iran and they were painted in an almost identical colour scheme to that applied to the T-38A Talons of the USAF *Thunderbirds*. The main difference was that the dark blue was replaced by Iranian dark green. A yellow crown appeared under the cockpit on both sides and *IIAF GOLDEN CROWN* lettering appeared down the fuselage port side. This was repeated in Arabic on the starboard side. This also applied to the team numbers with English serial numbers on the port side and Arabic numerals to starboard. The 1977 team was led by Major M. Khalili and the leader's F-5E was serialled 3-7099 coded '1' and another was 3-7106 coded '8'. As the name of the team is so inappropriate to the current Iranian regime, it is assumed that the *Golden Crown* team was disbanded in 1979 when the Shah was overthrown by the Islamic revolution. The F-5Es were probably returned to fighting duties against Iraq and it is doubtful whether an Iranian aerobatic team will ever exist again in the foreseeable future.

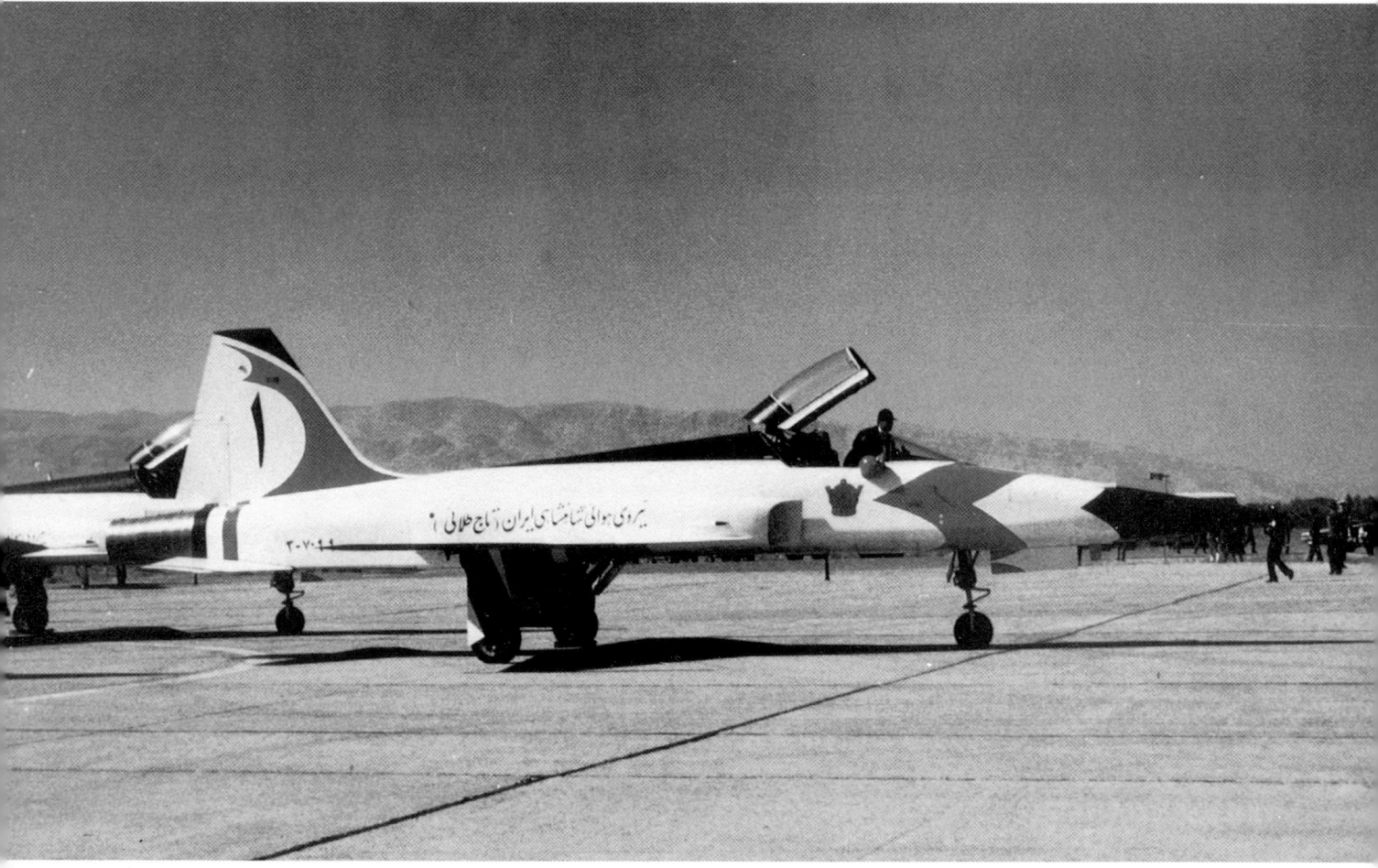

Northrop F-5E Tiger, 3-7099 of the Imperial Iranian Air Force *Golden Crown* team in 1977. Note the team name, serial number and tail code are all in Arabic. These were all repeated on the port side in English.
(Courtesy The Aviation Hobby Shop)

ISRAEL
Israeli Defence Force/Air Force

1950-to date: Israeli Defence Force/Air Force Aerobatic Team, Hatzerim

The first Israeli Air Force aerobatic team was formed in 1950 by Hugo Marom, who was a flight instructor. He led a team of four Stearman biplanes, doing loops and banks in 'box' formation. Although aerobatics could be done with the Stearman, due to its low horse power many manoeuvres were impossible to perform. When the Harvard was introduced into training, the aerobatic team re-equipped with this type. A few shows were performed with Harvards, but in 1952 it was decided that the dangers were too great in relation to the benefits. Therefore, the official aerobatic team was disbanded. However, a trio of P-51 Mustangs performed in formation at occasional ceremonies, but a stop was put to this following a terrible accident on 18th August 1954. The formation took off from Ramat David Air Base, but two of the aircraft collided in mid-air during the display, killing both pilots. This put a stop on aerobatics altogether, for the time being.

The Israeli Defence Force/Air Force aerobatic team is joined by more Fouga Magisters to provide this impeccable 30-ship formation of the Star of David.
(Israeli D.F./A.F.)

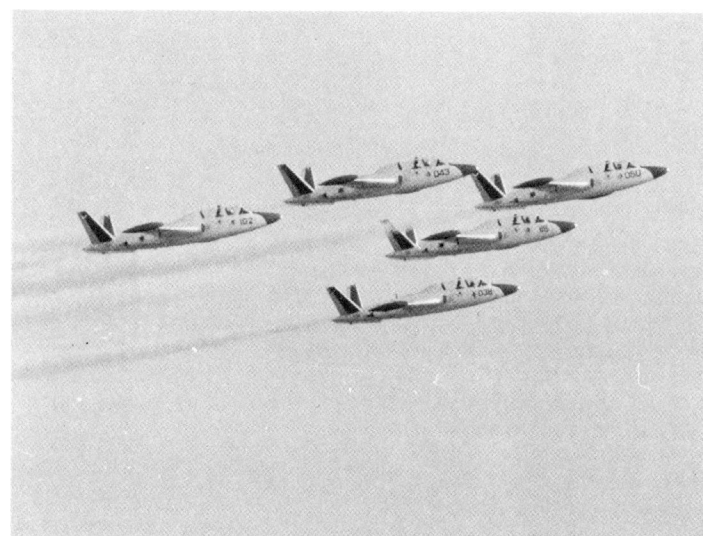

Above: Fouga Magisters of the Israeli Defence Force/Air Force aerobatic team in their current colour scheme of white and orange. Serials are 050 (leading), 043, 115, 038 and 102 (Israeli D.F./A.F.)

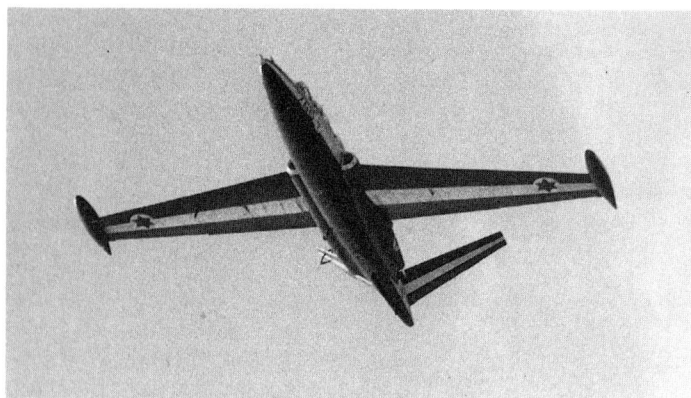

One of the Israeli aerobatic team's Fouga Magisters showing the dark blue and white colour scheme on wings and tails. (Israeli D.F./A.F.)

Below: A Fouga Magister of the Israeli Defence Force/Air Force team in 1967. Colour scheme is dark blue and white with red geese in badge.
(S. P. Peltz via R. Ward)

However, in July 1958, an official IAF team was permitted to be formed, called *Golden Harvards*. From then on, the aerobatic team had no major interruptions. A month later, Asaf Ben-Nun became the team's leader for 2½ years. The team was picked from the best of the flight instructors at the Flight School, using the better-equipped Harvards. The first exercises were simple loops, banks and formation changes, since the Harvard wasn't capable of difficult manoeuvres.

In 1960, the Fouga Magister came into service at the Flight School at Hatzerim. With its arrival, the aerobatic team began training on the type. In July 1964, Colonel "A" became the team's leader and Commander of the Flight School. Because of the latter appointment, he found it impossible to fulfil his duty as team leader, so handed the leadership over to Yaelo, an advanced squadron commander. Training was intensified and the team expanded from four aircraft, to six, then eight. Even nine aircraft were attempted in formation, but the commander felt this too hazardous, so the formation was reduced to six Magisters. It was planned to show the team at the 1965 Paris Air Show, but at the last moment the plans were cancelled. Finances were just too low to invest in such an operation.

By 1966, twelve Magisters were painted in the colours of the team. The aircraft were mainly dark blue overall, with blue/white/blue striped wings, top and bottom. The insignia of the team was two red geese flying back-to-back. The Magisters were equipped to make smoke and by the mid-'60s were comparable to the more famous teams. In this form, they flew at official engagements throughout Israel, but due to financial trouble, the aircraft could not be spared for sole aerobatic team use. The special colour scheme was removed and the team was reduced to a part-time basis, performing at a limited number of official ceremonies only. The team's aircraft retained the smoke-making capability, but were repainted in the Flight School's training colours of white and orange. In this severely limited form, the team continues to this day.

Fouga Magisters in the blue and white scheme included: 033, 044, 209, 212, 227 and 283.

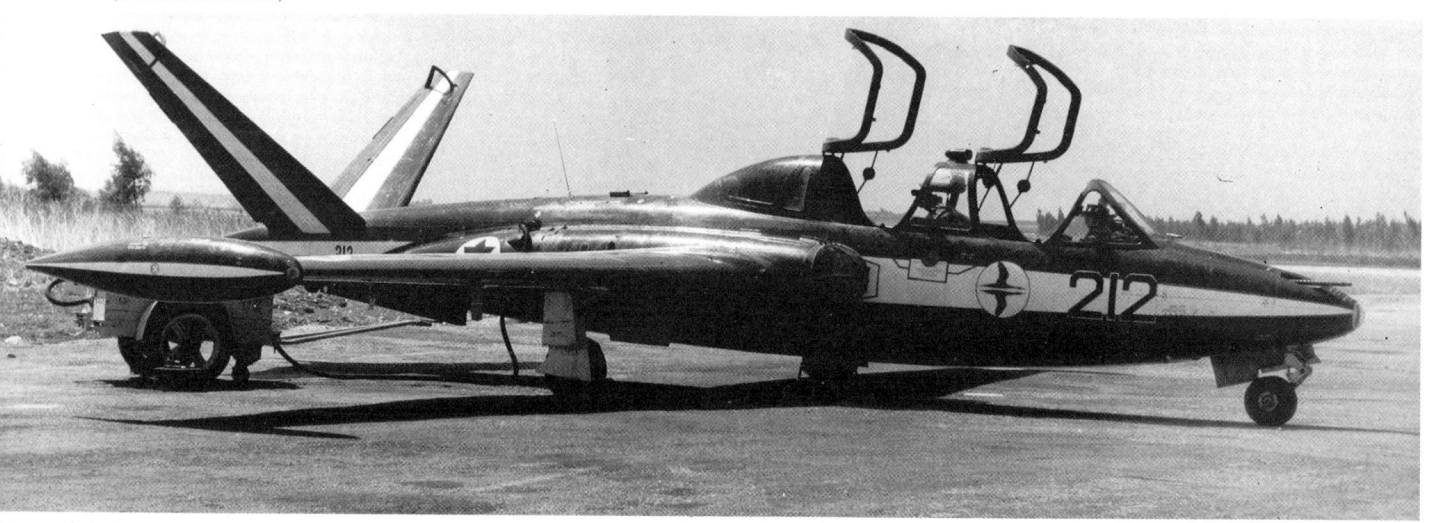

ITALY
Italian Air Force

1930-1939

The first school for aerobatic flight in formation was activated in 1930 at Campoformido. It was founded by Colonel Rino Corso Fougier, who convinced the Air Staff that a military pilot had to utilise the aircraft in war operations with the maximum efficiency and absolute control.

Consequently, the aerobatic flight was the result of a daily, severe and continuous training for air combat. Colonel Fougier trained a formation of 5 aircraft with a complete aerobatic programme. Furthermore, he studied the ground attack mode in formation. The attack was the final sequence of the programme and therefore it had to present the war effectiveness of the action.

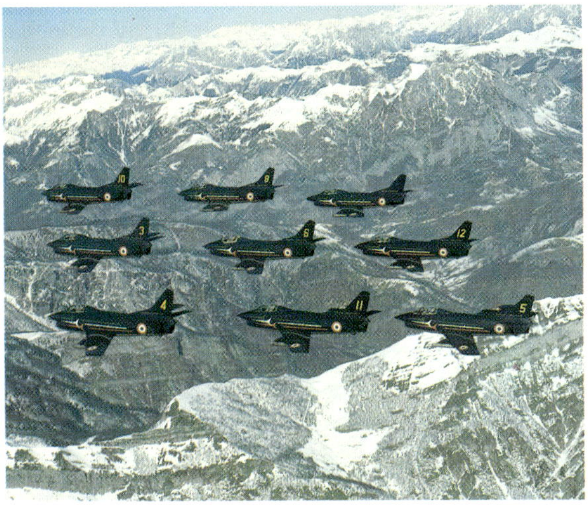

Fiat G-91 PANS of the *Frecce Tricolori* (Tricoloured Arrows) team over the Italian Alps. This type equipped the team during 1964-81. (Italian Air Force via R. Lamplough)

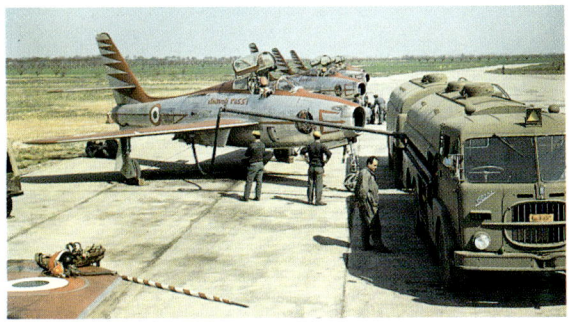

Above: Republic F-84F Thundersteaks of the *Diavoli Rossi* (Red Devils) team, being refuelled prior to a display in 1959. (Italian Air Force via R. Lamplough)

Below: The current Italian Air Force team, *Frecce Tricolori*, flying Aermacchi MB. 339 PANS. Nearest aircraft is MM54482 '3'. (Italian Air Force via R. Lamplough)

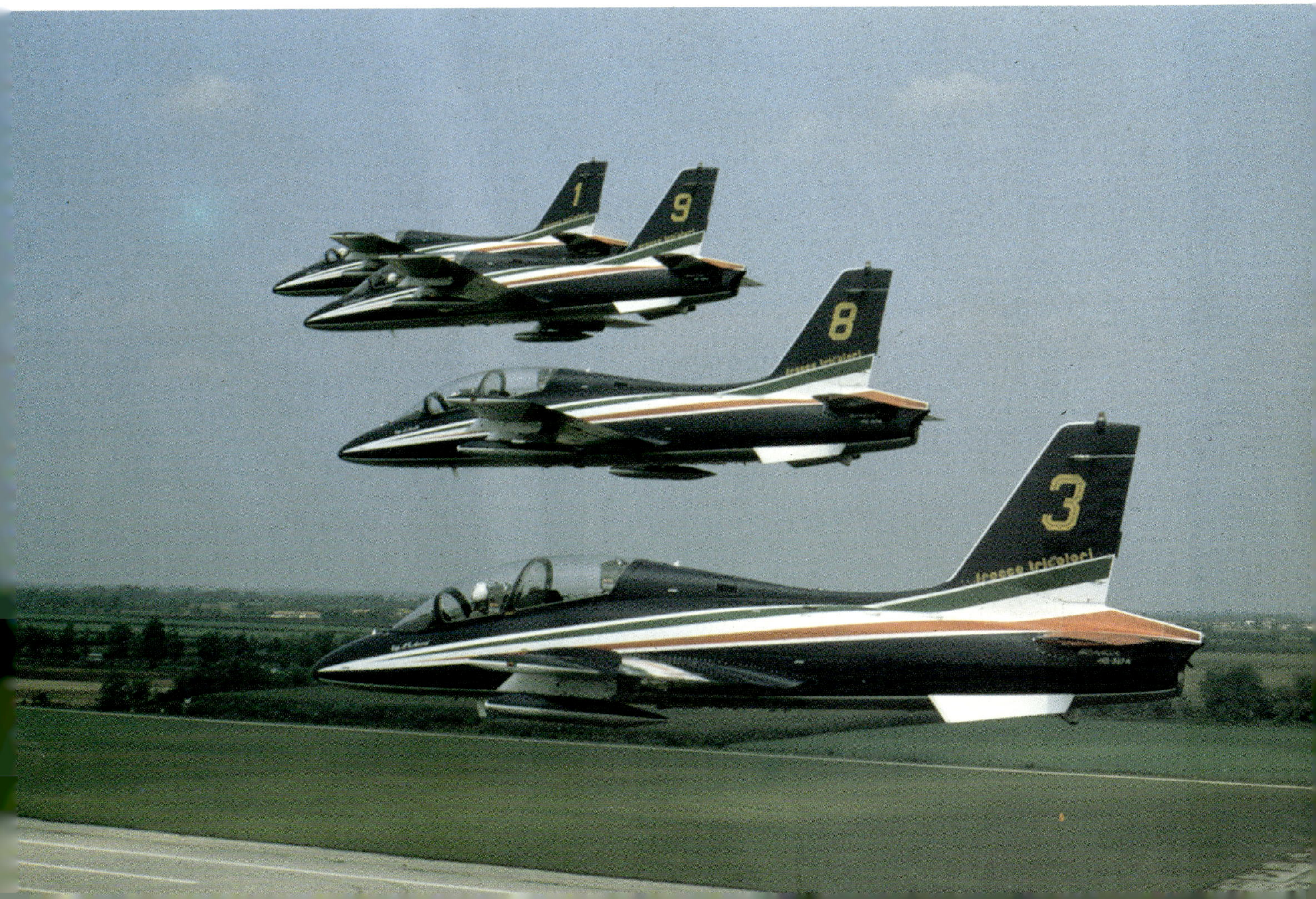

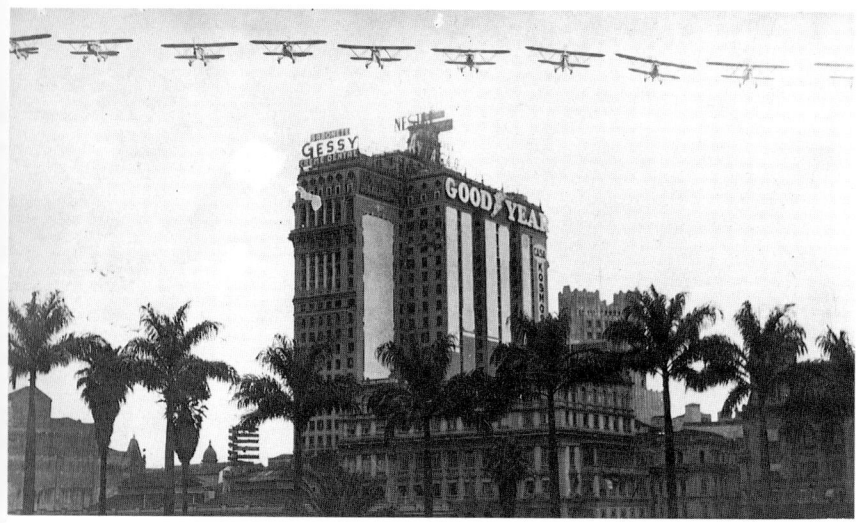

Italian Air Force aerobatic team's Fiat CR-32s in South America, 1937. (Italian A. F. via R. Lamplough)

Below: Four F-86E Sabres of the Italian Air Force's *Cavallino Rampante* (Rampant Horses) team from 4 Aerobrigata in 1956-57.
(Italian A. F. via R. Lamplough)

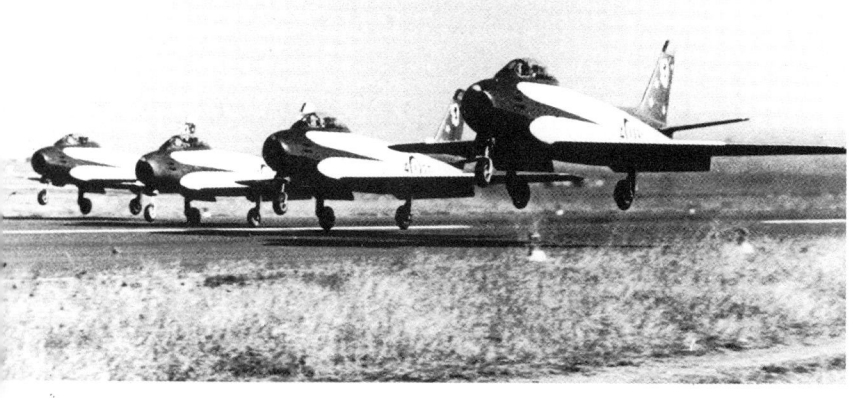

The 5 Fiat CR.20s, after having performed the programme in close formation, changed to 'wedge formation' diving on a vehicle on the ground. At a few metres from the target, the formation leader pulled up and performed a complete loop, while the right and left wingmen performed a tight pull-up turn and crossed right over the vehicle and repeated this manoeuvre three times. At the end of the display, the remotely-controlled vehicle was driven through a dynamite charge. Colonel Fougier presented his daring programme at the First Air Day, the 8th June 1930, raising waves of enthusiasm. His pilots were soon named the *Campoformido Boys*.

This daring and thrilling final carousel was named 'bomb-burst'. Since that day, this aerobatic manoeuvre, which was later called 'reaction test', has always been the finalé of all the Italian Air Force aerobatic teams.

From 1930 to 1939, the Italian Air Force Aerobatic Team has been represented by 1^0 Stormo flying Fiat CR 20s and BA 19s, followed by $4^0, 6^0, 1^0$ and 53^0 Stormos flying Fiat CR 32s. They participated in displays all over Europe and even undertook a South American tour in 1937, which included a display at Sao Paulo, Brazil.

The Second World War interrupted display flying and it was not until 1950 that Italian Air Force teams formed again.

1950-1952: "Cavallino Rampante" (Rampant Horses), 4 Aerobrigata, Naples

This was the first Italian Aerobatic Team to form after the war and comprised four De Havilland Vampires led by Ten. C. B. Ceoletta from 4 Aerobrigata. The aircraft were natural metal overall with unit markings and the team's displays included one at Brussels in 1952.

1953-1955: "Getti Tonanti" (Thunder-Jets), 5 Aerobrigata, Villafranca

This team comprised four Republic F-84G Thunderjets, hence the team's name, led by Major L. Deggiovanni. The aircraft were equipped to make smoke and represented the Italian Air Force at displays in Italy, Germany, France and Spain.

1955-1956: "Tigri Bianche" (White Tigers), 51 Aerobrigata. Treviso Istrana

This was the second team of four F-84G Thunderjets, led by Captain R. Di Lollo, which flew a similar display to *Getti Tonanti* and represented the Italian Air Force in Holland, France, Germany as well as in Italy.

1956-1957: "Cavallino Rampante" (Rampant Horses), 4 Aerobrigata, Pratica di Mare

This was the Italian Air Force's first Sabre aerobatic team, flying four Canadair-built F-86E aircraft painted primrose yellow with red nose trim. All tail surfaces and undersides of the wings were painted dark blue, with white stars on all blue-painted surfaces. The team was led by Capt. A. Melotti and participated in various shows in France and Italy.

In 1956, the Italian Air Staff decided to assign each year to a different Fighter Air Brigade to present the national aerobatic team.

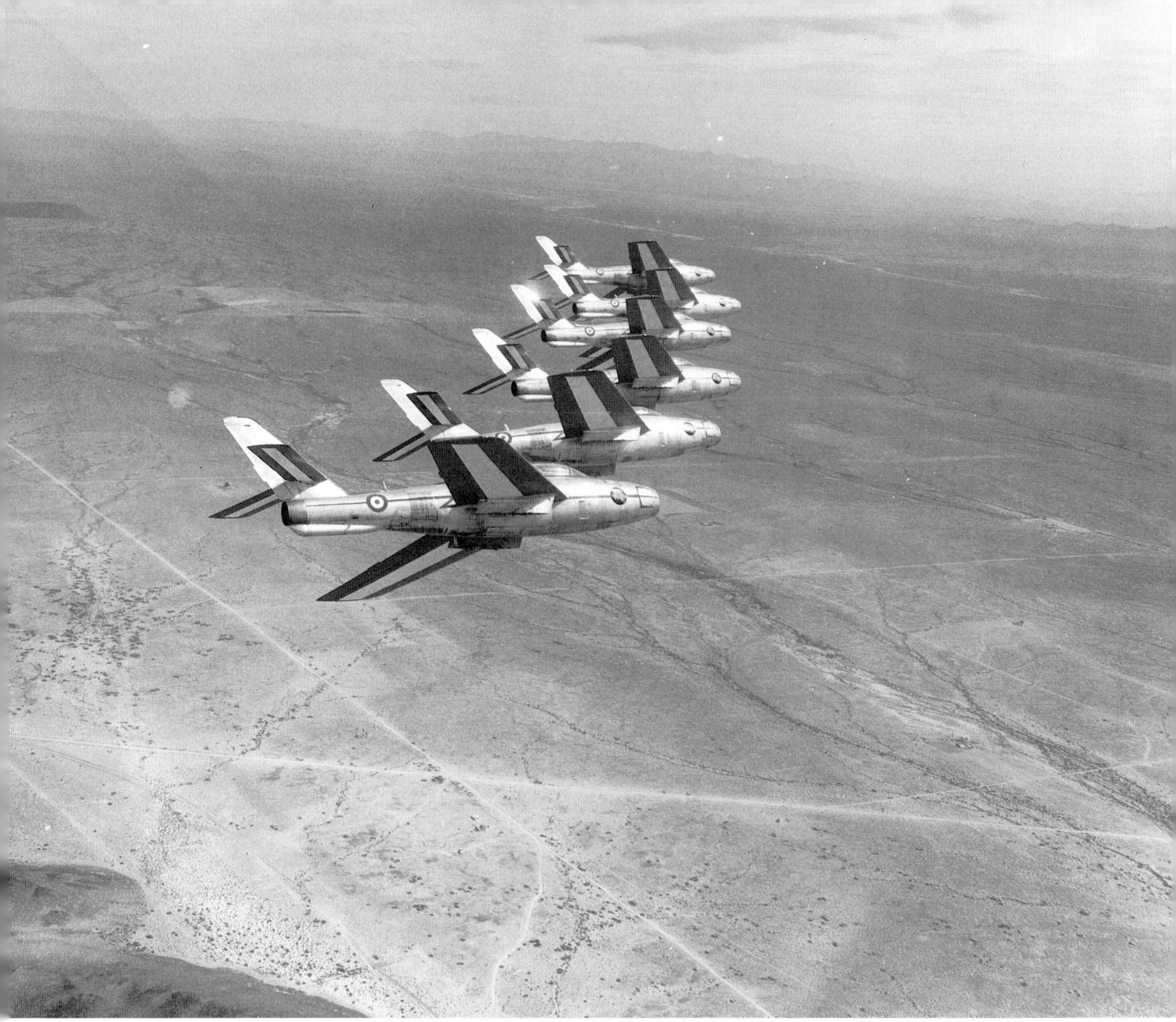

1957-1959: "Diavoli Rossi" (Red Devils), 6 Aerobrigata, Ghedi

This was a team of six Republic F-84F Thunderstreaks led by Captain M. Squarcina, which competed in air shows in Italy, Holland, Belgium, America and Spain. In 1959, it was invited to the United States where it participated in the First World Flight Congress among other events. The team also went to Las Vegas, Nellis AFB, Andrews AFB, McGuire AFB and Long Island. The aircraft were natural metal with red trim and Italian-coloured stripes under the wings and tailplanes.

1958-1959: "Lanceri Neri" (Black Lancers), 2 Aerobrigata, Cameri

Led by Captain A. Nencha, *Lanceri Neri* were a team of six black-painted Canadair Sabres, which also had red, white and green stripes under the wings and tailplanes. The team's name derived from the squadron badge, which comprised a lancer on a black horse mounted on a yellow sun rising above white clouds. This insignia appeared on the nose of the Sabres. The *Black Lancers* participated in Air shows in Italy, England, France, Germany and Persia (now Iran).

Above: The Italian Air Force *Diavoli Rossi* (Red Devils) team flying Republic F-84F Thunderstreaks during their tour of the USA in May 1959. (U.S. Air Force)

Below: Canadair F-86E Sabres of 2 Aerobrigata, *Lanceri Neri* (Black Lancers) in 1958.
(Italian Air Force via R. Lamplough)

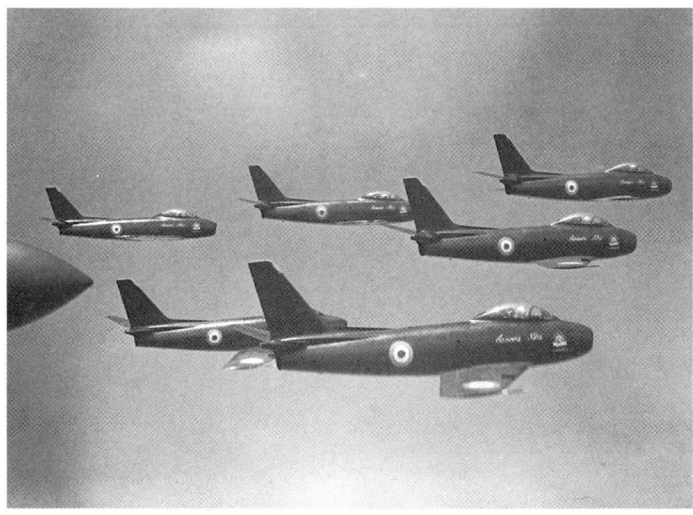

1959-1960: "Getti Tonanti" (Thunder-Jets), 5 Aerobrigata, Rimini

This was the second team with this name, but this time flew 5 F-84F Thunderstreaks led by Captain F. Picasso. This team participated in air shows in Italy, England, Germany, France and Spain. As 1959 was the year the Olympic Games were held in Rome, the aircraft wore the famous Olympic Rings design on their fins. The fuselage was natural metal and tops of the wings and tailplanes were painted in Italian red, white and green colours. Each of the five aircraft was given a different fin/spine/nose colour as follows: 5-648-black, 5-36591-orange, 5-619-pale green, 5-721-yellow and one with red trim. The 5 Aerobrigata badge appeared on the starboard nose and the team's name appeared in bold red letters on the port side of the nose.

1960-to date: "Frecce Tricolori" (Tricoloured Arrows) — 313 Gruppo Addestramento Acrobatico, Rivolto, Udine

At the end of 1960, the Italian Air Staff decided to form a National Aerobatic Team with permanent headquarters at Rivolto del Fruili. The pilots of the National Aerobatic Team, *Frecce Tricolori*, are recruited from all the Squadrons of the Air Force and are chosen after a selective screening. The first *Frecce Tricolori* team formed early in 1961 with nine Canadair F-86E Sabres, which were painted black overall with a pale blue diamond design on the fuselage and red/white/green stripes under the wings and tailplanes. Led by Captain M. Scala, who was relieved by Major M. Squarcina in October 1961, the Sabres retained this colour scheme until 1963, when they adopted the overall dark blue scheme with tri-coloured arrows insignia, as applied to the later Fiat G.91PANs. They appeared all over Europe, including the 1963 Paris Air Show. The aircraft wore yellow *letter* codes on their fins for most of 1963, but later changed to **number** codes. The 1963 team was led by Captain F. Pisano who relinquished the position to Captain V. Cumin towards the end of 1963.

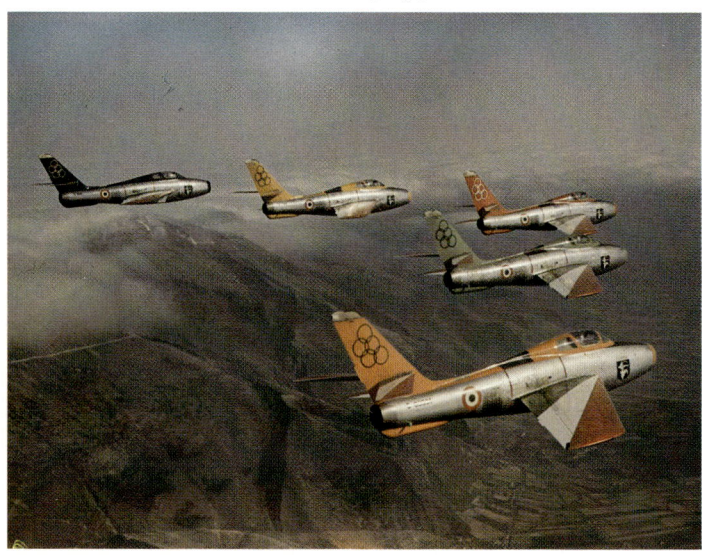

Republic F-84F Thunderstreaks of the *Getti Tonanti* (Thunder-Jets) team from 5 Aerobrigata. Each aircraft wore a different tail colour with the Olympic Rings insignia denoting that Italy was the host country for the Games in 1959. (Italian Air Force via R. Lamplough)

Canadair Sabres of the 1963 *Frecce Tricolori* team, in their second colour scheme as worn by the team's later Fiat G.91s. (Italian Air Force via R. Lamplough).

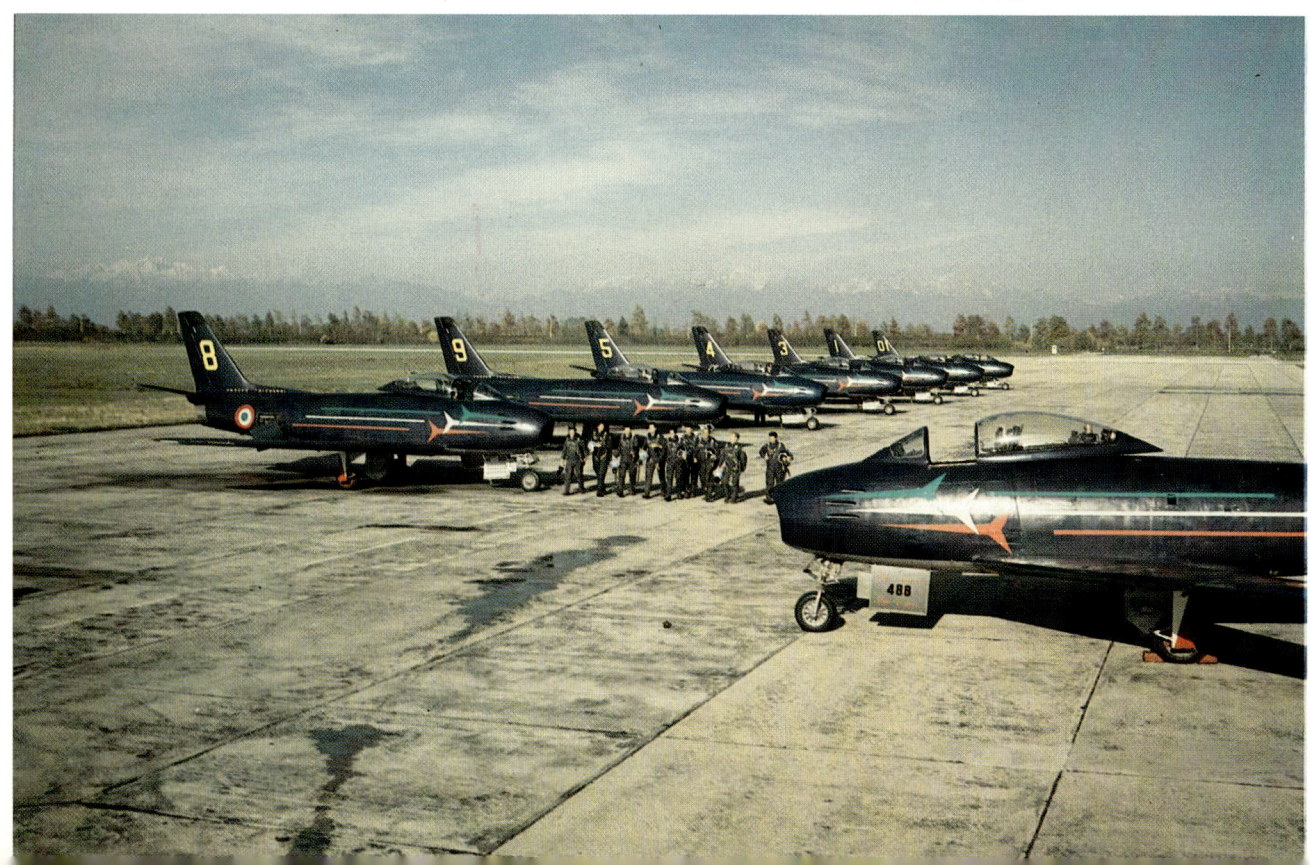

On 28th December 1963, the first Fiat G.91 assigned to the 313⁰ Gruppo Addestramento Acrabatico, arrived at Rivolto Air Base in *Frecce Tricolori* colours. The era of the Italian Air Force Sabre aerobatic teams had come to an end. The team converted to the Fiat G.91PAN during the early months of 1964, led by Captain V. Cumin, who took the team through the 1964 and '65 seasons participating in displays throughout Europe. Nine smoke-equipped Fiat G.91PANs were operated by the team, most of which were early production machines from the Fiat production line. In 1966, T. Colonel Roberto Di Lollo became the Commandant of 313⁰ A.A. and Major Vittorio Cumin continued to lead the team throughout the 1966, '67 and '68 seasons and the team operated the Fiat G.91 right up until the end of 1981. Over the last few years, some later model Fiat G.91Rs were added to the team to replace aircraft withdrawn or involved in accidents. The team flew two types of show, the 'high' programme, which required a minimum ceiling of 6000 feet to operate. Also, a 'low' programme, which is carried out horizontally thus enabling the formation to operate with low clouds and visibility. This team is most notable for their finalé, where all nine aircraft appear from nine different points on the compass and cross over in the centre of the airfield simultaneously. Slightly different heights are carefully calculated for each aircraft at the cross-over point, to avoid collision! Each aircraft had a yellow tail number code on its fin and these were changed around between aircraft as they went in for servicing. Fiat G-91PANs operating with *Frecce Tricolori* during the 1964-81 seasons included: MM6238'1', MM6239'15' became '8', MM6240'9' became '6', MM6242'12', MM6243'8' became '9', MM6244'2', MM6248'5', MM6249'16', MM6250'6', MM6252'4', MM6254'3', MM6260'10', MM6261'14', MM6264'1', MM6265'2', MM6241'4', MM6262 and MM6253'11'. Support aircraft was a Fairchild C-119G or 'J from 46 Aerobrigata at Pisa, which was replaced by a C-130H Hercules in the early 1970s. 1981 was the last season with the Fiat G-91 for the *Frecce Tricolori*. The team re-equipped with the Aermacchi MB-339PAN on 27th April 1982 and currently flies a display with nine aircraft of this type. MB-339s operated by *Frecce Tricolori* include: MM54475/1, MM544483/2, MM54482/3, MM54478/4, MM54486/5, MM54474/6, MM54481/7, MM54480/8, MM54479/9 MM54476/10 and MM54484/11 — the last numbers after each serial being the tail codes.

The 1959 *Getti Tonanti* team again, with their F-84F Thunderstreaks. This view shows the team's name, which appeared on the port side of the nose only. Also note the colour scheme under the wings compared with the photograph opposite.
(Italian Air Force via R. Lamplough).

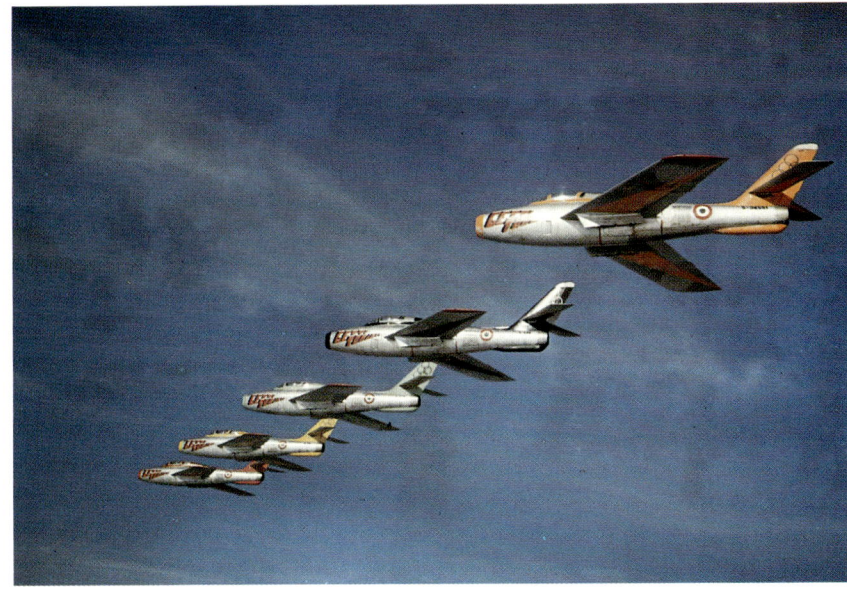

Fiat G-91PAN, MM6250/6, of the Italian Air Force *Frecce Tricolori,* seen landing at the Farnborough Air Show on 10 September 1972.
(Adrian M. Balch).

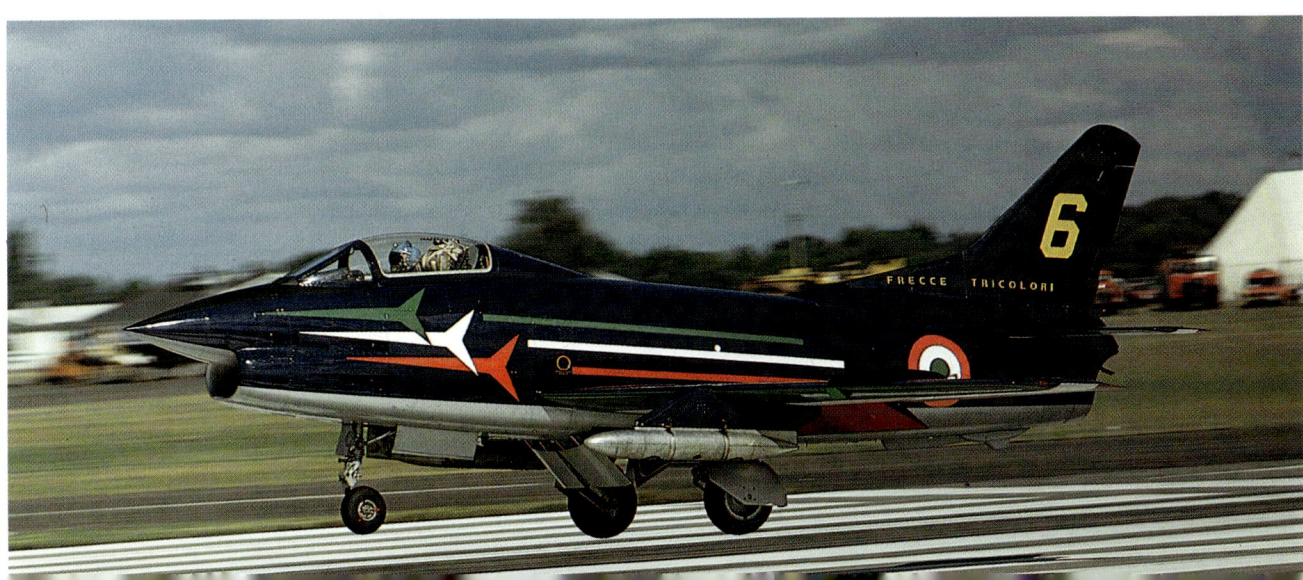

JAPAN
Japanese Air Self-Defense Force

1960-to date: 1st Air Wing, "Blue Impulse", Matsushima

In the Spring of 1958, it was decided to form a full-time aerobatic team to represent the JASDF at shows and events throughout Japan, for recruiting and public relations. Preparatory studies were started and conducted by four instructors on F-86F Sabres at Hamamatsu Air Base.

In the Spring of 1960, the *Blue Impulse* Aerobatic Team was formed and gave their first public demonstration on 4th March of that year. Five F-86F Sabres were used, of which one flew solo demonstrations while the main formation regrouped. Initially the Sabres retained their natural metal finish overall, with the Wing's black and yellow checkered band across the fin. The following year, 1961, the aircraft were painted in their own colour scheme, which was still basically natural metal but with blue and white trim. The leader's aircraft had the same scheme, but with gold and white trim. This scheme was retained for two years until 1963, when the second and final colour scheme was implemented. The aircraft were basically white overall, apart from the underside of the wings. Trim was medium blue with orange-red trim on the undersurfaces. This colourful scheme was retained right up until the F-86F was retired in 1981. If that wasn't attractive enough, the *Blue Impulse* team used blue, pink, white, yellow and green smoke during their display — a different colour from each of the five aircraft.

In 1964, Japan was the host for the Olympic Games. The *Blue Impulse* team opened the Games by making the famous Olympic rings symbol in smoke over the stadium. Five Sabres flew a ring each with a diameter of 6,000 feet and 1,000 feet separation between each ring.

A similar, but more intricate exercise was performed in 1970, when Tokyo hosted "Expo' 70". Through a complicated series of well-planned manoeuvres, the five Sabres wrote "Expo' 70" in white smoke over Tokyo.

These were just two highlights in over twenty years of safe operation with the F-86F Sabres. The final demonstration flights by F-86Fs of the *Blue Impulse* team were flown in the morning and afternoon of 8th February 1981 over Iruma Air Base, near Tokyo. Because of very limited air space in Japan, the team had been prohibited from demonstrating various aerobatic manoeuvres. What is more, they had to fly within a radius of approximately 5 miles. In the 21 years of operations, the *Blue Impulse* Sabres flew 545 performances. The *Blue Impulse* disbanded for about six months, but started practising on their new mount, the Mitsubishi T-2 on 26th July 1981.

The Japanese Air Self-Defense Force *Blue Impulse* team of F-86F Sabres in their 1962 colour scheme. Trim was blue and white, while the leader's aircraft was in gold and white trim. (D. Kasulka via R. Ward)

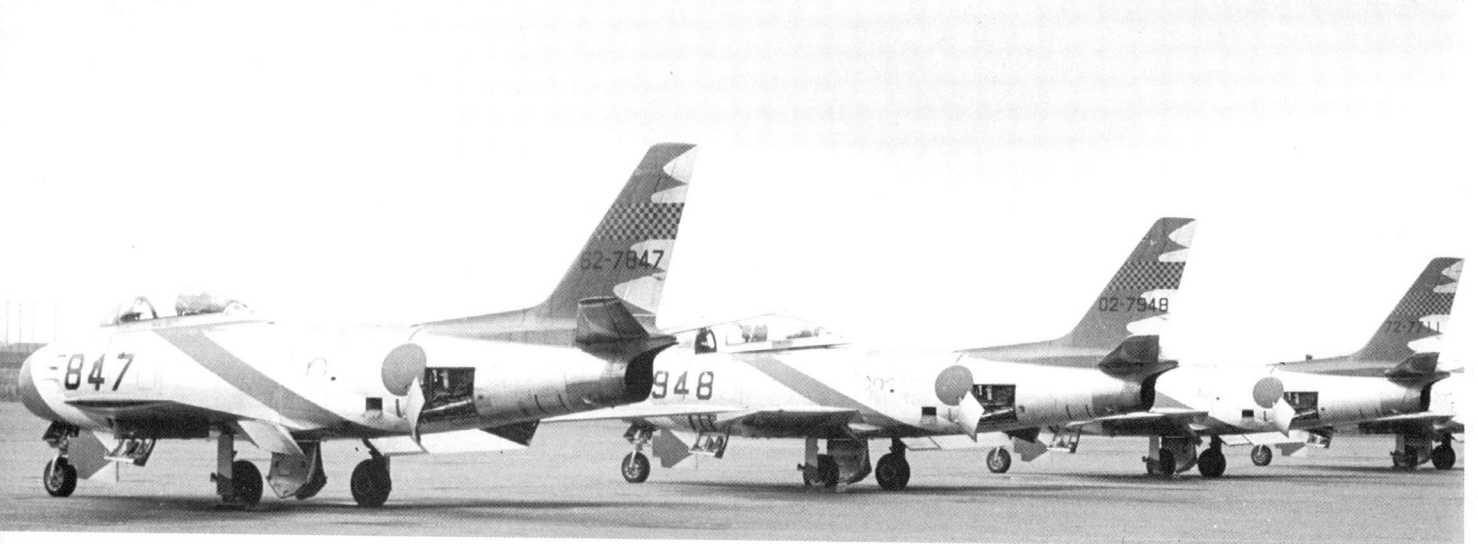

Looking like Jaguars, there are six Mitsubishi T-2s in the current *Blue Impulse* team, two solos with a main formation of four. Colour scheme is a very attractive design of dark blue, light blue and white. In 21 years, some 40 F-86F Sabres have appeared in the *Blue Impulse* team colours. Aircraft wearing the 1962 colour scheme included 92-7939, 92-7872, 92-7915, 02-7948, 82-7847, 72-7711 in the blue/white trim with 92-7937 in the gold/white trim denoting the leader's aircraft. F-86F Sabres known to have worn the white, blue and red scheme during 1963-81 are: 02-7960, 02-7962, 02-7966, 12-7993, 12-7995, 62-7439, 62-7510, 62-7512, 72-7709, 72-7772, 72-7773, 82-7809, 82-7832, 82-7834, 82-7847, 92-7873, 92-7894, 92-7901, 92-7913, 92-7927, 92-7929, 92-7931 and 92-7937.

The current team of Mitsubishi T-2s comprise: 29-5176 (leader), 19-5172, 19-5173, 19-5174, 59-5111, 29-5111, 29-5175 and 59-5112

F-86F Sabre, 92-7894, of the Japanese Air Self-Defense Force's *Blue Impulse* team seen taxying at Tsuiki Air Base in November 1973. (T. Hotta).

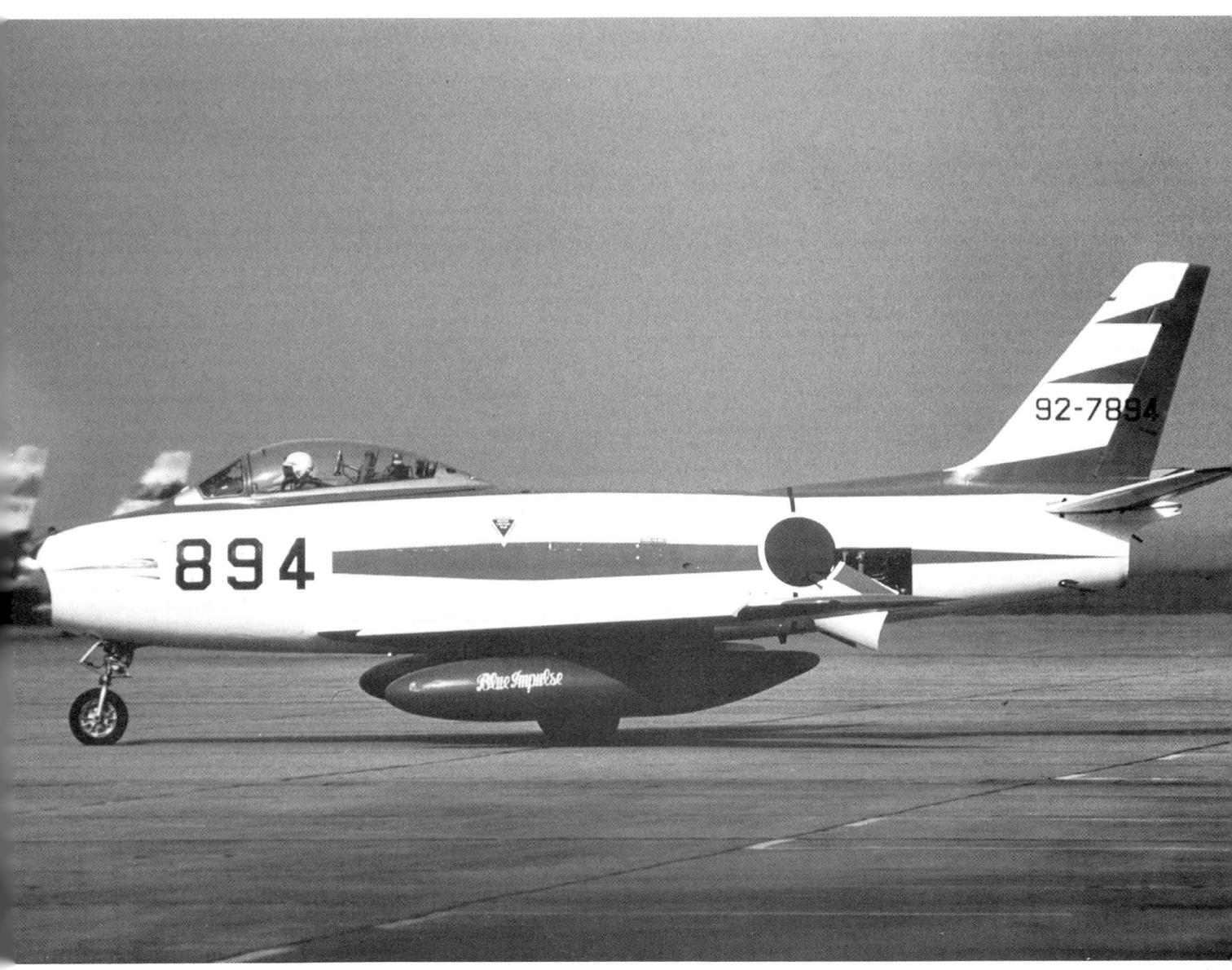

Right: F-86F Sabres of the Japanese Air Self-Defense Force aerobatic team *Blue Impulse*, August 1978.
(Author's Collection)

Below: Mitsubishi T-2, 29-5177 of the Japanese Air Self-Defense Force *Blue Impulse* team, seen taxying at Chitose in August 1982. (Akira Watanabe via J. M. Hughes)

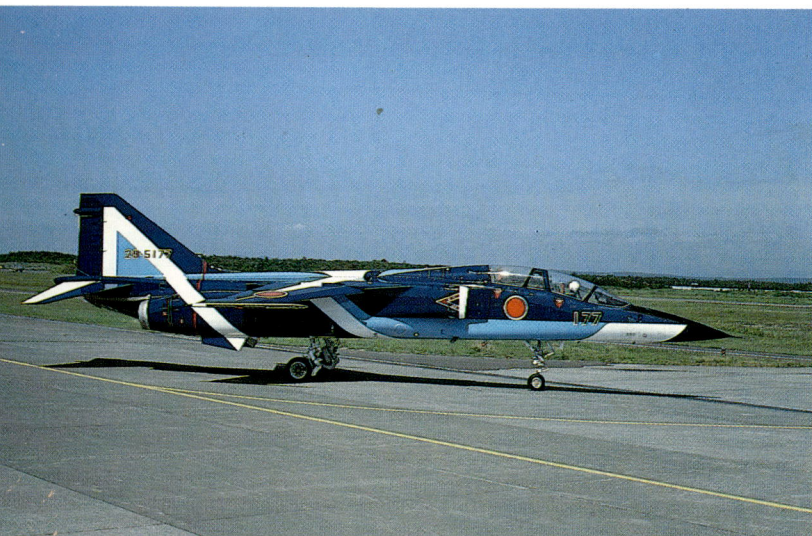
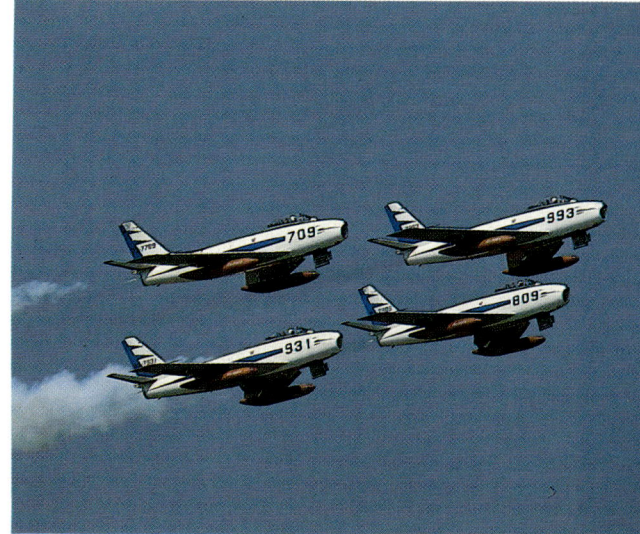

In 1967, the Royal Netherlands Air Force equipped their *Whisky-4* team with F-84F Thunderstreaks. With P-232 nearest, they are seen here in their smart pale green and black scheme with fins in Dutch national colours of red/white/blue.
(Royal Netherlands Air Force via R. Ward)

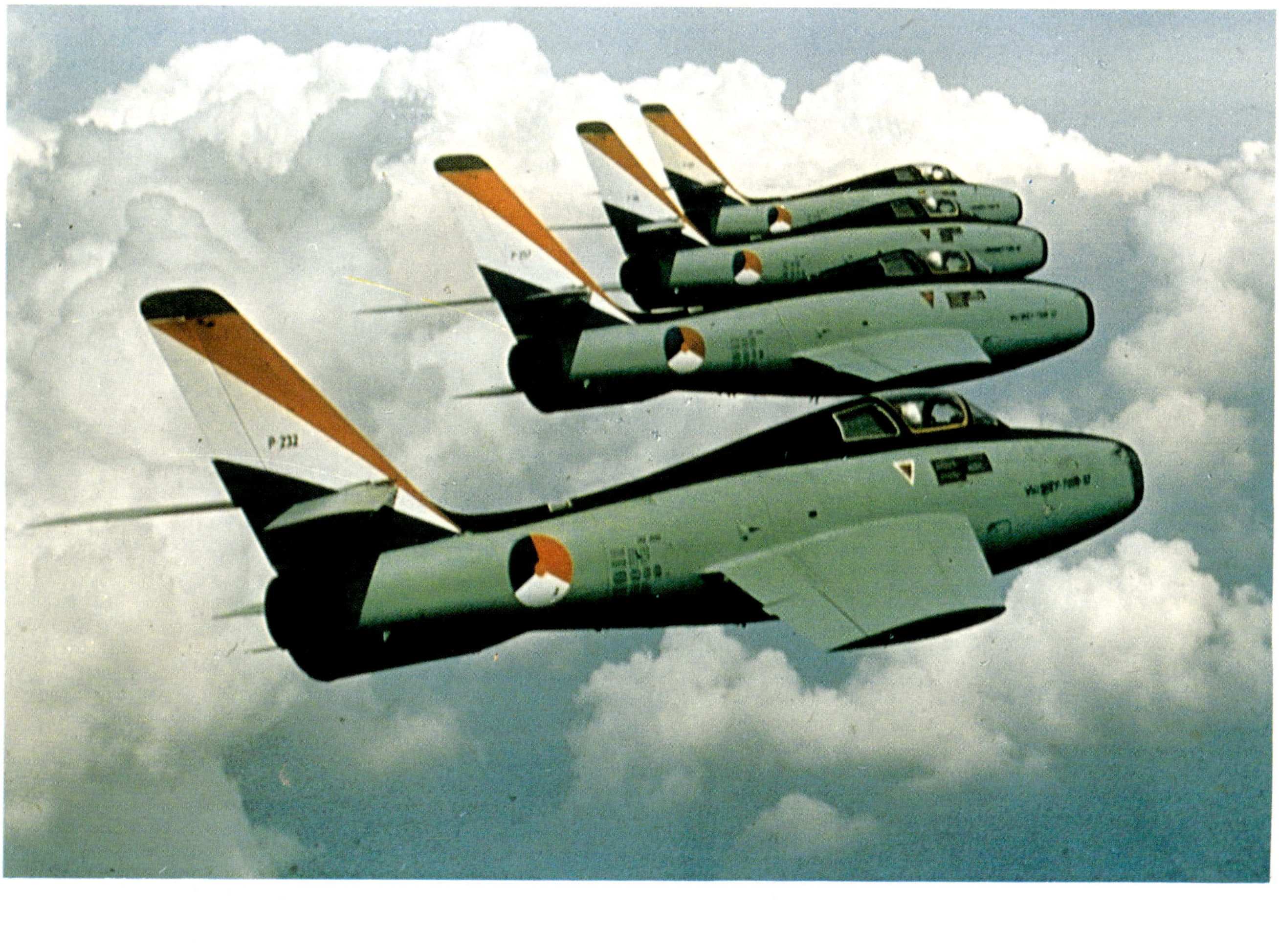

NETHERLANDS
Royal Netherlands Air Force

1952-53: 327 Squadron, "Red Diamonds", Soesterberg.
This was a team of four Gloster Meteor F.8 fighters, which was formed in 1952 at Soesterberg. In 1953, it performed at a display to mark the 40th anniversary of Dutch military aviation and was dissolved at the end of that year. Their Meteors were in a silver and red colour scheme with a large 'four-of-diamonds' playing card on the engine nacelle.

1955: 311 Squadron "Skyblazers", Volkel
This was the third aerobatic team to form in Europe with this name and flying four F-84G Thunderjets. The USAF team of the same name obviously made quite an impression during 1951-52, as teams of the same name were subsequently flown by Greece and then The Netherlands. The Dutch team lasted for the one season only and no special colour scheme is known to have been carried by the aircraft.

1956: 313 Squadron, "Dash-4", Twenthe
This was another quartet of F-84G Thunderjets, whose first public display was at Soesterberg. Later in the year, they went on to win an aerobatic competition at Las Vegas, Nevada. Little is known about this team, which lasted for the one year only.

During the same year, 313 Squadron formed a team of four T-33s at Woensdrecht, called the *Skysharks*, which disbanded at the end of 1957.

1956-67: "Whisky-Four", Woensdrecht
This team was formed in 1956 by an RAF instructor, Flight Lieutenant G. R. Wilson, who was stationed at Woensdrecht. The team's name was derived from the NATO Phonetic Alphabet, in which 'Whisky' stands for the letter 'W'. This was the first letter of Woensdrecht air base and also Wilson. *Whisky-Four* flew four Lockheed T-33s, the pilots being instructors at the Transition Flying Training School. The team was called just *Whisky* until 1963, when *Four* was added. In January 1964, Captain H. J. J. van Dommelen became the leader and took the four T-33s to displays throughout Europe, including RAF Colerne's Battle of Britain display in September 1964. Until 1966, the team's aircraft were in the standard silver and dayglo orange training colours. For the last season with the T-33, 1966, a smart colour scheme was adopted of pale green and dark green. Four T-33s that appeared in this scheme were: M-47 (51-6661), M-51(51-6528), M-52(51-6953) and M-55 (51-6531). The team appeared in England at RAF Gaydon's Battle of Britain display in September 1966 and disbanded shortly afterwards. They reformed in 1967 with four F-84F Thunderstreaks, which were painted in a pale green and black scheme. Two of the aircraft in this scheme were P-228 (53-6611) and P-232 (53-6608) of which the latter was written-off on 5th June 1967 in an accident, which killed the pilot. *Whisky-Four* were immediately disbanded by the Minister of Defence and no jet aerobatic teams have since been formed in the Royal Netherlands Air Force.

Below: Meteor F.8s of the Royal Netherlands Air Force *Red Diamonds* team from No. 327 Squadron in 1953. (R. Neth A. F. via R. Ward)

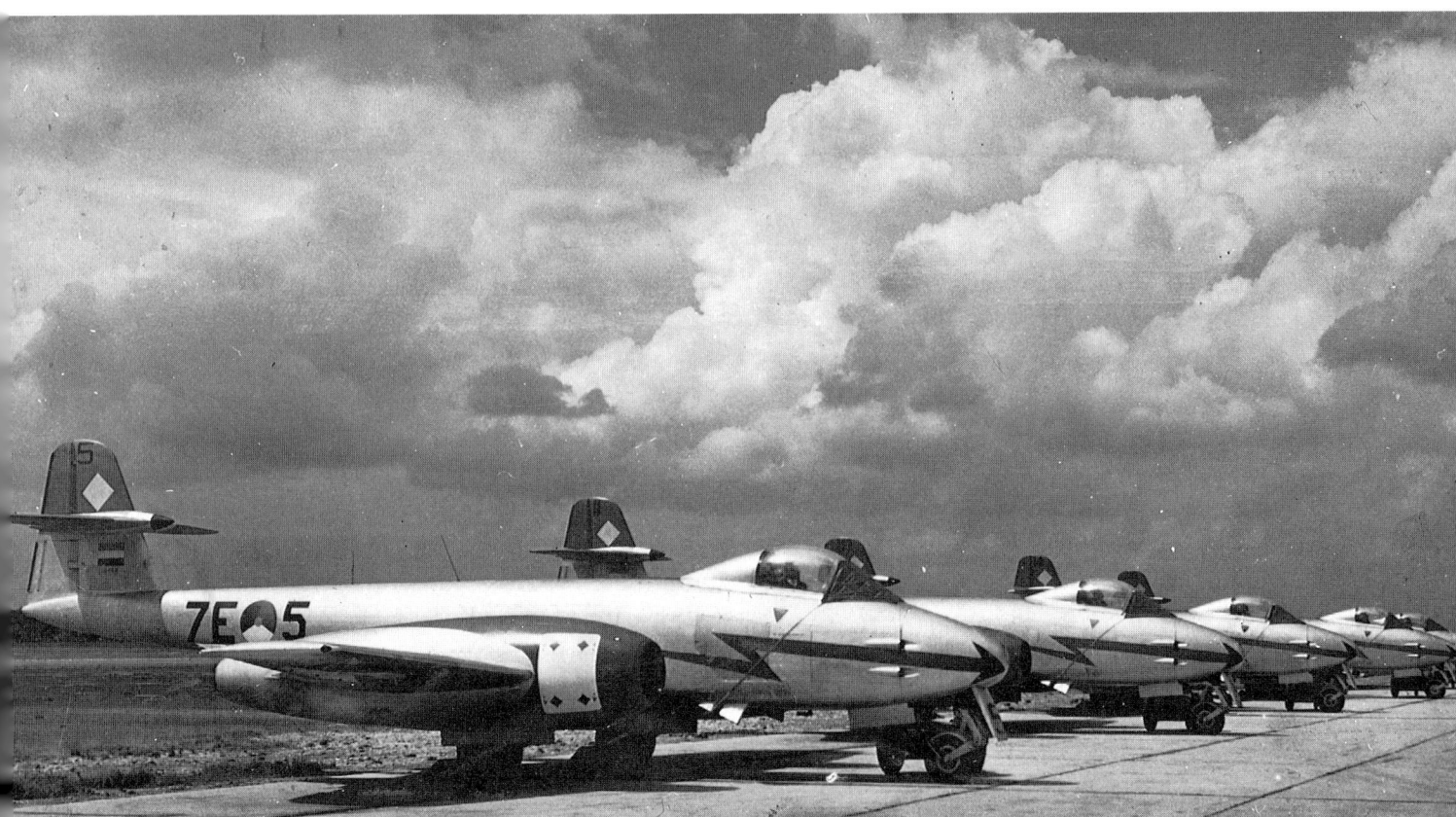

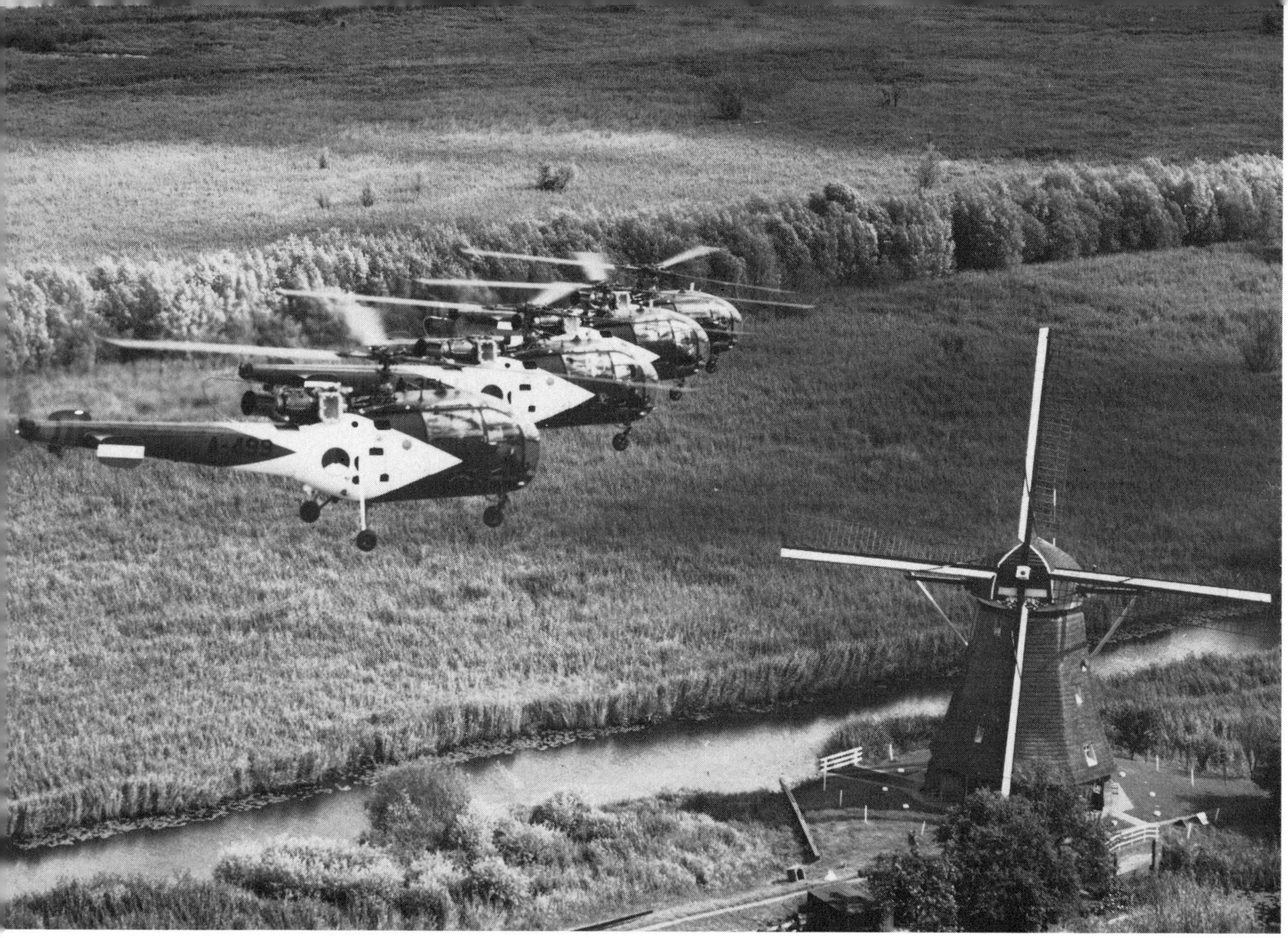

Above: The *Grasshoppers* — the current Royal Netherlands Air Force display team flying four Alouette 3 helicopters. They are seen here during 1982 with a typical Dutch backdrop. (R. Neth. A.F.)

Below: The Royal Netherlands Air Force *Whisky-4* team of T-33s seen in 1966 wearing their smart colour scheme of pale green with holly-green trim. Note smoke-making pipes at rear. (R. Neth. A.F)

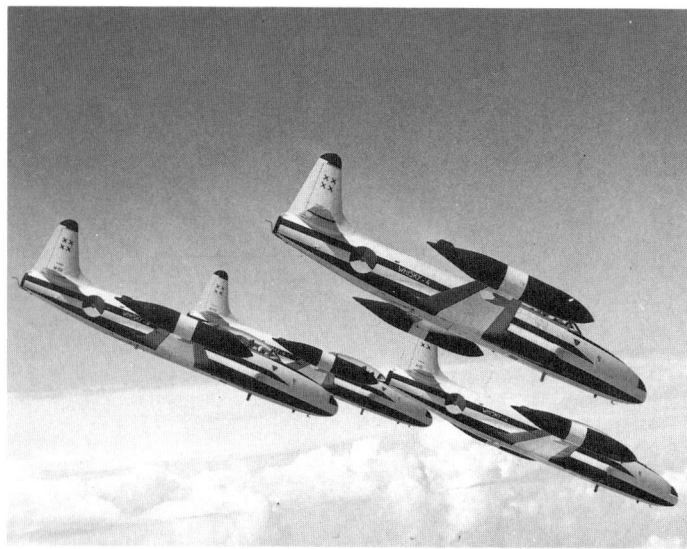

1963: 315 Squadron, "Sandbag Diamonds", Twenthe

This was the first team of F-84F Thunderstreaks, of which there were four. The origin of the team's unusual name is unknown, but the following aircraft were flown by the *Sandbag Diamonds* for the one season only: P-125, P-128, P-133, P-155 and P-165.

1973-to date: 299/300 Squadrons. "Grasshoppers", Deelen

On the occasion of the 50th anniversary of the Royal Netherlands Air Force, a helicopter demonstration team was formed by pilots of 299 Squadron at Deelen. This team was called the *Grasshoppers* and comprised four Alouette 3s. Until 1977, the team did not perform on a regular basis, but after the Open House at Gilze-Rijen in 1977, the team became the official helicopter demonstration team of the RNLAF. Since then, they have performed in Belgium, Germany, England and the Netherlands.

In 1981, the team started with a new crew of instructors from 300 Squadron and a new display sequence. The Alouettes were painted overall in Dutch national colours of red, white and blue for the 1980 season onwards. The team's four Alouettes in this scheme are drawn from: A350, '351, '390, '398, '406 and '499. During the 1981 season, the *Grasshoppers* took part in the largest military air show in the world — the International Air Tattoo at Greenham Common and won the UK Shell Oil Trophy for the best overall flying performance. The team's Alouettes are equipped with smoke-making canisters attached to the undercarriage legs and the *Grasshoppers* have appeared at many displays throughout Europe to date.

NEW ZEALAND
Royal New Zealand Air Force

During the years 1947-49, there were trios of Harvards formed for specific events, but these were short-lived anonimous teams. The RNZAF's original jet aerobatic team, flying Vampire jet fighters, made its public debut over thirty years ago.

This team was formed in Cyprus in 1952, where No.14 Squadron was operating as part of New Zealand's contribution to the then Middle East Air Force of the RAF. During the Coronation celebrations of 1953, three five-man teams gave many aerobatics displays throughout the Middle East and in Tanganyika, Uganda and Kenya.

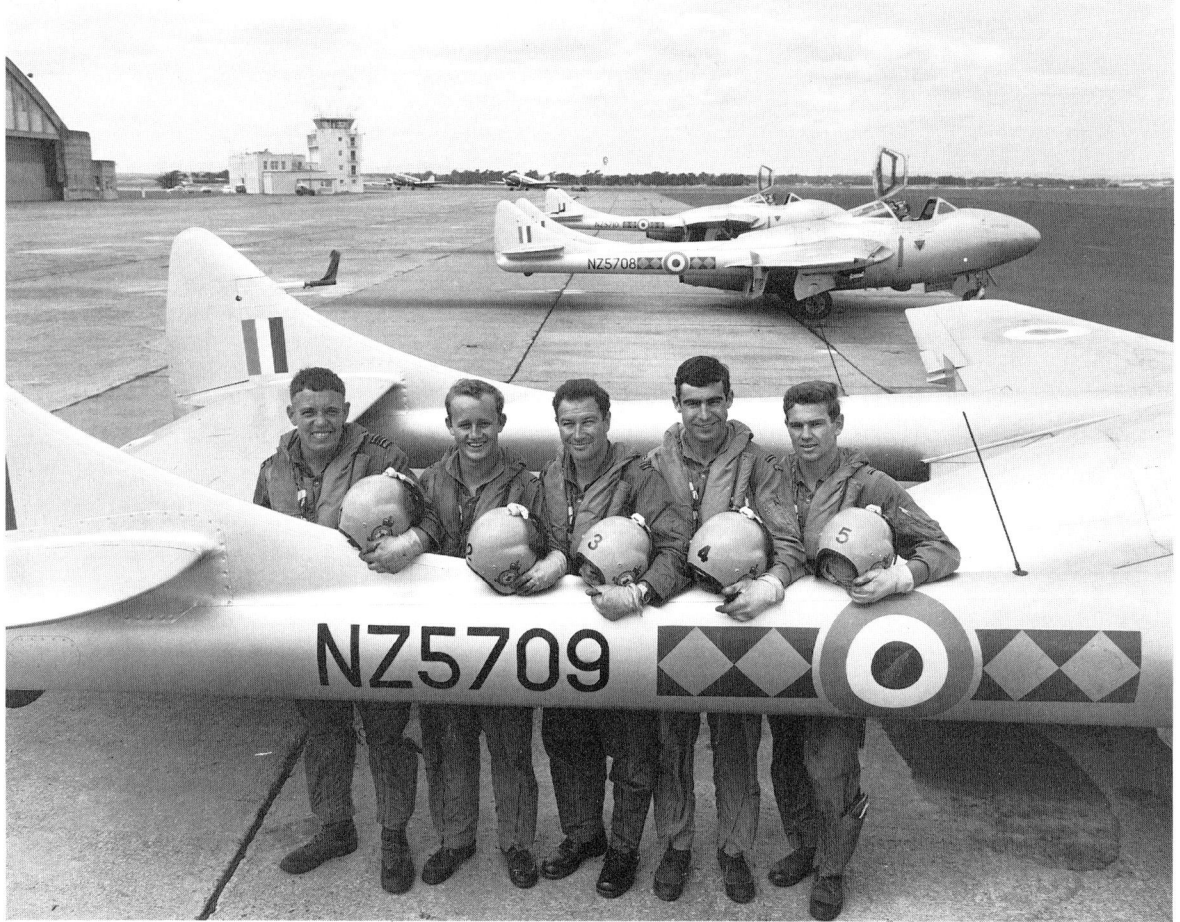

1958-60 and 1964-69: No. 75 Squadron, the "Yellowhammers", Ohakea

This Vampire team was formed in 1958, when the RNZAF celebrated its 21st anniversary and performed before a crowd of 100,000 at the Air Force Day that year. Later, that same team captured the imagination of audiences throughout the world as they performed before cameras of the National Film Unit. The award-winning film, 'Jetobatics' became a household word, just as the Vampire team became an institution in the RNZAF.

The team was disbanded in 1960 and reformed four years later to appear at the Air Force Day in 1964. The team was given the name *Yellowhammers* from the emblem of their squadron badge. Following the introduction of the Strikemasters into service in 1970, the team was disbanded and the Vampires withdrawn from service. No. 75

Above: The *Yellowhammers* team from No.75 Squadron, Royal New Zealand Air Force with Vampire T.11 NZ5709 in January 1969 — the team's last year. This view shows the markings well, the diamond markings being red and yellow. Note old-style roundel with silver fern leaf in centre.
(RNZAF via P. Harrison)

Squadron re-equipped with A-4K Skyhawks and formed a team with this type for the 1981 Air Force Day, but they did not continue with the name *Yellowhammers* and disbanded.

The *Yellowhammers* comprised four Vampires, usually three single-seat FB.9s and one T.11 two-seater. Colour scheme was silver overall with standard red/yellow squadron markings on the booms. The only team marking was a pair of yellow crossed hammers under the cockpit. The aircraft were equipped to make smoke and included: NZ5767, NZ5755, NZ5774, with examples of T.11s being NZ5707 and NZ5709.

1966-75 and 1981-to date: C.F.S. "Red Checkers", Wigram

Another RNZAF aerobatic team that attracted the admiration of young and old wherever they appeared were the *Red Checkers* from the Central Flying School at Wigram, flying Harvard training aircraft.

Formation aerobatics with Harvards were first carried out in 1947. The highlight of this quartet's display was having their wingtips tied together throughout their routine.

In 1966, a fifth Harvard was added to the team for solo aerobatics and the following year, at the time of the 50th anniversary of flight at Wigram, the team took the name of *Red Checkers* and appeared with distinctive red and white checks on the engine cowls of the aircraft.

On 15 March 1970, led by Flight Lieutenant L. A. Olsen, the *Red Checkers* had the distinction of being the first RNZAF aerobatic team to perform before Her Majesty The Queen during her visit to Picton.

The *Red Checkers* team was disbanded in 1975 and the Harvards were subsequently withdrawn from service and replaced by CT4 Airtrainers. In 1981, a team of four Airtrainer aircraft performed before 100,000 people at Air Force '81. This team continued and has adopted the name *Red Checkers*. A spectacular aspect of their display is the 'mirror' formation by two of the team. Since their reformation, the team has been led by the officer commanding the RNZAF's Central Flying School at Wigram, Squadron Leader Bruce Ferguson. The five Airtrainers in the team wear their standard light grey and red training colours, as worn by the Harvards in their final years. In addition, a band of red/white checks adorns either side of the nose.

The *Red Checkers* Harvards have worn three colour schemes. The first was silver overall with yellow training bands around the wings and fuselage and the original RNZAF roundel, which was similar to that of the RAF with a silver fern leaf in the red centre. This scheme was during the team's un-named period from 1947 to about 1965. The second colour scheme was worn between 1966 and 1970 and retained the same roundel but dispensed with the yellow training bands. The rear fuselage, fin, tailplanes and wingtips were dayglo red. The entire engine cowl was painted in red and white checks. In 1970, the roundel centre was changed to a red Kiwi and this was when the *Red Checkers* adopted their third and final scheme. Silver was replaced by light grey and the whole rear fuselage, tailplanes and fin and rudder were painted red, as were the wingtips. The checks on the cowl were enlarged four times, so there were less of them, but they stood out from a greater distance. Examples of *Red Checkers* Harvards were: NZ1065, NZ1066, NZ1079 and NZ1080.

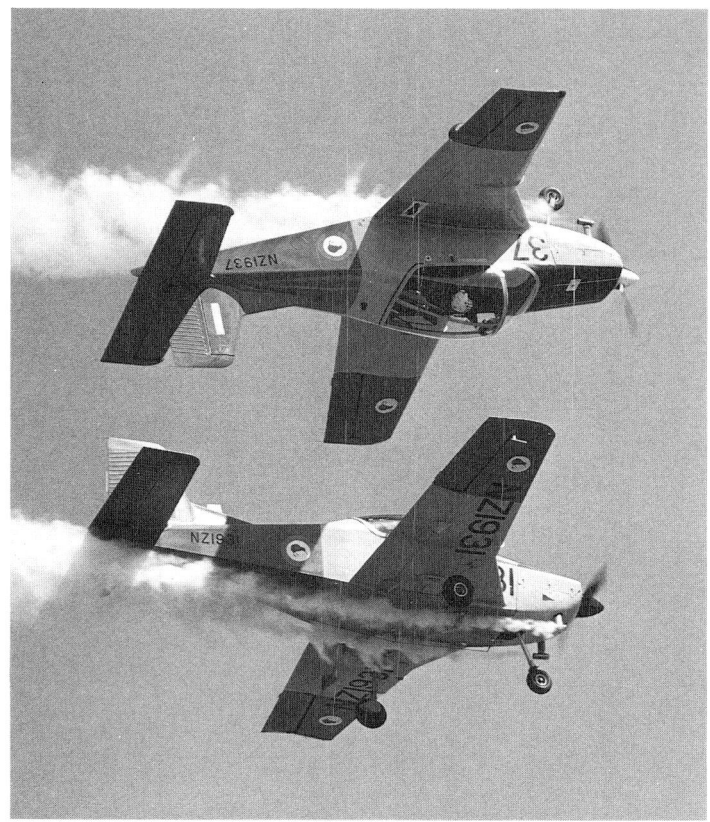

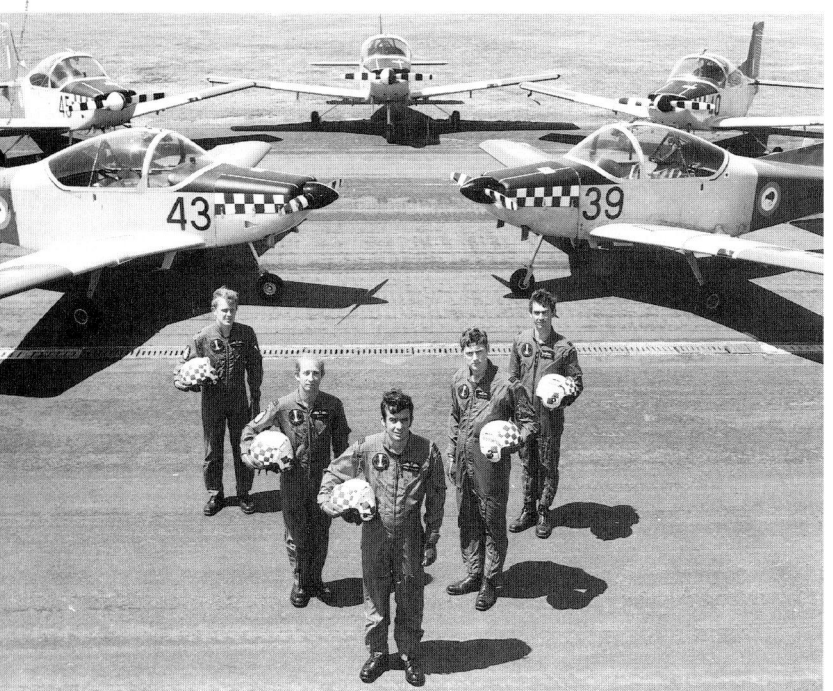

Above: The Royal New Zealand Air Force's *Red Checkers* aerobatic team with their Airtrainer aircraft. The team members are, from left, Flight Lieutenant Colin Pearce (No 4) from Lower Hutt, Flight Lieutenant Steve Bone (No 2) from Wellington, Squadron Leader Bruce Ferguson (leader) from Tauranga, Flight Lieutenant Malcolm Knox (No 3) from Dunedin and Flight Lieutenant Roger Read (No 5 and solo) from Auckland at Wigram, January 1983. (RNZAF)

Top: A dramatic view of two CT-4 Airtrainers of the Royal New Zealand Air Force's *Red Checkers* team in 'mirror' formation. (RNZAF)

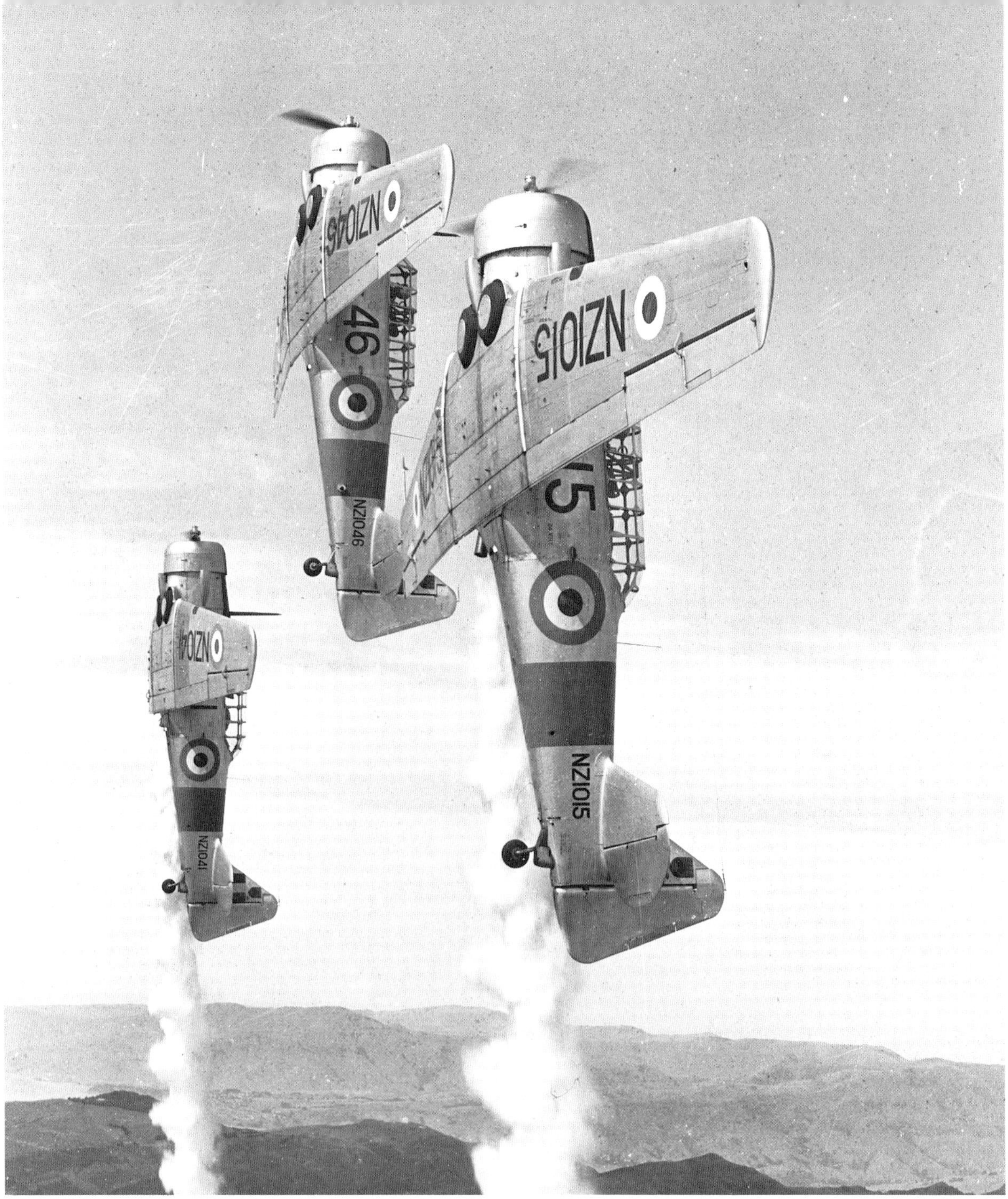

The first Royal New Zealand Air Force Harvard team from CFS in 1959/60 before being named *Red Checkers*. Colour scheme is silver overall with yellow training bands. (RNZAF via P. Harrison)

Harvard, NZ1080, of the RNZAF *Red Checkers* team in the second scheme of silver and dayglo with red and white cowl checks. Note the exhaust pipe extension to aid smoke-making. Photo taken at Wigram in Jan 1969.
(Paul A. Harrison)

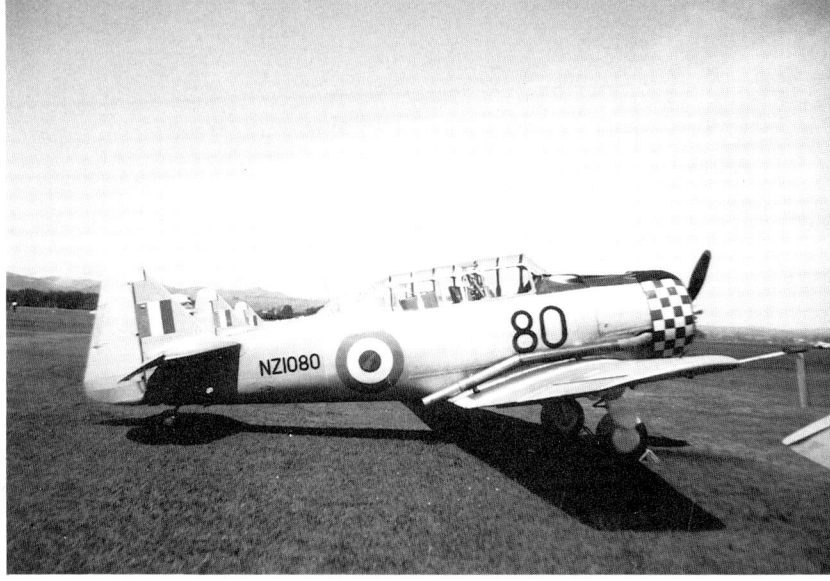

NORWAY
Royal Norwegian Air Force

1957-77: "Flying Jokers", No. 332 Squadron, Rygge.
The *Flying Jokers* aerobatic team was formed in January 1957. Originally the team flew with four F-84G Thunderjets, but in May the same year, the team changed to F-86F Sabres, also increasing in number to six aircraft. At one time, they even flew with nine Sabres. In 1959, the F-86Fs received special 'Joker' markings on the wings and tail and began to use smoke during their performances.

In 1963, the F-86Fs were replaced by F-86Ks. The size of the team was now reduced to five aircraft. The *Flying Jokers* was the first team to fly 'Card Five' formation, but their F-86Ks carried no special markings.

The *Flying Jokers* were not a permanent aerobatic team and have been activated and de-activated at regular intervals, whenever the aircraft could be spared from operational duties with 332 Squadron. The team was disbanded in the autumn of 1964, when the squadron disbanded and the aircraft were transferred to 334 Squadron. In 1967, No. 332 Squadron was reformed again, at Rygge, with F-5A Freedom Fighters. However, the *Flying Jokers* team was not resurrected during the period until the squadron disbanded again in 1972. It was not until 1977 that No. 336 Squadron activated the team once again, now with three Northrop F-5As. All rehearsals were carried out alongside normal training duties and the aircraft were equipped to make smoke. The *Flying Jokers* appeared at the International Air Tattoo at Greenham Common in June 1977 and, at the end of that year, the team disbanded once again. The F-5As wore the standard silver scheme overall, with the addition of a 'Joker' playing card insignia on the fin. The aircraft used were 156 (67-21156), 207(66-9207), 905(67-14905) and 372(64-13372) — one aircraft being used as a spare.

At the end of the 1970s, No. 332 Squadron was reformed once again and equipped with F-16A Fighting Falcons during 1980. During the squadron's 40th Anniversay celebrations in June 1982, the Officer Commanding No. 332 Squadron Major Trond Moltzau, flew his F-16 with *Flying Jokers* markings, indicating that the team will probably reform in the near future with F-16s.

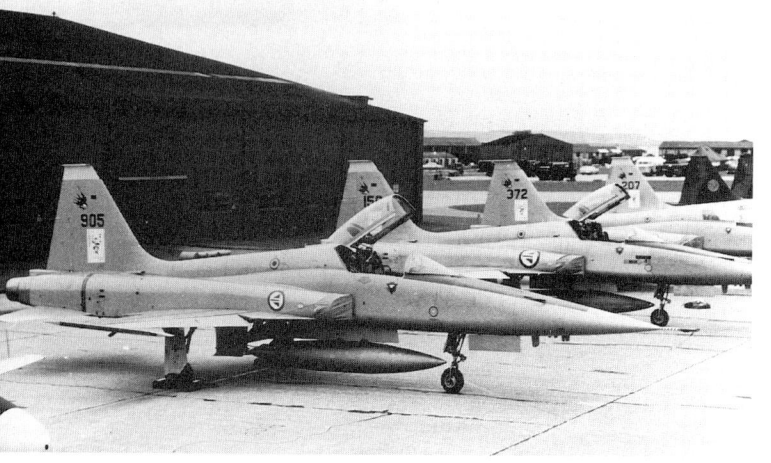

Above: F-5As of the Royal Norwegian Air Force *Flying Jokers* team lined up at Greenham Common in June 1977. Note the 'Joker' playing card insignia on the fins and the variation in roundel size. (Adrian M. Balch)

Below: Royal Norwegian Air Force F-86F Sabres of the *Flying Jokers* team from No. 332 Squadron, in 1958 before special team markings were applied. (R. Nor. A.F.)

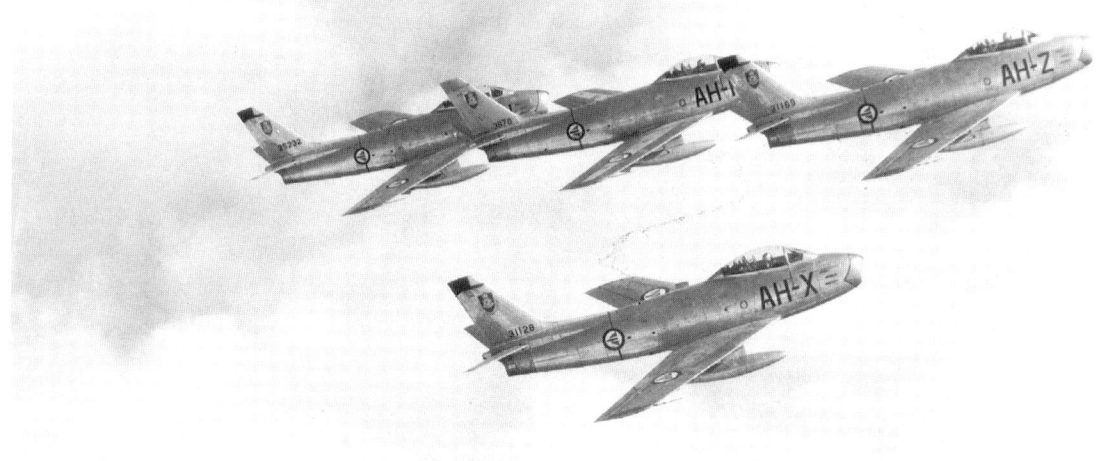

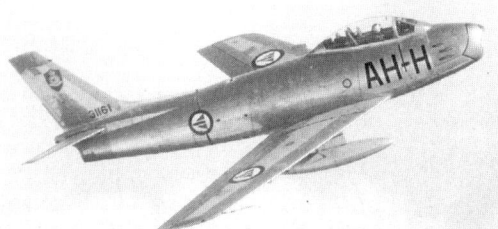

PAKISTAN
Pakistan Air Force

The first public performance of formation aerobatics in the Pakistan Air Force was given in December, 1950 at Risalpur when two Tempests, flown by the then Flight Lieutenant (later Air Marshal) Rahim Khan and Flight Lieutenant (later Air Commodore) M. Z. Masud, executed loops, rolls and wing-overs during an air display held for distinguished visitors. Aerobatic teams were formed by Nos. 9 and 14 Squadrons at the time, flying Hawker Furies, but they performed on few occasions. The first jet team was formed by No. 11 Squadron in 1952 with Supermarine Attackers. They used the name *Paybill*, which was the Squadron's call-sign.

1956-64: 11 Squadron, "The Falcons", Mauripur then Sargodha

In 1956, No. 11 Squadron had just been equipped with F-86F Sabres and formed the most famous of the Pakistan Air Force's aerobatic teams — *The Falcons*. Starting as a 4-man team, *The Falcons* increased to 7 aircraft in 1957 and were thought to have had the largest number of jet aircraft in an aerobatic team worldwide. However, they were not content with this and gradually increased the numbers until they had 16 Sabres. At a huge air display held at Karachi on 2 February 1958, *The Falcons* made history by looping all 16 Sabres in perfect 'diamond' formation in the presence of the then King of Afghanistan and the Chiefs of Staff of the Turkish, Iranian, Iraqi, Jordanian and Afghan Air Forces. This historic loop, which was the first part of a 3-part demonstration, was performed by pilots drawn from 11, 15, 5 and 4 Squadrons, led by Wing Commander M. Z. Masud.

This world record was short-lived, however, as in September of the same year, the RAF's *Black Arrows* broke the looping record with 22 Hunters, which stands today.

After its 16-aircraft display in 1958, *The Falcons* reverted to a 4-member team for several years. In 1963, No. 11 Squadron moved to Sargodha, when they increased their number to nine and were led by Wing Commander (now Air Chief Marshal) Anwar Shamin. Following a display at Peshawar in 1964, the team disbanded.

Other PAF Teams

Although the PAF does not operate a full-time aerobatic team, mention should be made of some of the part-time teams.

When *The Falcons* disbanded in 1964, the PAF's Flying Training Wing at Risalpur formed a team of Cessna T-37 jet trainers, called the *Sherdils*. For the past 20 years, they have operated this 4-man team at RAF Academy Graduation Parades, official functions and at the annual Air Force Day. The other team worthy of mention is the Combat Commanders School Aerobatic Team flying Shenyang F-6s, which are Chinese-built MiG-19SFs. This team operated during the 1970s, their aircraft having an overall red and yellow colour scheme. One of this team's aircraft was serialled 7723.

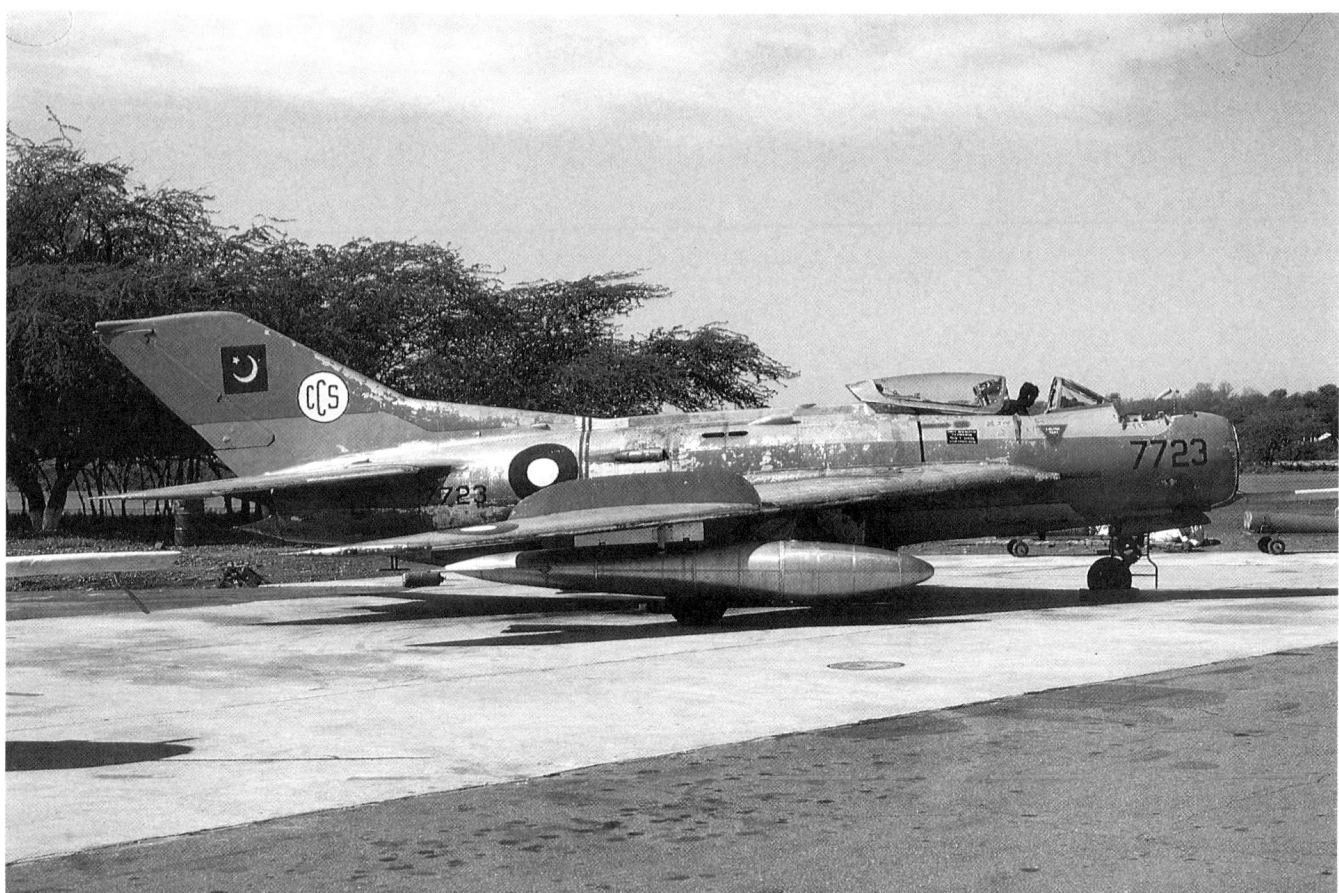

A Pakistan Air Force Shenyang F6 (Chinese-built MiG-19) serial 7723 of the Combat Commanders' School still retaining the red and yellow colour scheme of the disbanded aerobatic team, photographed at Peshawar on 22 March 1981. (L. T. Peacock)

PHILIPPINES
Philippine Air Force

There have been several part-time teams formed with F-86F Sabres during the late 1950s and early '60s including the *Falcons* and *Sidewinders*, which formed within the 5th Fighter Wing at Basa Air Base. The only official team is as follows:

1953-to date: 6 FS,5 FW, "Blue Diamonds", Basa
The *Blue Diamonds* were organised in 1953 by First Lieutenant José F. L. Gonzales of the 6th Fighter Squadron with four members using the F-51D Mustang. The *Blue Diamonds* made their initial public appearance during the Philippine Aviation Week in November of the same year. This debut of the aerobatic team was led by the commander of the 6th Fighter Squadron, the Major José L. Rancudo.

In 1957, with barely 50 hours of flying time in F-86F Sabres, the team switched to jet aircraft with a team of seven. The team was then led by its organiser, Lieutenant Gonzales.

Subsequent appearances of the team during air shows assured the success of the annual Philippine Aviation Week, as well as the celebration of Philippine Air Force Day.

The *Blue Diamonds* made their transition to the Northrop F-5A supersonic jet fighter in 1968, four years after the Philippine Air Force acquired this type.

The team members received the 'Kahusayan Award' in 1969 from the PAF Commanding General in recognition of their outstanding accomplishments beneficial not only to the Philippine Air Force, but also to aviation in general.

Below: Northrop F-5A, 66-9150, of the 6th TFS, 5 FW at Basa Air Base on 23 November 1980. Note the *Blue Diamonds* aerobatic team nose markings and the target drogue under the port wing. (Adrian M. Balch)

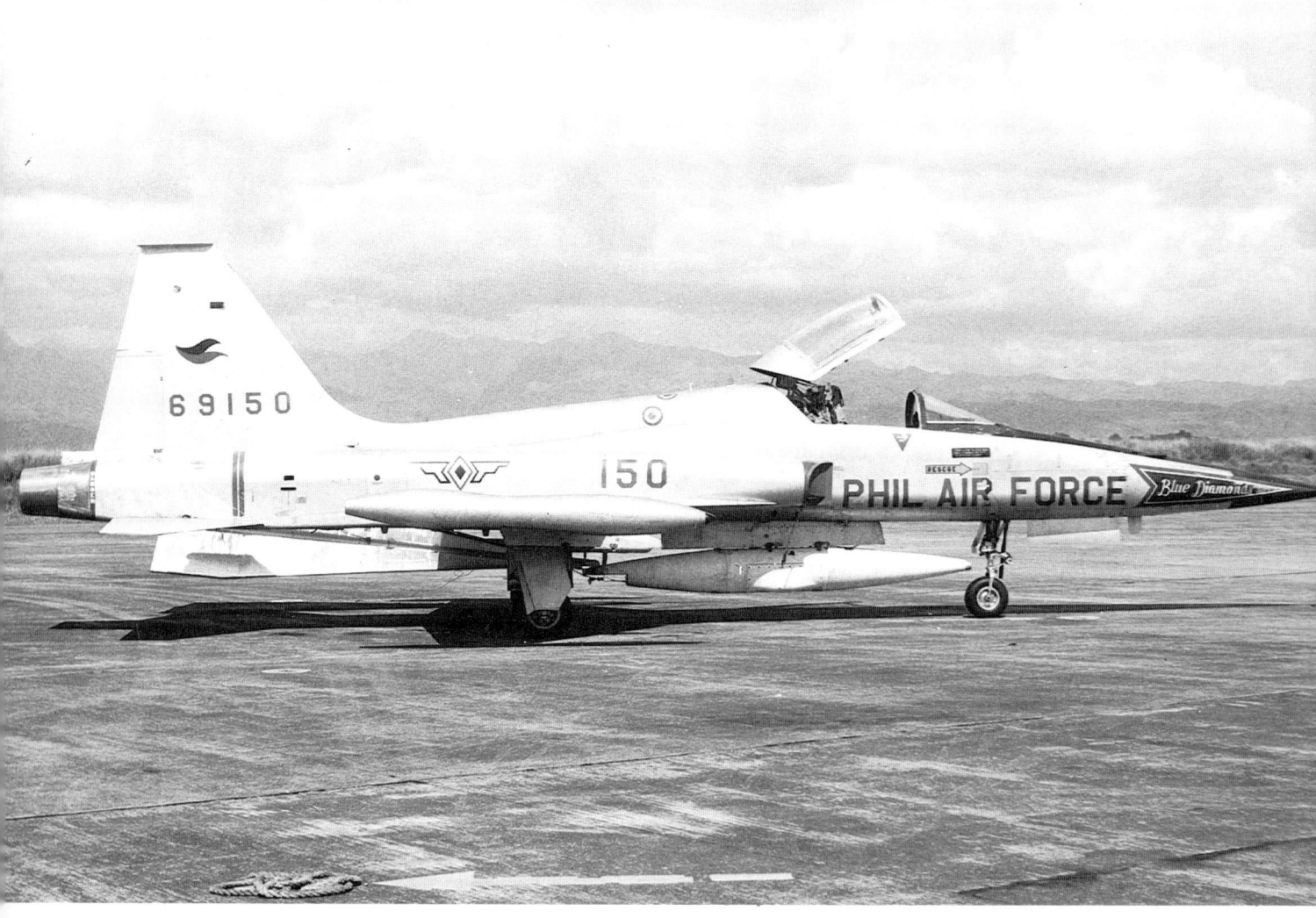

The F-51D Mustangs used by the team were silver overall with standard national markings and the Wing's badge on a diamond-shaped background on the fin. No special team markings were known to have been carried and serial numbers included 44-43733, 44-72933 and 44-72821.

The F-86F Sabres were natural metal overall with red, white and dark blue trim. Individual code numbers were allocated to team aircraft, worn on the fin in a red, white and blue design. Only two aircraft that wore these markings are known: 113468'1' and 113432'4'.

When the team changed to the F-5A, similar markings were adopted with the leader's aircraft being 10507'1'.

During the early 1970s air shows were banned in the Phillippines as an economy measure. The team's tail markings were replaced by the 6th FS markings of a black Cobra's head on a white disc mounted on a broad dark blue band. About 1978, the C.O. of the 5th FW ordered the removal of all colourful markings, so all squadron insignia was removed but the F-5As still carry *Blue Diamonds* in script on the nose and practices are maintained for any official function or when air shows are permitted.

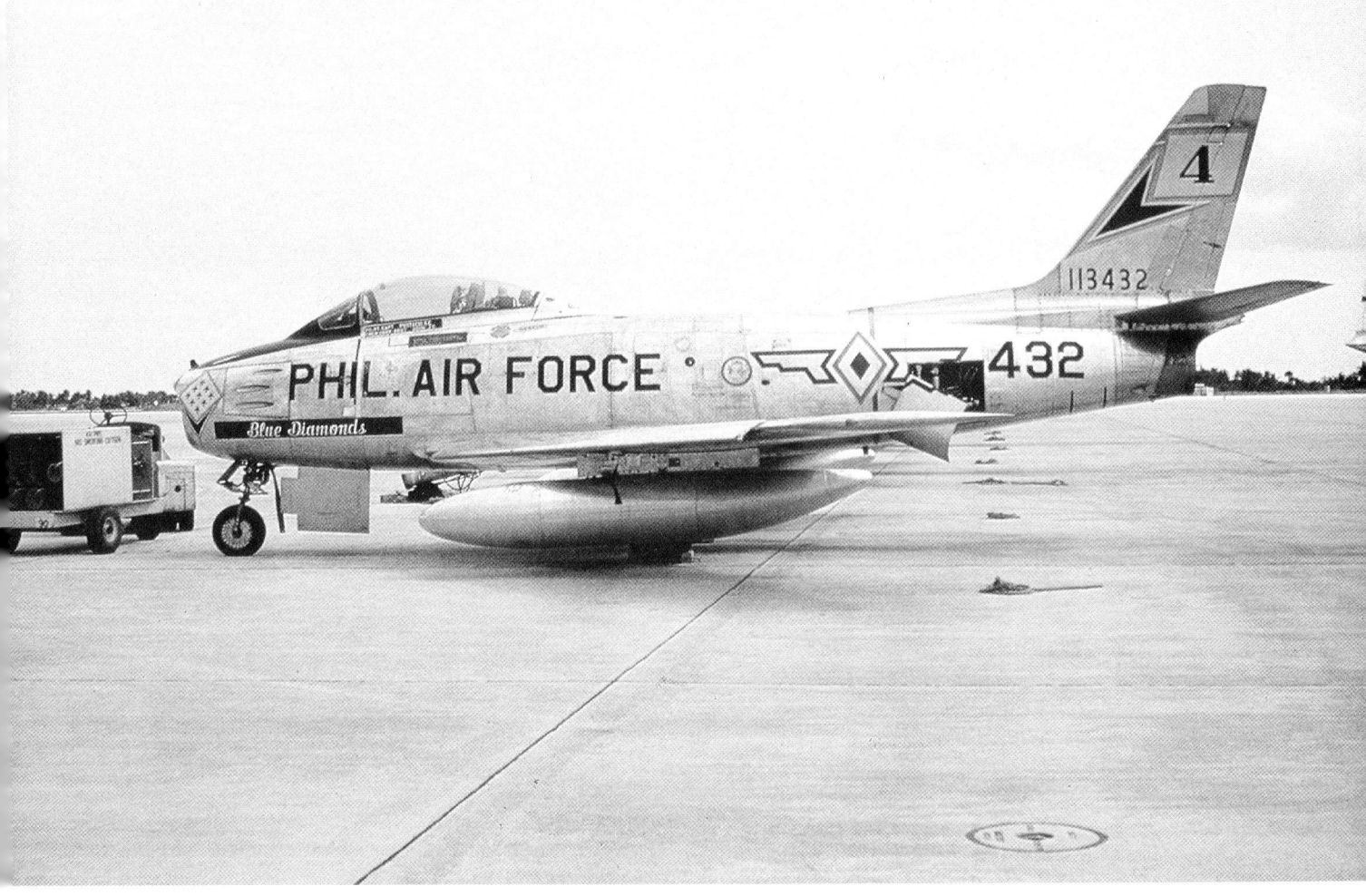

Below: F-86F Sabre of 5 FW Philippine Air Force aerobatic team the *Blue Diamonds* at Mactan Air Base in November 1965. (David W. Menard)

PORTUGAL
Portuguese Air Force

1977-84: "Asas de Portugal" (Wings of Portugal), Sintra

The Portuguese Air Force aerobatic team was formed in 1977, when the Air Force Chief of Staff accepted an RAF invitation for the participation of the PAF in the Air Tattoo '77 at Greenham Common. Based at Sintra Air Base, the team flew six Cessna T-37Cs, and have displayed in France, United Kingdom, West Germany, Belgium, Luxembourg and Italy.

The Portugese Air Force doesn't have a tradition in aerobatic teams. There was a demonstration team in the mid-1950s, flying F-84G Thunderjets and in the late 1950s another with one with F-86F Sabres. In the mid-1960s, there was an attempt at forming an aerobatic team comprising T-37 instructor pilots called *Diabos Vermelhos* (Red Devils). None of these teams lasted more than a couple of years.

Asas de Portugal was formed within 102 Squadron, whose primary mission is the undergraduate pilot training. For this purpose, the Squadron is equipped with 25 Cessna T-37C trainers, that have been operating since 1963. The Squadron has 18 Instructor Pilots and graduates an average of 25 pilots a year.

Below: Cessna T-37Cs of the Portuguese Air Force aerobatic team *Wings of Portugal* lined up at Greenham Common in July 1977 during their public debut.(See page 98 for colour photograph).(Adrian M. Balch)

Since its formation in 1977, the aerobatic team have carried out nearly 100 displays, 20 of which were at international displays. In 1981, all displays by *Asas de Portugal* were cancelled for economical reasons, but the team reformed for the 1982 season.

The only modification introduced in the basic aircraft for the aerobatic team, was the smoke system. One of the fuel cells in the right wing was isolated and used to carry approximately 180lbs of diesel oil. When smoke is required, this is injected into the exhaust of the engines. 10 of the 25 T-37s in service with the PAF were modified for smoke, and the team made the Portuguese red, white and green colours in smoke throughout its routine.

The T-37Cs of *Asas de Portugal* were painted basically white overall, with a smart design in the Portugese colours of red and dark green. The PAF liked this colour scheme so much, that they painted their entire fleet of some 25 T-37s in the aerobatic team's colours.

Unfortunately, due to economy, *Asas de Portugal* was forced to disband again at the end of the 1984 season and it is not known if they will reform once more.

The following T-37Cs were seen with the team during the 1977-83 seasons: 2404, 2406, 2407, 2408, 2414, 2415, 2421, 2423, 2426, 2427, 2428, 2429, 2430 and 2437. Support aircraft was either a CASA Aviocar for internal displays, or a C-130H Hercules when deployed to other countries.

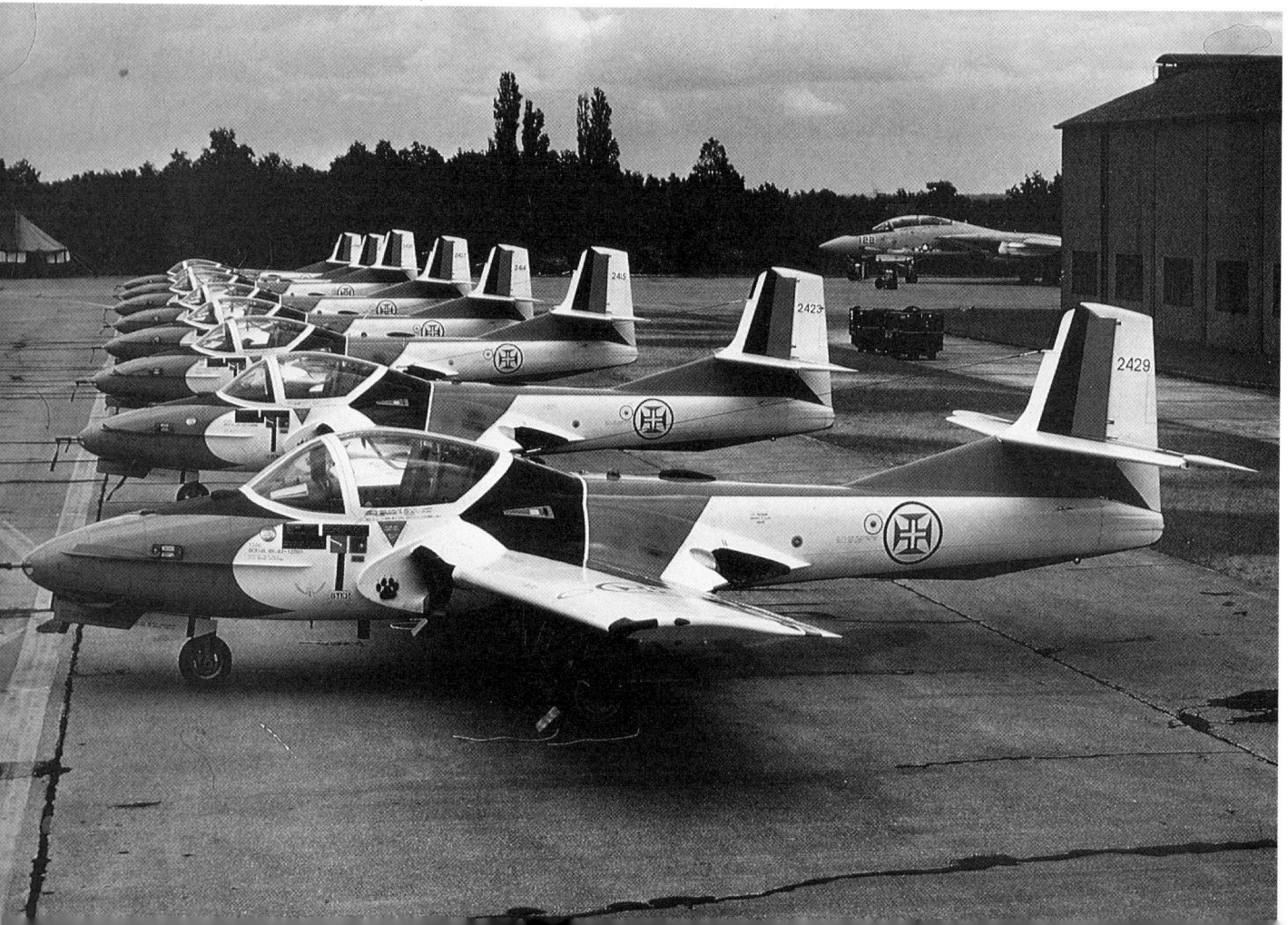

SOUTH AFRICA
South African Air Force

1967-to date: "The Silver Falcons", Langebaanweg
The Silver Falcons, the S.A. Air Force's official formation aerobatic team, has been entertaining crowds at various functions throughout the Republic of South Africa since 1966, when the SAAF received its first MB-326 Impala.

Although the team was initially formed at Flying Training School Langebaanweg in 1966, under the leadership of Commandant Chris Prins, it was not until the following year that the team was named *The Silver Falcons*, or in Afrikaans *Silver Valke*, a name that was readily translatable in both official languages. Before this, the aerobatic team was named the *Bumbling Bees* and flew D. H. Vampires.

Traditionally, the SAAF's aerobatic teams have consisted of four pilots, usually instructors from FTS Langebaanweg. This has been the case since 1953, when a four-ship Vampire formation under the leadership of Captain "Horse" Sweeny was established. The team included the present Chief of the Air Force, Lieutenant-General A. M. Muller.

Prior to 1953, formation aerobatics were performed by instructors from Central Flying School, Dunnotter, in AT-6 Harvards.

In 1959, the Vampire aerobatic team at Langebaanweg was disbanded and formation aerobatic displays were given by teams of Canadair Sabres from Nos.1 and 2 Squadrons. Lieutenant-General Muller led the SAAF's largest jet formation aerobatic team which comprised nine Sabres.

The Silver Falcons team made its first public appearance under its new title at the opening of the Atlas Aircraft Corporation, where the Impala is built, on 24 November 1967. Since this date, *The Silver Falcons* have performed at air displays throughout South Africa and some 41 pilots have become members of the team, each serving for approximately one year. There have been 24 teams so far. In 1983, the team was led by Colonel O. W. (Ollie) Holmes, who was the Officer Commanding of the Air Force Base Langebaanweg and has led the team from 1982 to date.

Unlike other aerobatic teams, *The Silver Falcons* are not employed full time as a team. Practices take place when work allows and after working hours. The team are all drawn from the Staff Instructors at 83 Jet Training School at AFB Langebaanweg and selection is made by the current leader, whenever a vacancy occurs.

The aircraft used is the MB326M Impala manufactured by Atlas Aircraft Corporation under licence from Aermacchi. The aircraft used are all standard finish aircraft. However each fin has the number of the team painted on it, and the pilot's name appears just above *The Silver Falcons* badge on the fuselage below the front cockpit. For show purposes, smoke tanks are fitted in place of the rear seat, giving the team the facility to use white smoke. Although the sequence has changed with each change in leadership, with various variations from season to season, the present sequence included a high number of formation changes. Highlight of the present display is the individual barrel-roll in which the formation does an upward break, followed by individual barrel-rolls with a join up in a wingover ready for the final 'bomb-burst'.

The MB-326 Impalas normally used by the team are 524'1', 492'2', 491'3' and 489'4', but these are often changed as the aircraft go in for servicing.

Below: Atlas Impala Mk.IIs (licence-built Aermacchi MB-326s) of the South African Air Force *Silver Falcons* aerobatic team seen in line-abreast. (SAAF)

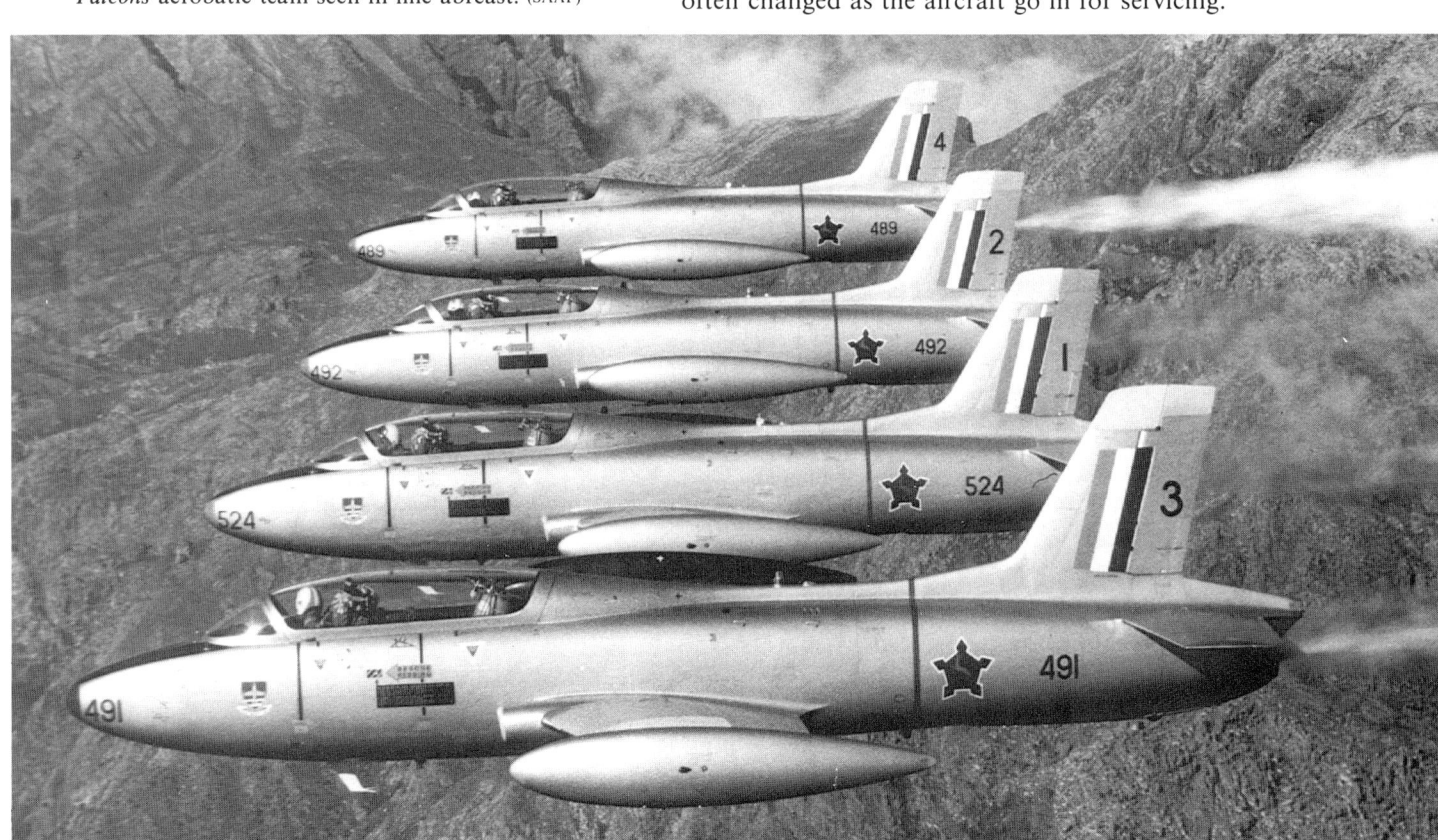

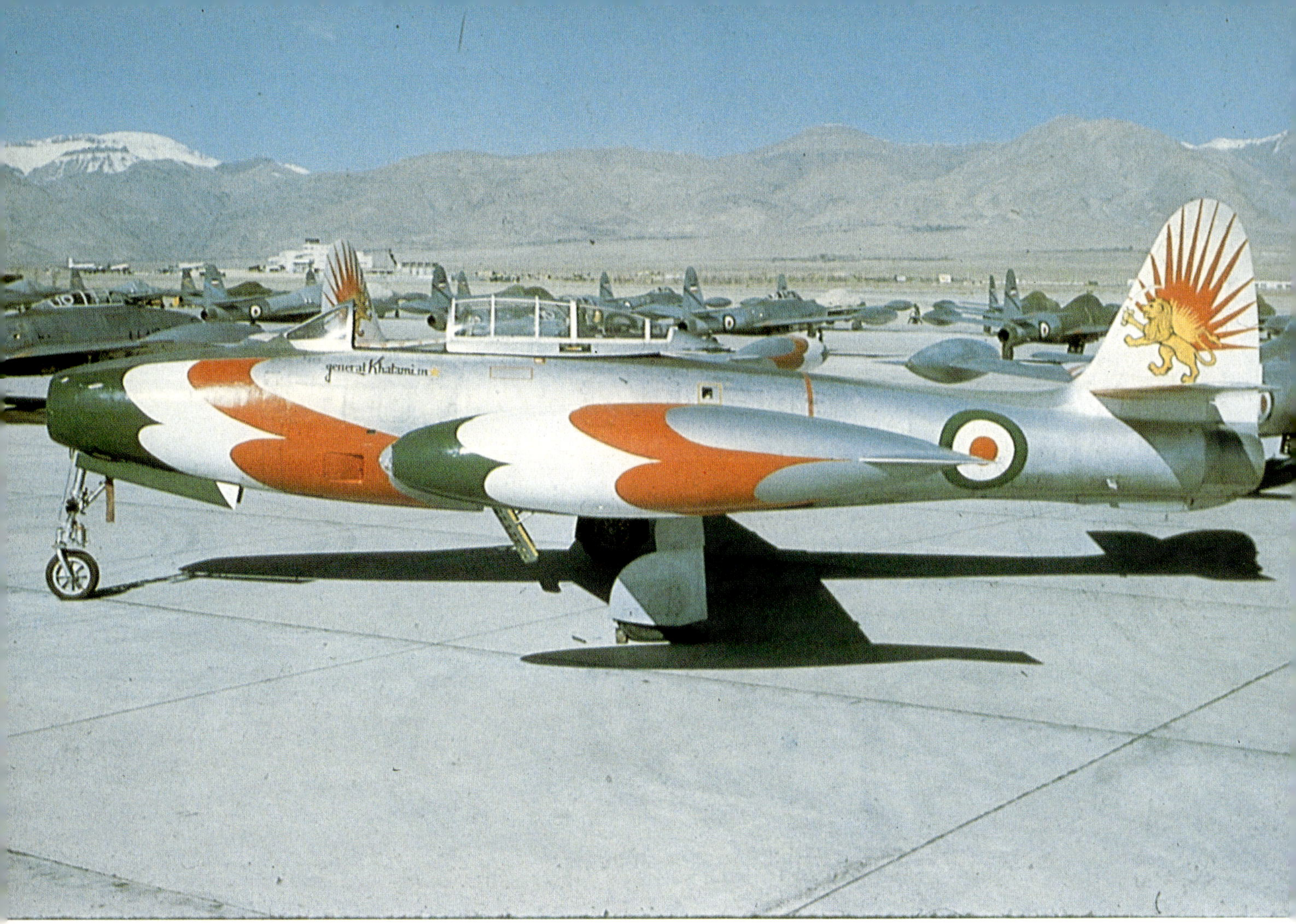

Above: Very rare shot of a Republic F-84G Thunderjet of the Imperial Iranian Air Force aerobatic team *Golden Crown* at Shiraz in 1959. The name under the cockpit, General Khatamin, is thought to be the team's leader. This team's history appears on Page 75.

Cessna T-37Cs of the Portuguese Air Force *Asas de Portugal* (Wings of Portugal) seen performing at Greenham Common on 24 June 1979.
(Adrian M. Balch)

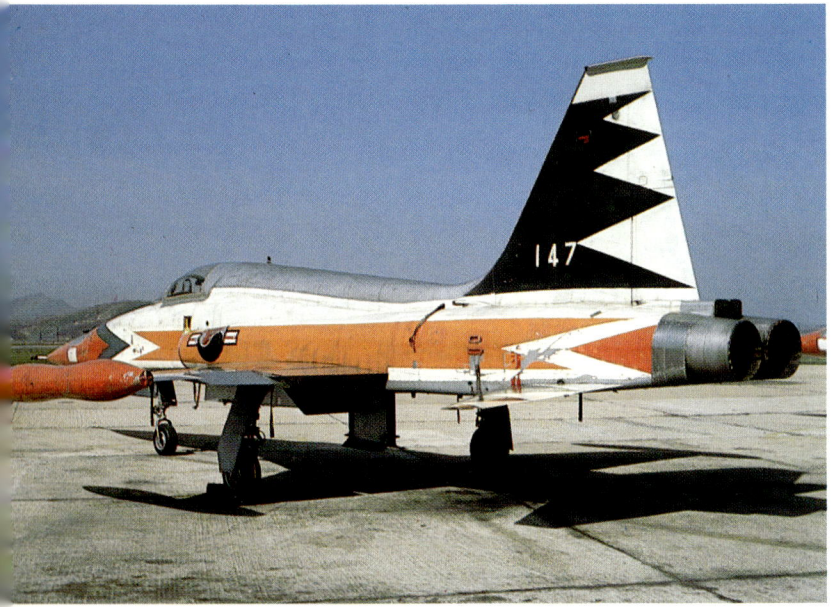

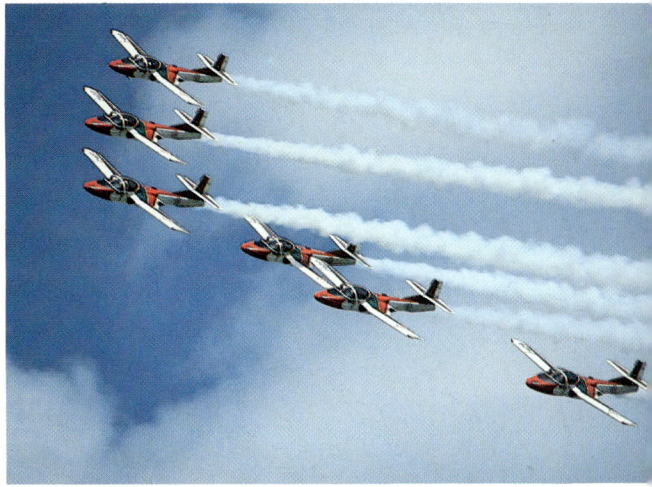

Above: Northrop F-5A, '147' (66-9147) of the Republic of Korea Air Force team at Suwon Air Base in May 1968. (S. H. Miller via D. W. Menard)

SWEDEN
Royal Swedish Air Force

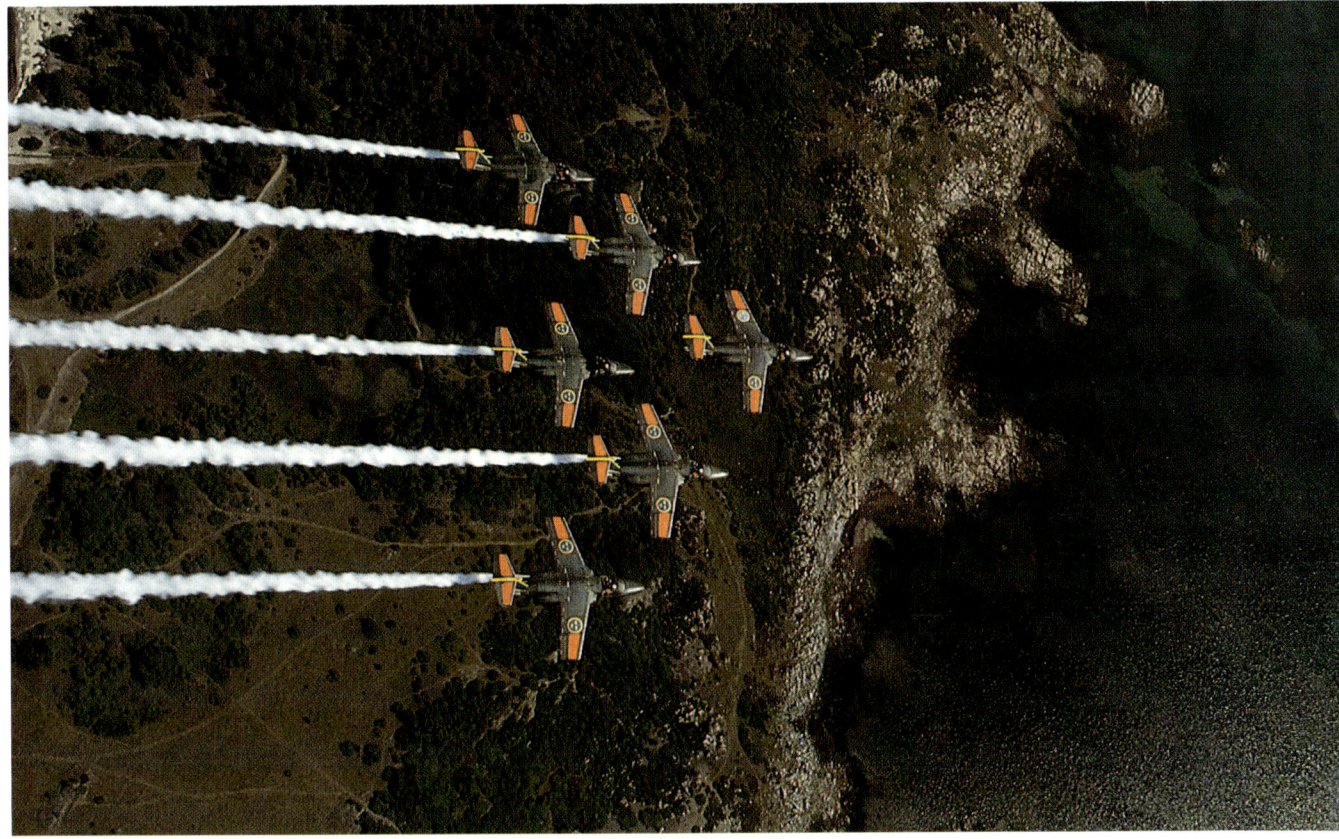

SAAB Sk.60As of F-5 Wing, Royal Swedish Air Force *Team 60* during rehearsals in 1983.
(Bo Dahlin via Gosta Norrbohm)

Organised aerobatics started in the RSAF at F5 Wing, Ljungbyhed — the Central Flying School. During the early 1940s, a team of three Focke-Wulf FW-44 Steiglitz (Sk12) trainers was led by the then Lieutenant Graels Näslund, who later became Colonel and C-in-C of F13 Fighter Wing, but was unfortunately killed in a J28 Vampire accident. His wing-men in this original team were Lieutenant Sten Ahlfors and Lieutenant Sigge Lundgren.

The first jet team
Shortly after the Swedish Air Force bought the de Havilland Vampire (J-28) in 1946, it was decided that a team from F9 Wing at Säve, near Göthenburg, should be formed for the 25th Anniversary of the Swedish Air Force on 3rd June 1951. Squadron Leader Kurt Wikner formed the team, whose Vampires used coloured smoke for the first time in Sweden. The, then, Swedish Air Force General Bengt Nordenskiold heard about this team and flew to F9 Wing at Säve to watch the training. They had planned their programme without his permission! However, when he saw their show, he was delighted and gave his permission for most of it, except rolling in column or changing places during rolls.

The J-29 'Flying-Barrel' Teams
The SAAB J-29 was the next aircraft to be used by Swedish aerobatic teams — the first Swedish-built aircraft to be used for that purpose in fact. Several Wings formed teams on the type, but two were most notable, as they represented the Swedish Air Force at home and abroad. These were the *Fogde-team* and the *Haglind-team*.

1956-59: F13 Wing, "Fogde Team", Nörrkoping
This was the first J-29 team, led by Squadron Leader Per-Olof Fogde — hence the team's name. Coming from F13 Wing at Nörrkoping, Squadron Leader Per-Olof Fogde led a team of four J-29s at a show at Waterbeach, England in 1953 — before the team was officially formed. Early in 1956, Squadron Leader Fogde's three other team members left to join Swedish airlines, so three new team members were selected on an official basis. Proper training began in the spring of 1956 and the team continued until the end of the 1959 season, when Squadron Leader Fogde was transferred to Draken training. The team's overseas displays included one at Dubendorf, Switzerland, in May 1956, which they shared with one of the RAF's Hunter teams, Mystere IVAs of *La Patrouille de France* and F-86 Sabres of the USAF *Skyblazers*.

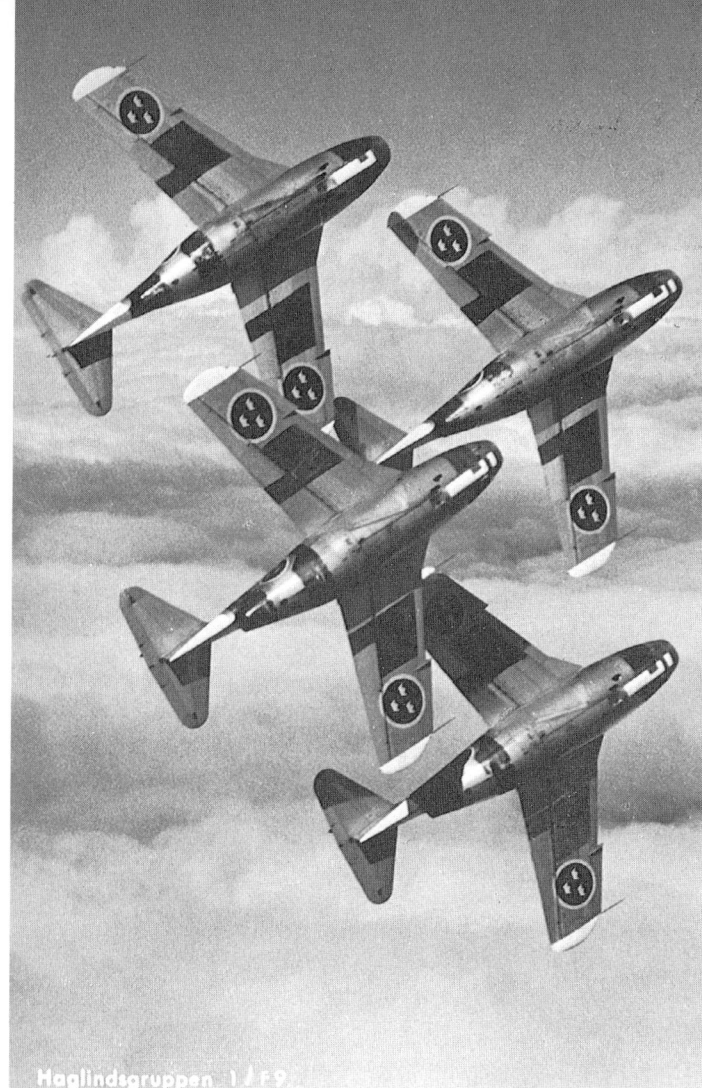

SAAB J-29Fs of the *Haglind Team* from F9 Wing, Royal Swedish Air Force 1954-58.
(Swedish A.F. via Gösta Norrbohm)

Below: Hunter F.51s of the Royal Swedish Air Force *Acro Hunters* team from F18 Wing, seen taking off for a display in 1961. (Bo Dahlin via Gosta Norrbohm)

1954-58: F9 Wing, "Haglind Team", Säve

Responsibility for forming a second J-29 team was given to F9 Wing at Säve. Lieutenant Per Axel Haglind was the leader, thus the name *Haglind Team*. He put the team of four aircraft through a series of loops and rolls with coloured smoke. This was usually in Swedish blue and yellow colours, but they used red and white smoke during a display at Geneva, Switzerland, in June 1955. The team lasted for five years, disbanding at the end of the 1958 season. The aircraft were natural metal overall with wide black bands round the wings and fuselage.

1957-62: F18 Wing, The "Acro Hunters", Tullinge

The *Acro Hunters* formed in the spring of 1957 at F18 Wing, Tullinge and were led by Squadron Leader Sven Lampell. The team of four Hunter F-51s retained their standard Swedish A. F. colour scheme of olive green upper surfaces with PRU blue undersides, but had the *Acro Hunters* insignia in yellow on the nose and red letter code on the fin. There were four different displays, depending upon weather, venue and aircraft serviceability. Sometimes, the fifth aircraft was incorporated in the displays as a solo performer, but was usually retained as a spare aircraft. The *Acro Hunters* disbanded at the end of the 1962 season.

1963-65: F18 Wing, The "Acro Deltas", Tullinge

The SAAB J-35 Draken first entered service in 1960 with F13 Wing, so it was natural that this unit should be the first to form an aerobatic team on the type. There were several different leaders during the first years, but most notable was Lieutenant-Colonel Tore Persson.

The F13 team disbanded at the end of 1962 and the following year, the *Acro Deltas* were formed at F18 Wing, Tullinge to continue the popularity of the *Acro Hunters*. Led by Squadron Leader Claes Jernow, the team comprised four J-35A Drakens which retained their natural finish overall apart from the tail fin, which was painted light blue with yellow trim. One of the team's machines was serialled 35223 and the *Acro Deltas* made their overseas debut at the 1965 Paris Air Show at Le Bourget. The team disbanded at the end of the 1965 season and Squadron Leader Claes Jernow was assigned to F16 Wing at Uppsala, where he formed another J-35 team.

Below: Good close-up of the nose markings on a Hunter F.51 of the Royal Swedish Air Force *Acro Hunters* team 1960-61. (via Gosta Norrbohm)

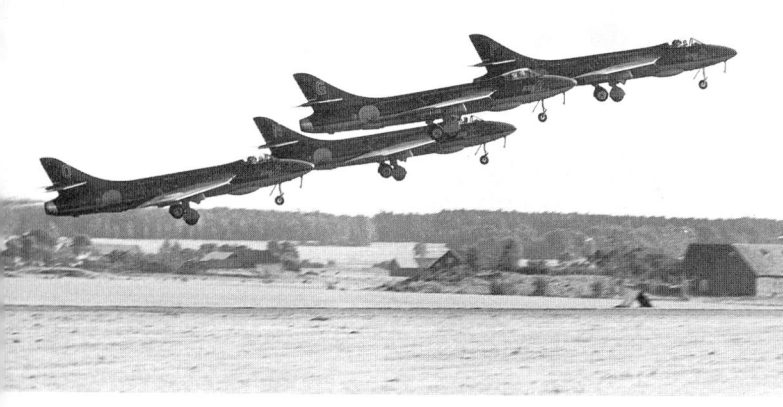

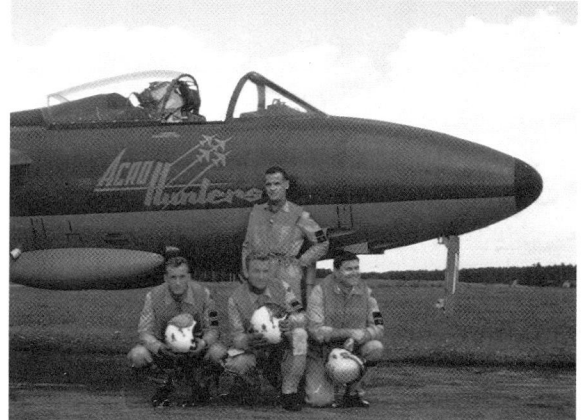

1964-78: The F16 Team, Uppsala

In 1964, it was decided that F16 Wing would continue to provide a Draken aerobatic team after the *Acro Deltas* disbanded. Squadron Leader Claes Jernow started training the team, then handed over to Major Boris Bjuremalm who had flown the Draken since 1962. The J-35A Drakens were natural metal overall, but were camouflaged about 1968. Squadron Leader Hans Hagman became the leader in 1967 and around this time, the team converted from the J-35A to the J-35F Draken. With white smoke, the F16 Team performed many displays in Sweden and made visits to Denmark in 1971, Moscow in 1972 and participated in the 50th Anniversary of the Swedish Air Force celebrations at Malmslatt in August 1976. The team's Drakens could only be identified by a small yellow 'flat fish' insignia called a "Rocka" at the top of the fin. The rest of the aircraft was in standard camouflage and markings. The F16 Team disbanded at the end of 1978 and the aircraft were retired from service. One of the team's aircraft went to the Musée de l'Air at Paris, where it can be seen today. Serials of the J-35F Drakens were: 35066/30, 35067/31, 35068/32, 35069/33, 35074/38, 35089/51 and 35090/52.

1973-to date: F5 Wing, "Team 60", Ljungbyhed

This is the current Swedish Air Force aerobatic team, flying six SAAB 105s (Sk60As) from F5 Wing at Ljungbyhed.

F5 Wing operated a team with Sk60s during 1967-68 and their venues included the Paris Air show in May-June 1967. The aircraft were natural metal overall with light blue and yellow fins. This team was unofficially called the *Vikings* in some circles, although this title was never officially adopted. This team disbanded at the end of 1968, but it was not until the autumn of 1973 that Captain Christian Muller-Hansen decided to revive F5 Wing's Sk60 aerobatic team.

With a team of four aircraft, training began in August 1974 and in the spring of 1975 the team made its official debut. After initially flying displays with four aircraft, Captains J. Å. Brandmyr and A. Wahlstrom increased the team to six after much pressure. They initially formated with the other four, but later broke off to perform a separate display synchronised with the main formation. 1976 was the 50th Anniversary of the Swedish Air Force and *Team 60* participated in the celebrations at Malmslatt in August of that year. The team's Sk60s are equipped with smoke emitters. The smoke is generated by diesel-oil from a separate tank being injected into the exhausts of the engines, forming a white, strongly contrasting and rapidly dissolving trail, against a hopefully blue sky. Loops and rolls are flown in four basic formations, which are interspersed by the synchro-pair. Major Jan Å. Brandmyr has been with the team since 1975 and has led *Team 60* from 1979 to the present day. The tail colours of the aircraft are the same as on the 1967-68 team; i.e. pale blue and yellow, but the rest of the aircraft is camouflaged in two-tone dark green with medium grey undersides. Dayglo-red panels appear on the nose, tailplanes and above and below the wingtips. SAAB Sk.60As of *Team 60* include: 60040/40, 60078/78, 60096/96, 60098/98, 60104/04, 60112/112 and 60116/116.

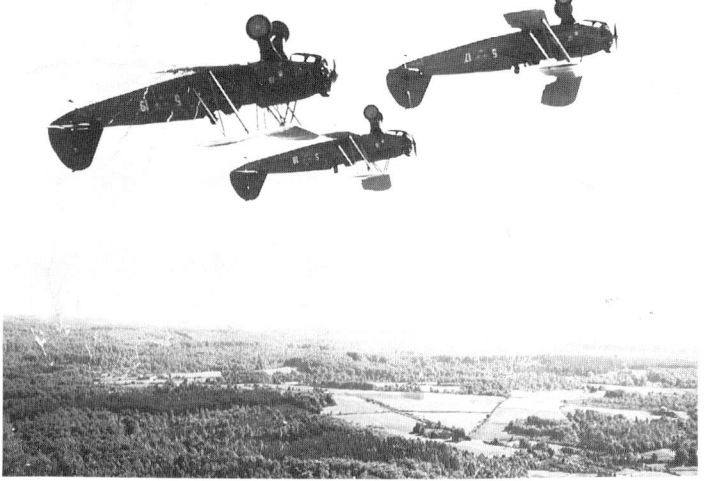

Above: The first Swedish aerobatic team with three Focke-Wulf FW-44 Steiglitz (Sk12) trainers during the 1940s. This team was from F-5 Wing and led by Capt. Graels Näslund. (Swedish Air Force via Gösta Norrbohm)

Below: J-35A Drakens of the *Acro Deltas* team from F-18 Wing, Swedish Air Force in 1965. The fins were the same colours as the roundels — light blue with yellow trim. Nearest aircraft is 35223.
(Swedish Air Force via Gösta Norrbohm)

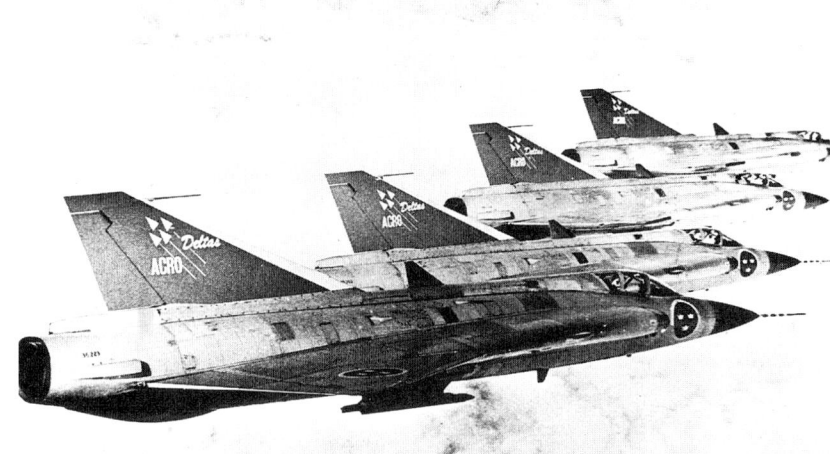

Below: A J-35F Draken of the Royal Swedish Air Force F-16 team. The only team marking is the yellow 'Rocka' fish marking at the top of the fin.
(RSAF via Gosta Norrbohm)

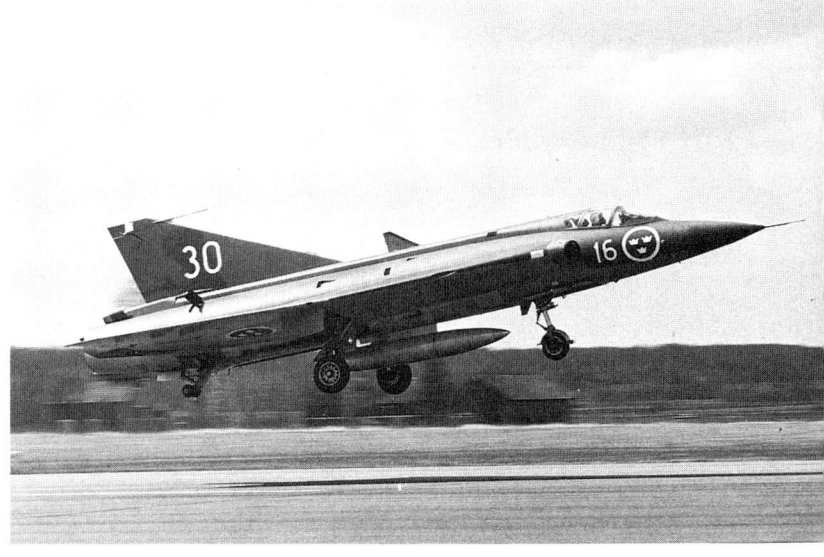

SWITZERLAND
Swiss Air Force

1964-to date: "La Patrouille Suisse", Dubendorf
Founded in 1964, *La Patrouille Suisse* is enlisted from military pilots of the Surveillance Wing, who also serve as instructors in their respective squadrons. The team consists of 6 pilots, 1-2 reserve pilots and 1 ground supervisor officer, a former pilot of the team.

Six smoke-equipped Hawker Hunter F.58s are flown by *La Patrouille Suisse,* operating from Dubendorf Air Base. The leader chooses one of three different programmes which best suits the actual weather situation. The aerobatic display in close formation lasts about 16 minutes. It is the result of a once-weekly training flight over a period of 8 months. As the team is only part-time, they perform in only 5-6 displays each year. The Hunters retain their standard grey and green camouflage, with silver undersides. Since 1981 a silver and black badge has been added to the nose of the team aircraft. Hunters in the team include: J-4022, J-4023, J-4027, J-4021, J-4031 J-4047, J-4025, J-4072, J-4020 and J-4053. These are just a few that have been seen with the team, but they can be drawn from any of the 150-odd Hunters in service with the Swiss Air Force. The team's leader in 1982 was Hptm. B. Morgenthaler.

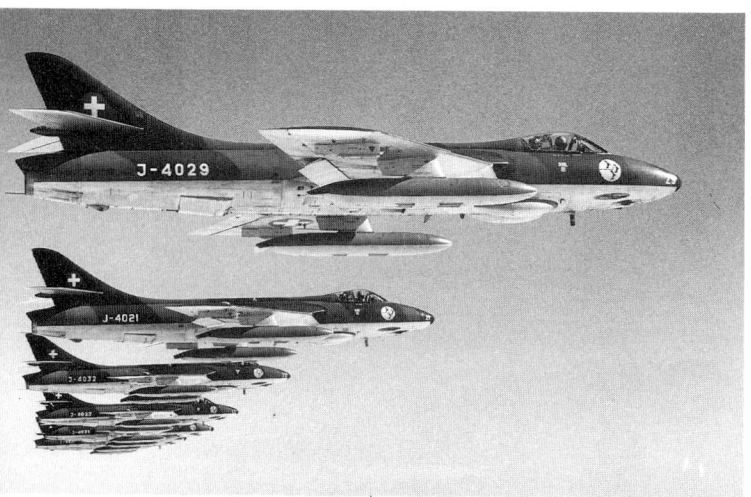

Left and below: Hunter F.58As of the Swiss Air Force aerobatic team *La Patrouille Suisse* in 1982. (Swiss A.F.)

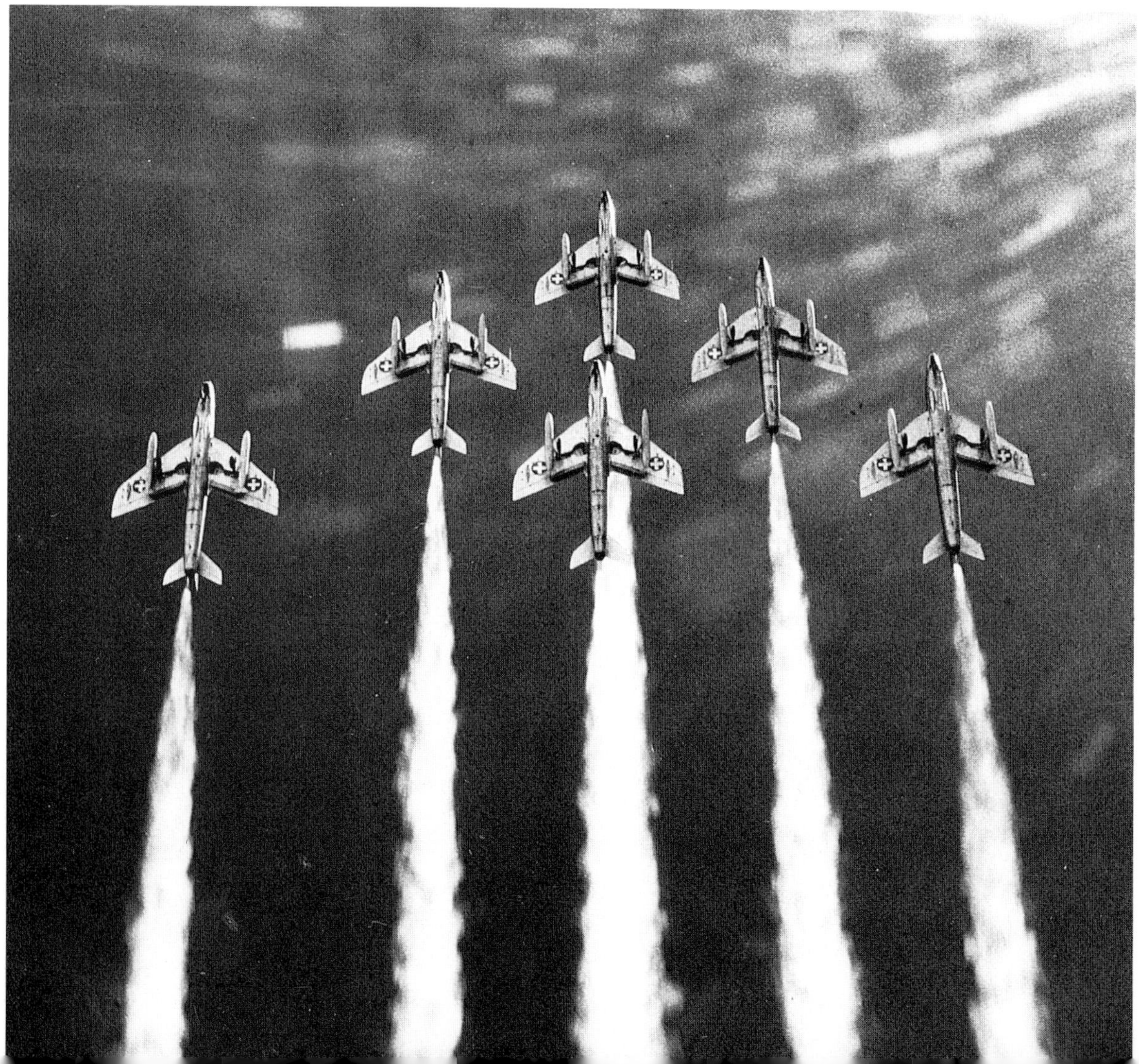

UNITED STATES OF AMERICA
U.S. Air Force

1953-to date: USAF Air Demonstration Squadron, "The Thunderbirds", Luke AFB, Arizona, then Nellis AFB, Nevada

It was decided to establish an official U.S. Air Force display team in early 1953, this being intended to fulfil the purpose of demonstrating the Air Force's undoubted skill to the general public whilst, simultaneously, acting as an aid to recruiting future personnel. They were originally known as the *3600th Air Demonstration Team,* when they formed at Luke Air Force Base, Arizona during May 1953. The team was declared operational on 1 June 1953 and gave their first display just eight days later.

The team's first aircraft type was the Republic F-84G Thunderjet, of which they were assigned five. The basic display lasted some 15 minutes, mainly involving manoeuvres by four aircraft in diamond formation. The Thunderjets were modified for their demanding aerobatic role, this work entailing the removal of the integral gun armament and the addition of ballast. The name *The Thunderbirds* was not chosen until well after the first season. To find a suitable name, a competition was held at Luke in June 1953, this generating a quite considerable response. The Thunderbird is associated with Indian folklore. Indian legend attributes thunder and lightning to an enormous bird. The thunder was supposed to have been caused by the flapping of the bird's wings. Lightning was explained as the opening and closing of the bird's eyes. The choice of colour scheme was made when the team formed and variations on the same theme have been applied to all the types used by the team. Major Dick Catledge was appointed as the first team leader, who led the team through some 50 demonstrations by the end of the 1953 season.

Below: The original *Thunderbird* team in 1953, with four Republic F-84G Thunderjets, based at Luke Air Force Base, Arizona. (US Air Force)

In 1954, the display routine remained much the same with such a good serviceability record, that the team used the spare aircraft for a solo slot. The first overseas tour was made in 1954, this involving a visit to South America during January and February, one of the eleven countries being Cuba. The practice of painting the flags of nations visited by the team on the aircraft began after this tour.

During the winter of 1954-55, a visit was made to Central America, by which time a Lockheed T-33A support aircraft was obtained to provide orientation flights to VIPs and members of the Press. In the early days, logistic support was provided by a C-47 Dakota, but *The Thunderbirds* colour scheme did not adorn this type. The increasing demand placed upon the team soon required the services of a larger and more versatile transport and so, in 1955, a pair of C-119s were acquired, one being painted in the team's colours whilst the other remained basically natural metal overall.

In October 1954, Major Jacksel Broughton took over as leader and this was followed by re-equipment for the team in 1955. The F-84G Thunderjet gave its 132nd and last performance at Webb AFB, Texas during February. The replacement aircraft came in the form of six new Republic F-84F Thunderstreaks, which were delivered in April and gave their first demonstration just one week later. A smoke-making system was devised to make the aircraft more visible to the crowd during the display.

Close-up of *Thunderbirds* Fairchild C-119F support aircraft, 51-8146, with F-84F Thunderstreaks behind, in 1955. The flags show the 12 countries visited at that time and 'Luke' above the badge denotes the team's base. This was later changed to 'Nellis'. (Fairchild-Republic)

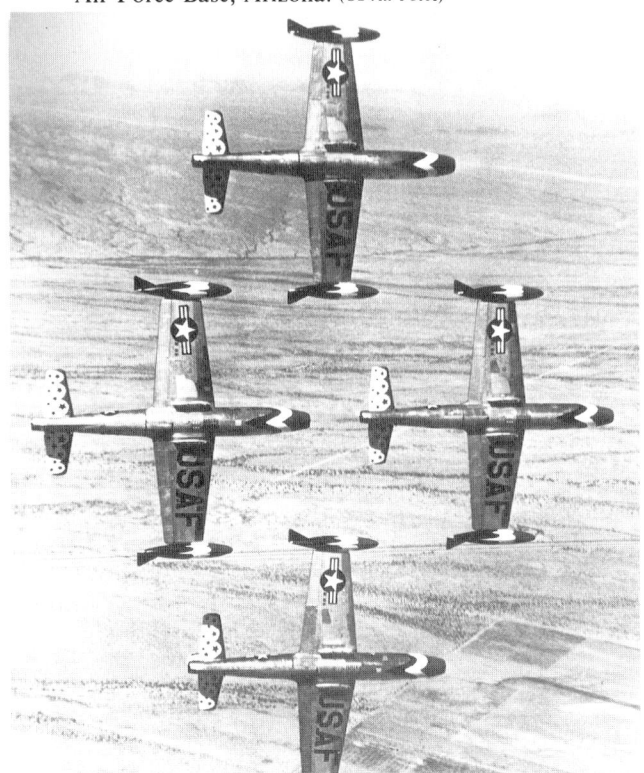

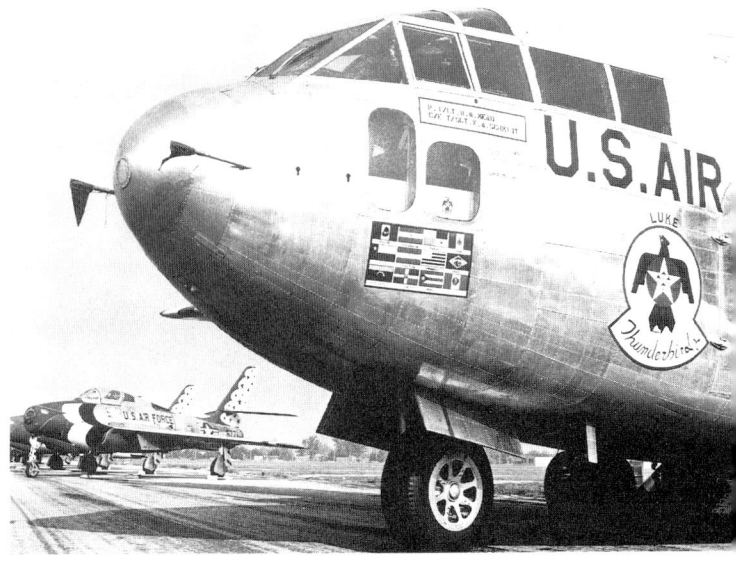

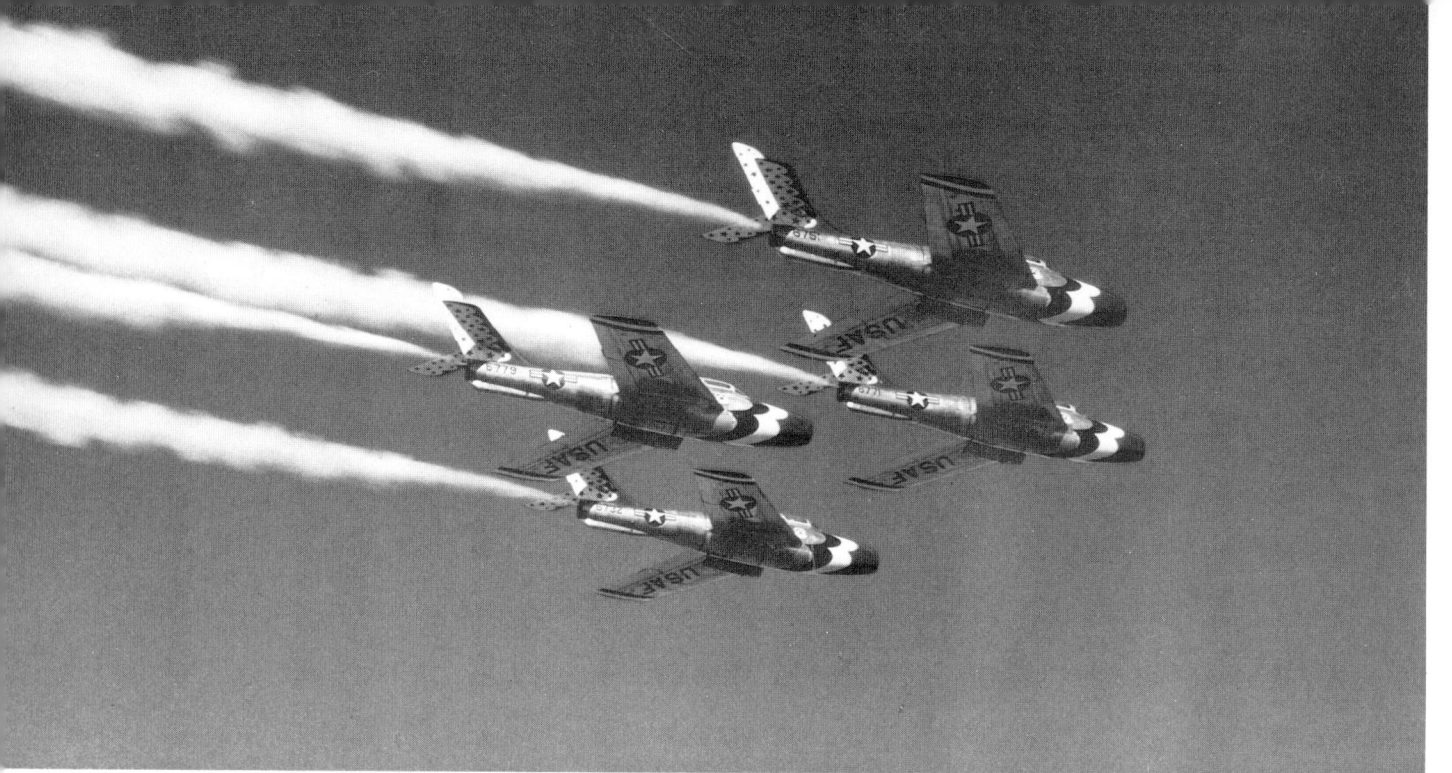

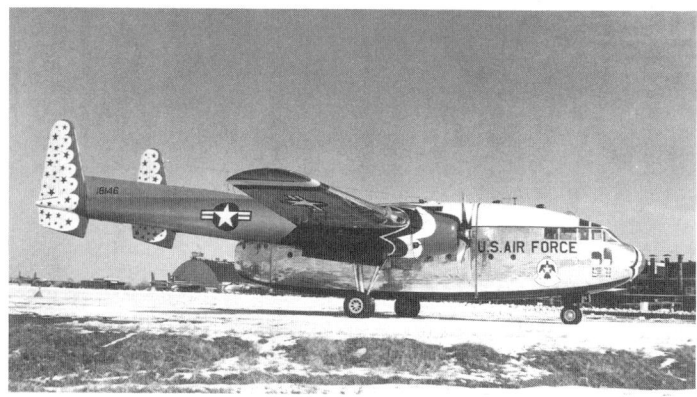

Republic F-84Fs of the USAF *Thunderbirds,* shown in diamond shape formation at Luke Air Force Base, Arizona, 27th February 1956. (US Air Force).

Above: Fairchild C-119F, 51-8146, photographed in late 1955. Although the *Thunderbirds* operated three C-119 support aircraft, this was the only one finished in their colours. (Fairchild-Republic)

A Republic F-84F Thunderstreak of the USAF Aerial Demonstration team, the *Thunderbirds,* comes in for a landing at Luke Air Force Base, Arizona, 27th February 1956. (US Air Force)

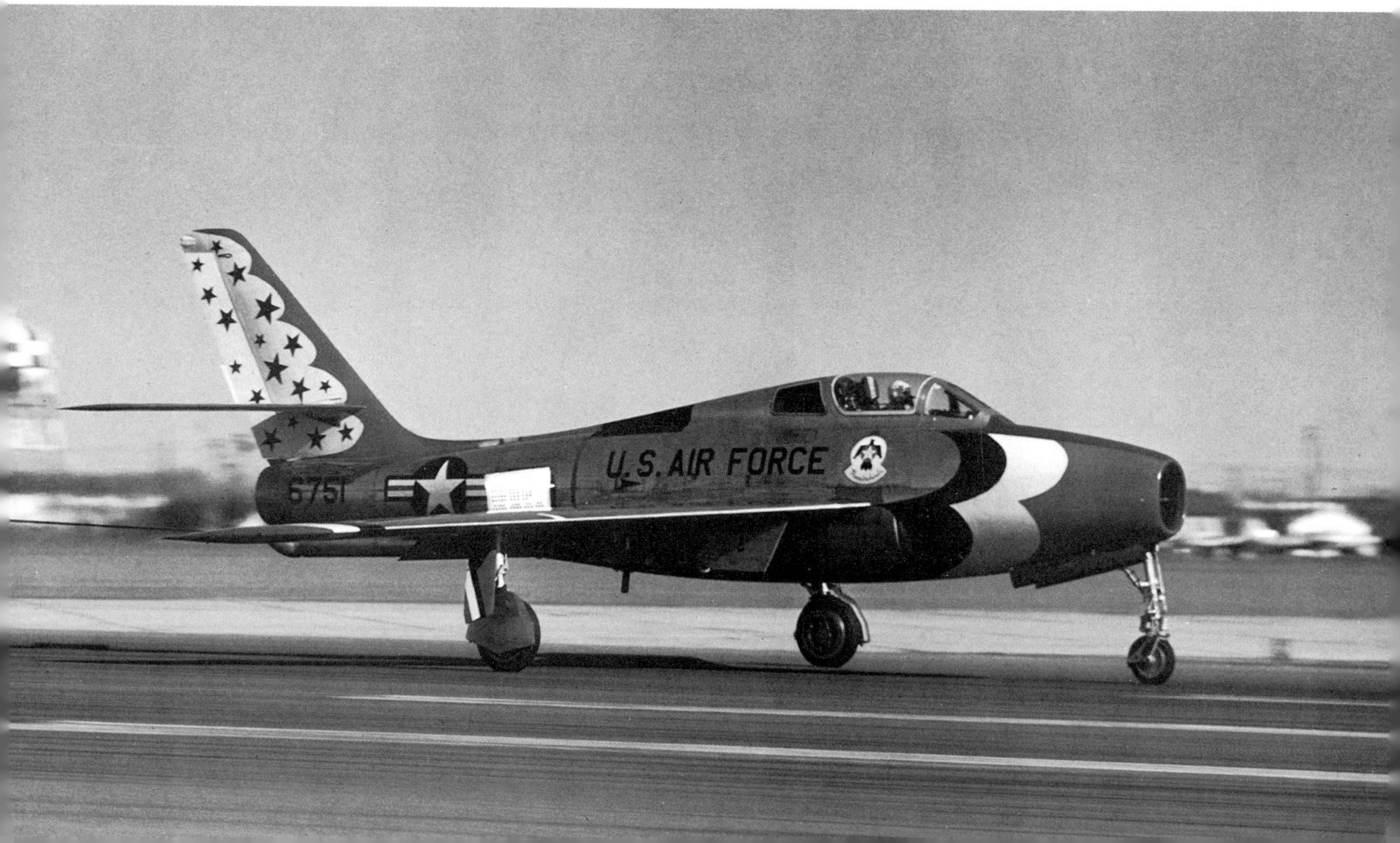

The display programme was gradually extended to 19 minutes and more use was made of the solo aircraft, which kept the spectators interested while the main formation repositioned. In addition to the basic diamond formation, the team introduced several 'in-trail' manoeuvres and also began their display with a 'finger-four' take-off routine. On 20 May 1956, at Bolling AFB, Washington, D.C., *The Thunderbirds* flew their last performance with the F-84F Thunderstreak, after a total of 91 shows with the type.

At this time, it was decided that the F-100 Super Sabre would make an admirable mount for the team. A change of type came with a change of base and *The Thunderbirds* moved from Luke AFB, Arizona to Nellis AFB, Nevada. The F-100C Super Sabre transformed *The Thunderbirds* from a subsonic to a supersonic team, making them the first Supersonic Air Demonstration Team. The 1956 show season saw the beginning of the maximum performance take-off, followed by the team's behind-the-crowd entrance, with the diamond cutting in the afterburners with a deafening roar as they sped overhead. The new afterburner allowed the solo a full stage to show the power and manoeuvrability of the F-100. At that time, show regulations were much less strict than they are today and it was not unusual for a Mach One-plus pass to be made by the solo aircraft. The high-speed solo pass with the repetitious booming of the afterburner rapidly became a crowd pleaser.

The team flew their first performances in Canada in 1957. The same season also saw them perform in Argentina, Uruguay and Brazil on another South American tour, the team leader being Major Robby Robinson. Major Robert Fitzgerald was appointed team leader in March 1959 and took *The Thunderbirds* on the first Far East tour. As the F-100Cs did not have an in-flight refuelling capability, a number of F-100Ds were borrowed from the 18th Tactical Fighter Wing at Kadena, these being repainted and prepared by an advance party of Thunderbirds technicians and mechanics. The tour took them to Okinawa, the Philippines, Taiwan, South Korean, Japan and Hawaii. Earlier, in 1958, the venerable C-119Fs had been replaced by another type from Fairchild, the C-123 Provider, which was also finished in *The Thunderbirds* scheme. Further airlift capability was gained in 1959, when the team acquired a C-54D Skymaster, which was used mainly to transport Press and media personnel around in airline-style luxury. The C-54 was painted in a variation of *The Thunderbirds* colour scheme and remained in use until the Spring of 1963 bearing the name 'City of Las Vegas' in the summer of 1960. A two-seat F-100F Super Sabre was added around this time, which replaced the T-33A during 1960. Immediately before the start of the 1960 season, flight refuelling equipment was installed in the F-100s, permitting the team to travel further afield and so visits to Alaska and South America were made. During the following year, the team made another visit to South America and extended their show to 23 minutes. The nose of the aircraft was no longer allowed to be aimed at the crowd, so the team had to revise their programme. 1961 was also the last year for the C-123 Providers, whose supporting role was now taken by a C-130

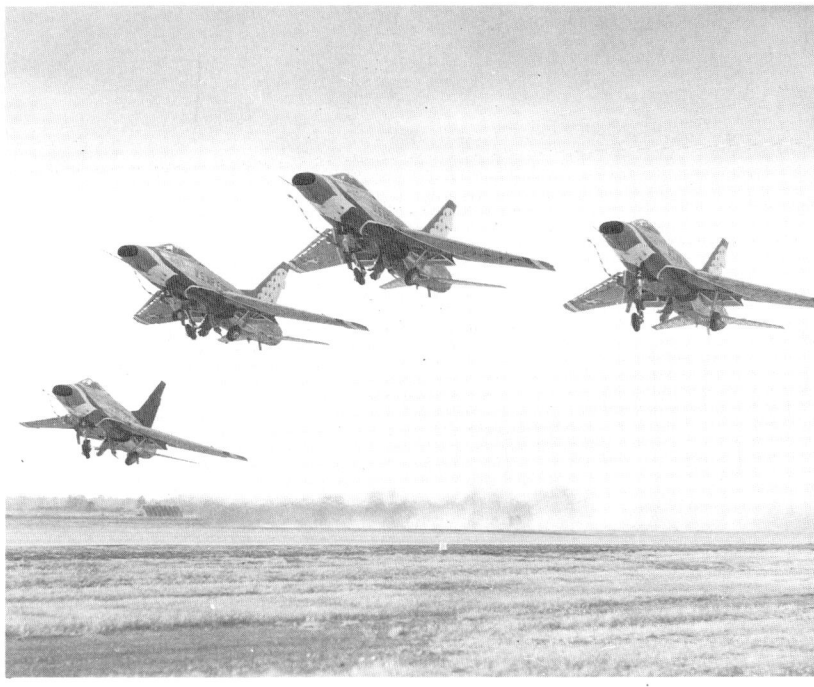

Four F-100D Super Sabres of the *Thunderbirds* taking off in 1964, shortly after the team's F-105s had been grounded (USAF)

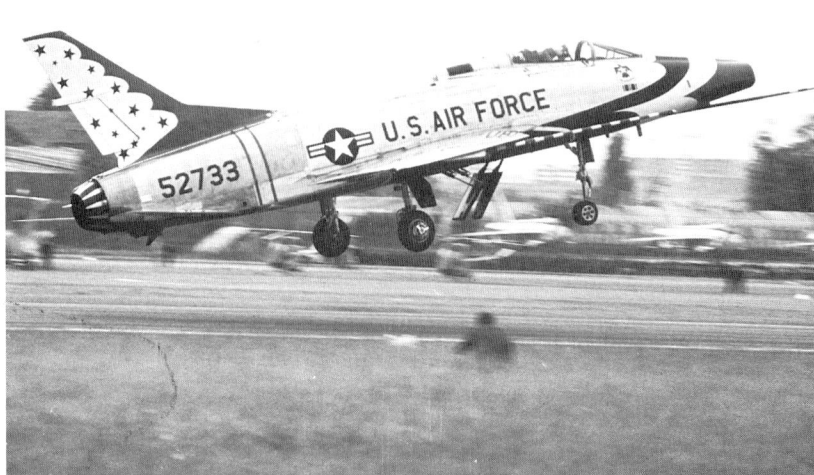

Dramatic landing shot of *Thunderbirds* F-100C, 55-2733, at the 1963 Paris Air Show during the team's first European Tour. (Werner Gysin)

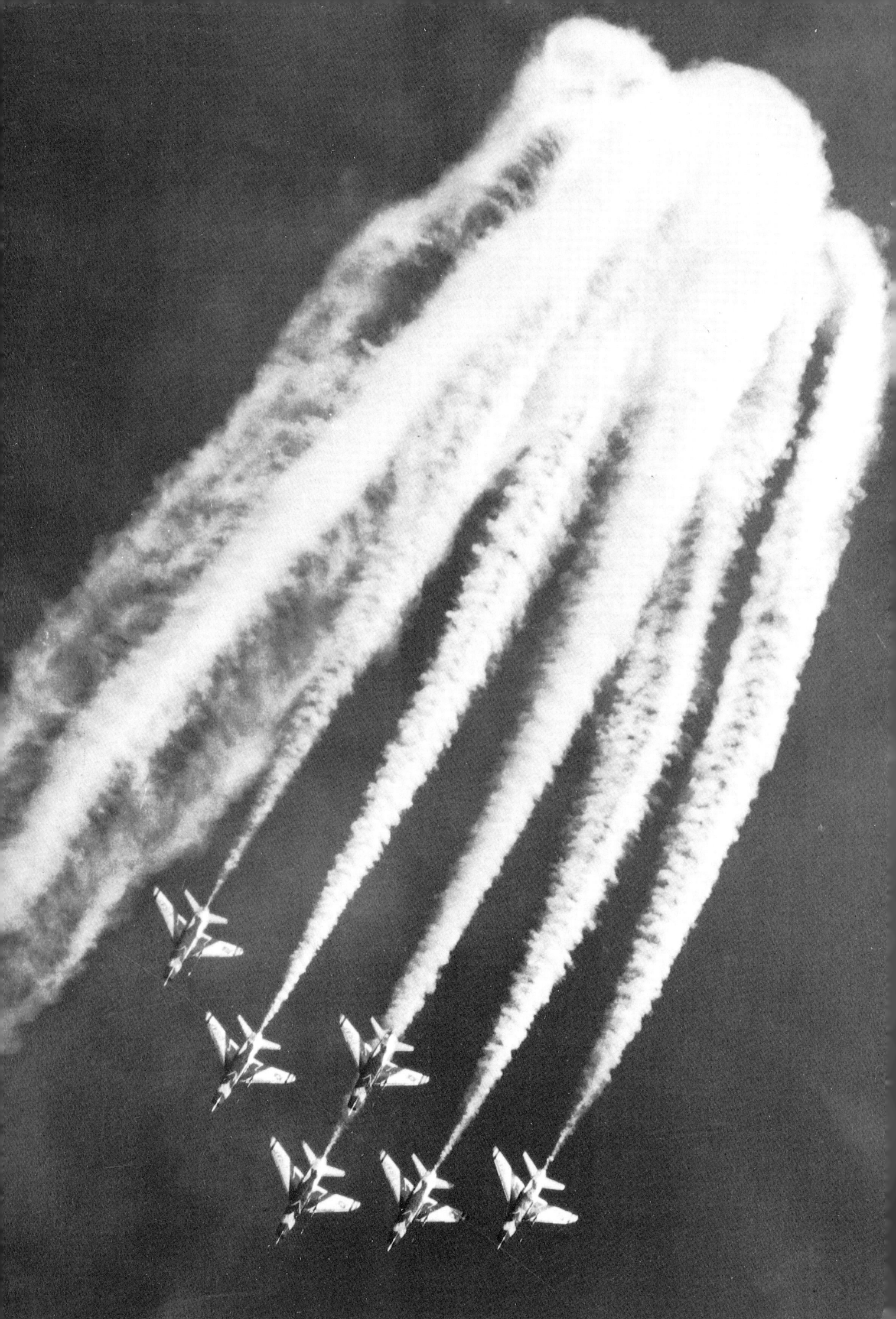

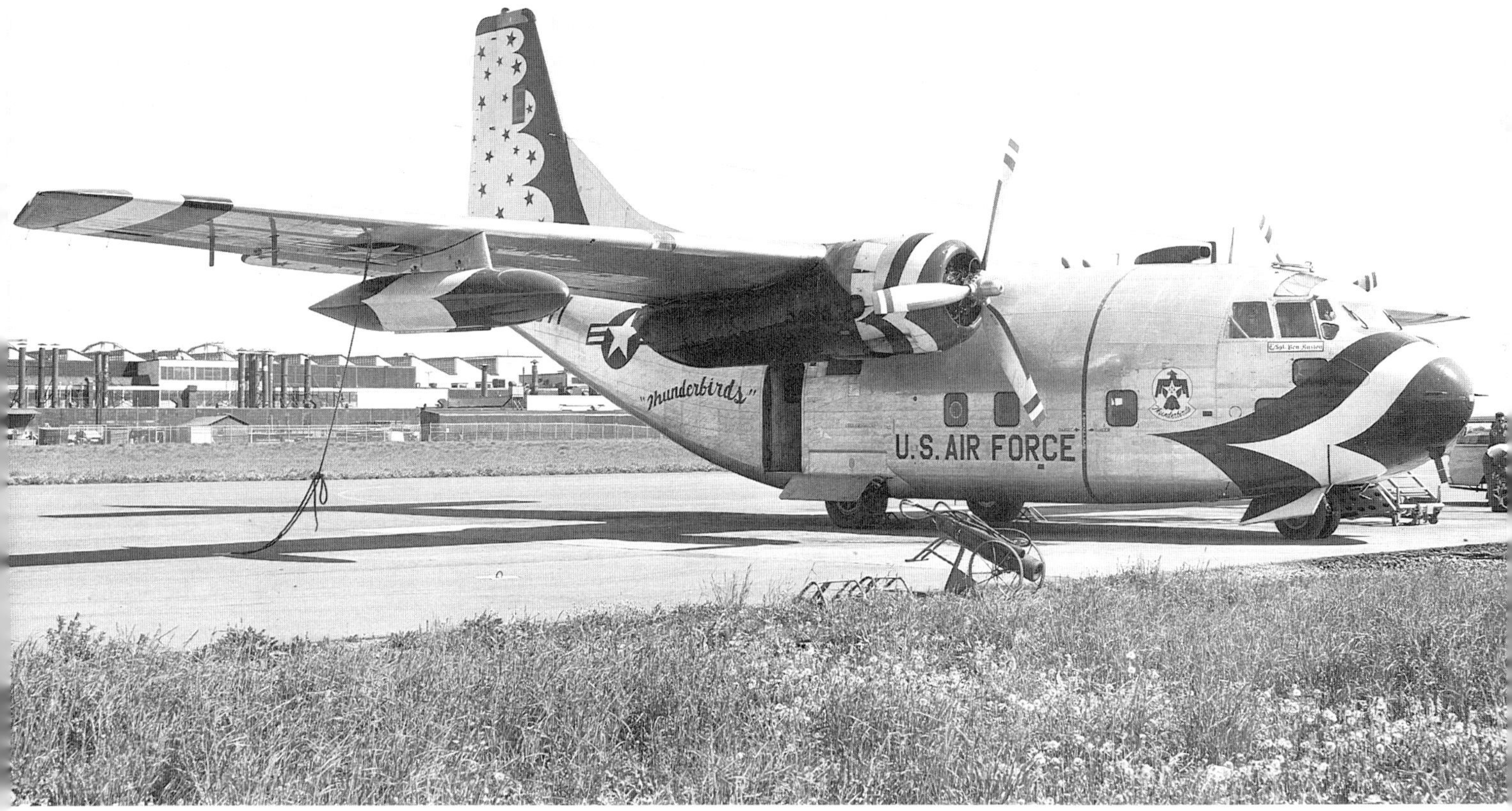

Hercules aircraft seconded from Tactical Air Command from 1962. The C-130s did not adopt the star-spangled *Thunderbirds* scheme, but retained their normal finish during deployment. At least one was known to have carried *The Thunderbirds* badge on the nose, together with the code '14' for a brief spell.

A second solo aircraft was added in 1962 and in 1963, the team made its first European tour, taking in nine countries including the United Kingdom, France, Germany, Italy and Portugal. This was the last year of the F-100C, the 641st and last demonstration taking place shortly before Christmas.

As a replacement, the team adopted the F-105B Thunderchief for the 1964 season. From the same stable that produced the Thunderjet and Thunderstreak, the Thunderchief was a huge aircraft — the largest single-seat, single-engined fighter to be produced at that time. Transition was fairly smooth and the first display was at Norfolk, Virginia on April 26th. Several modifications were necessary to convert the Thunderchiefs to their aerobatic team role. There were changes in the rudder and flap systems and the fuel system required modification for extended inverted flight. The gun armament was removed, together with the Doppler navigation equipment. Ballast was added to replace these and aid manouevrability. The life of the F-105B with the Thunderbirds was destined to be short-lived, only six displays being given before an accident, in May 1964, resulted in the decision to ground the team temporarily whilst further modifications were made to the aircraft. It was decided to revert to the F-100 Super Sabre for the remainder of the season, in the hope that the F-105Bs could be re-introduced for the 1965 season.

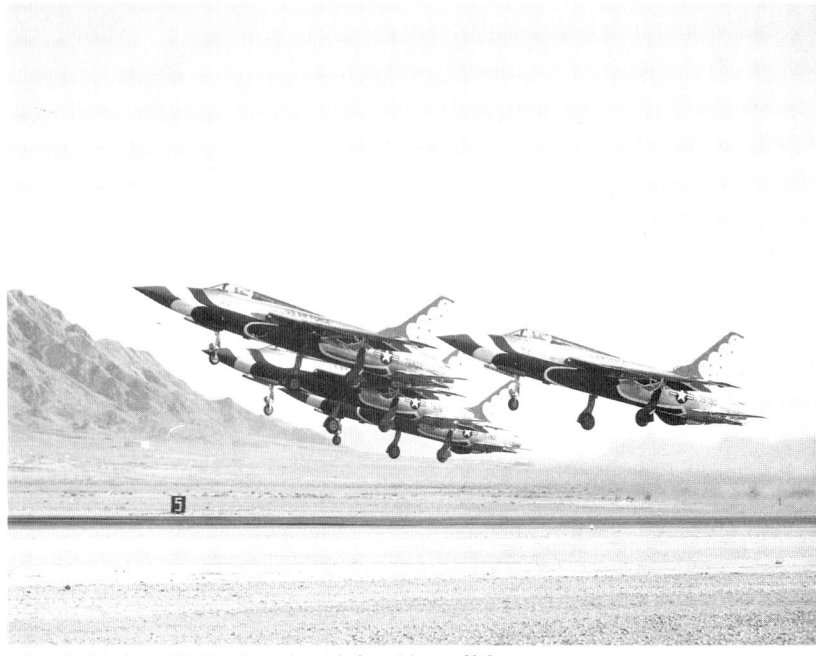

Thunderbirds F-105B Thunderchiefs taking off from Nellis Air Force Base, Nevada, early in 1964. This type only gave six public performances, as it was found unsuitable for aerobatics. (US Air Force).

Top: Thunderbirds support aircraft in 1958 was this Fairchild C-123B Provider, 54-0671. It is shown here in its original *Thunderbirds* livery. (Fairchild-Republic)

Opposite: Classic loop with smoke on, by F-100D Super Sabres of the USAF *Thunderbirds* in 1964. (US Air Force)

Opposite top: The original USAF *Thunderbirds* — four Republic F-84G Thunderjets seen rehearsing near Luke Air Force Base, Arizona on 19 August, 1953.
(US Air Force)

Opposite bottom: Republic F-84G Thunderjet, 51-16719, of the USAF *Thunderbirds,* seen taxying at Detroit in October 1954. Note the flag panel, which appeared port side only.
(W. J. Balogh via D. W. Menard).

Bottom: The F-105B Thunderchief was only retained for six shows during 1964, due to several problems. 57-5787 and 57-5793 are seen here in the team's 'calypso' routine, over Nellis Air Force Base in early 1964. (US Air Force)

F-4E Phantoms equipped the *Thunderbirds* during 1969-73 seasons. (Harry Gann)

However, the increasing demands on the F-105 for duty in Vietnam and the extensive modification requirements for the type to continue with the team resulted in *The Thunderbirds* returning to the Super Sabre, with the F-100D model for the 1965-68 seasons. 471 displays were given on this variant and several overseas tours were made, including European tours in 1965 and 1967 as well as visits to Latin America and the Caribbean Islands. In 1965, ther 1,000th demonstration was given in Illinois, which was just one of a record 121 shows mounted that year. By the beginning of 1966, the flag panel painted under the cockpit had increased to forty-five flags. The 1968 season included performances in Alaska, Hawaii, Canada and the Bahamas. On 30 November 1968, at Nellis AFB, *The Thunderbirds* performed their last show with the F-100D. With her sister model, the F-100C, the Super Sabres had carried *The Thunderbird* emblem for thirteen show seasons.

By the beginning of the 1969 season, *The Thunderbirds* had converted to the sixth type of aircraft to be used by the team. This was the McDonnell F-4E Phantom, of which a total of eight were acquired. Again, these were extensively modified with the gun-sight, cannon and ammunition drum all being removed as were certain items of the fire control and weapons systems. Dummy Sparrow missiles containing smoke oil were fitted and modifications were also made to the afterburner system so that this could be introduced at somewhat lower power settings. For the first time, a basically gloss-white overall colour scheme was adopted, which replaced the natural metal finish on previous types used.

Training was carried out on standard TAC F-4Es in camouflage paint. Individual aircraft were identified by black numbers on white discs applied to the engine intake sides, whilst small red, white and blue scallops adorned the top of the fin.

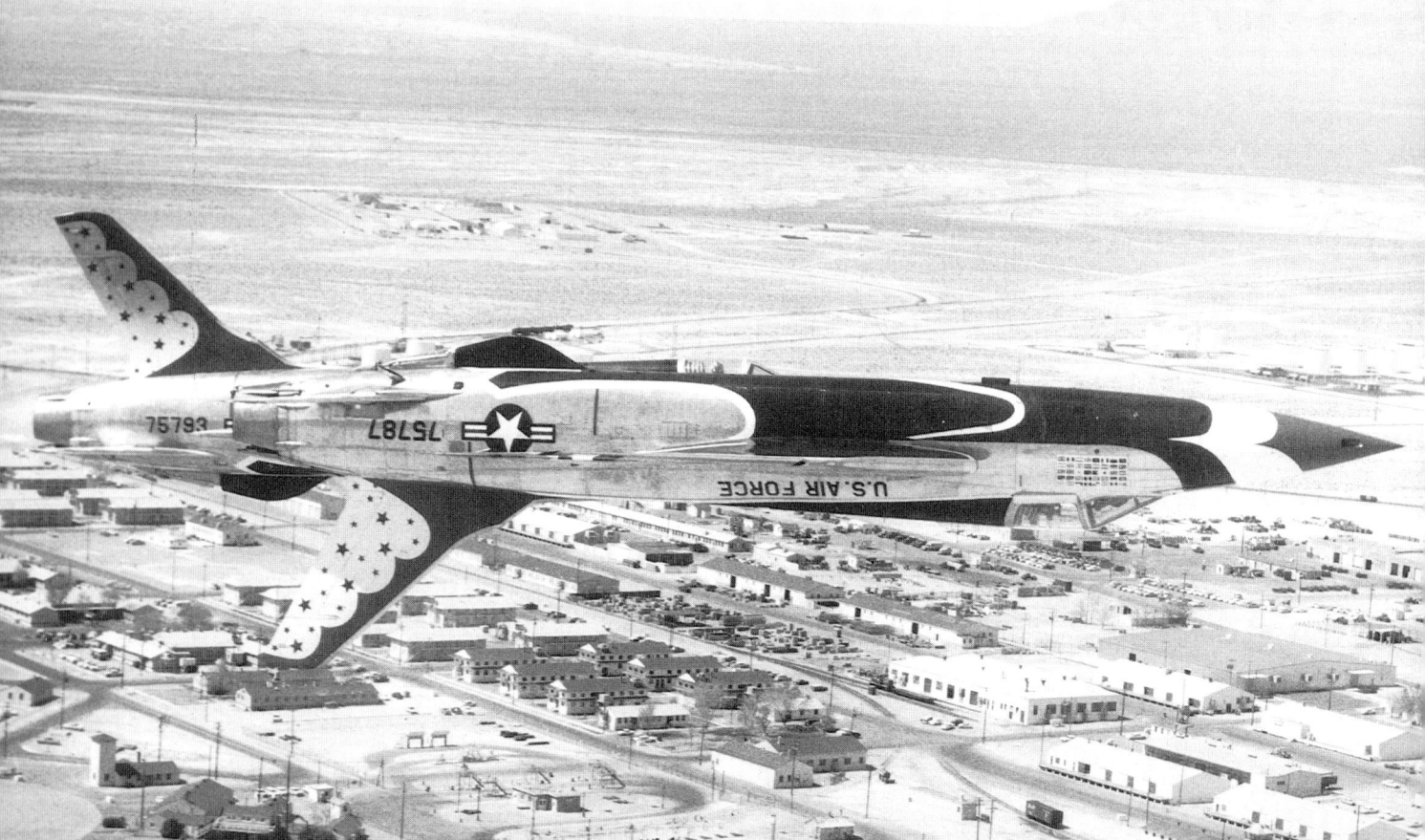

USAF
USAF
USAF
USAF

UNITED STATES AIR FORCE
116719

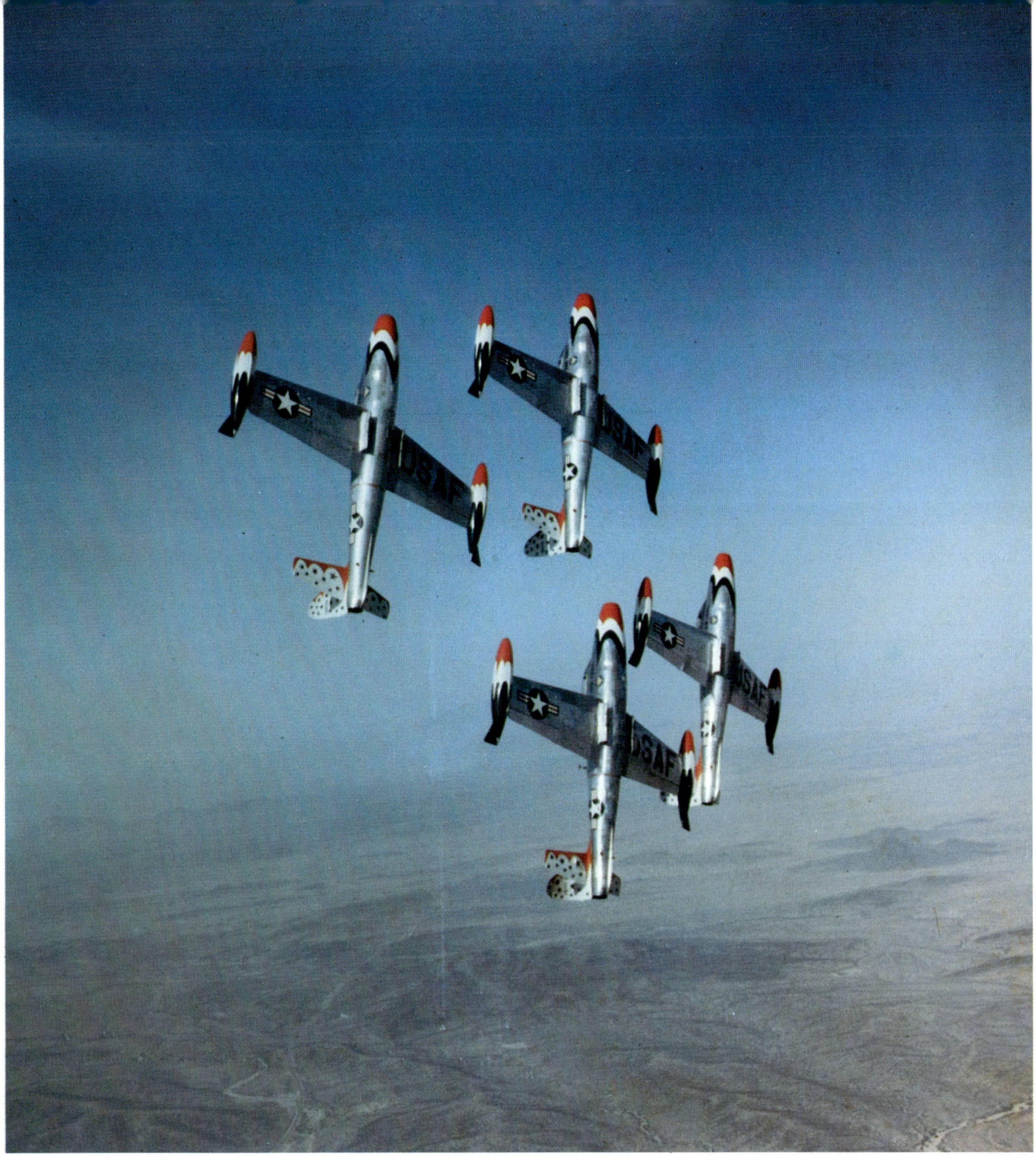

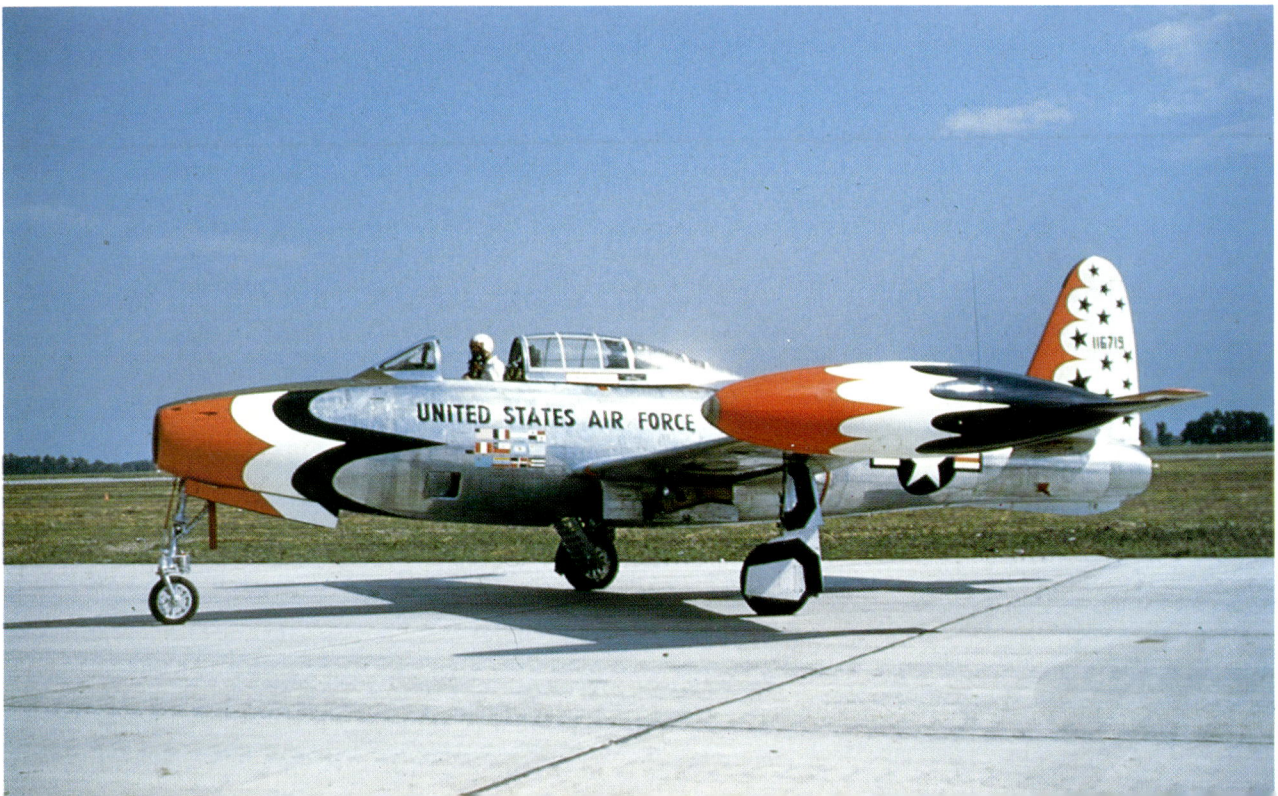

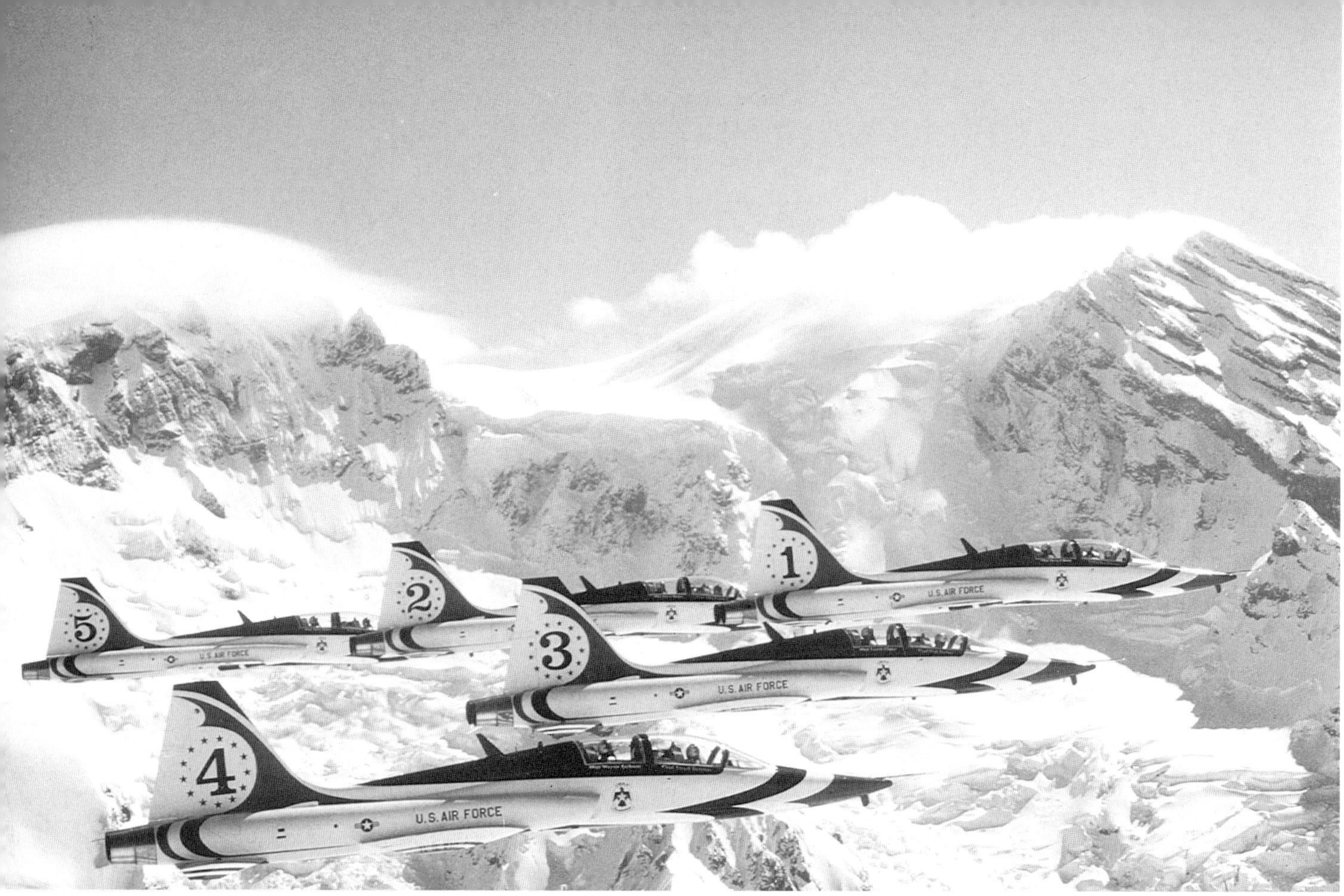

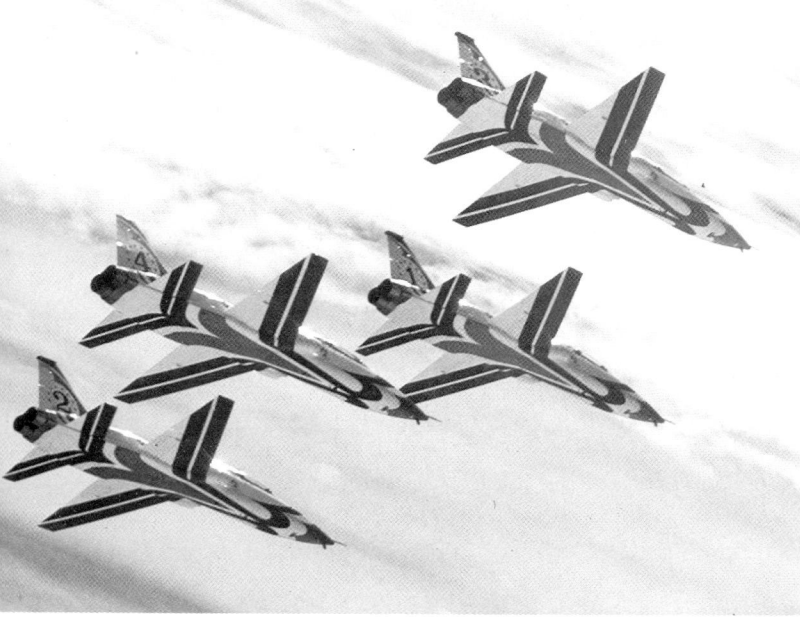

Above: Good view showing the underside colour scheme on the *Thunderbirds* Northrop T-38A Talons during 1974. (US Air Force).

Top: 1975 *Thunderbirds*, flying T-38A Talons over mountainous terrain. (US Air Force)

The team flew six Phantoms, a formation of five with a single solo performer. The first F-4E display took place on 1 June 1969 at the Air Force Academy and a tour of Alaska was also made later in the year. During 1970-71, overseas tours were made to South America, Canada, the Caribbean and Europe. By the end of the 1973 show season, the port flag panel numbered 48 flags. With the increasing pressures due to the energy crisis, the decision was made to change to a more economical aircraft type, as the Phantom was very much a thirsty bird. In November 1973, the F-4E gave its final performance at New Orleans, Louisiana, this being the team's 518th appearance with the type.

For the 1974 show season, *The Thunderbirds* switched from the impressive and awesomely noisy Phantom to the Northrop T-38A Talon, a much smaller but nevertheless handsome aircraft. The colour scheme adopted was very similar to that applied to the Phantom, although the underwing Thunderbird motif was somewhat modified. The T-38A was not capable of in-flight refuelling, so the team's performances were restricted to the United States and Canada. Some modifications to the aircraft were necessary, but these were by no means as extensive as in the past. The rear-cockpit control columns were removed, VHF radio equipment and stress recorders were added, as was smoke-making gear. In 1976, the team participated in the Bicentennial Year celebrations by altering the colour scheme to include a large Bicentennial emblem on the fin. With a performance at Mountain Home AFB, Idaho, on 8 May 1976, *The Thunderbirds* recorded their 2,000th official demonstration. After the 1976 show season, the colour scheme reverted to the original finish. The team continued with the T-38A until a tragic accident involving four of the aircraft occured during a practice session in January 1982 at Nellis AFB.

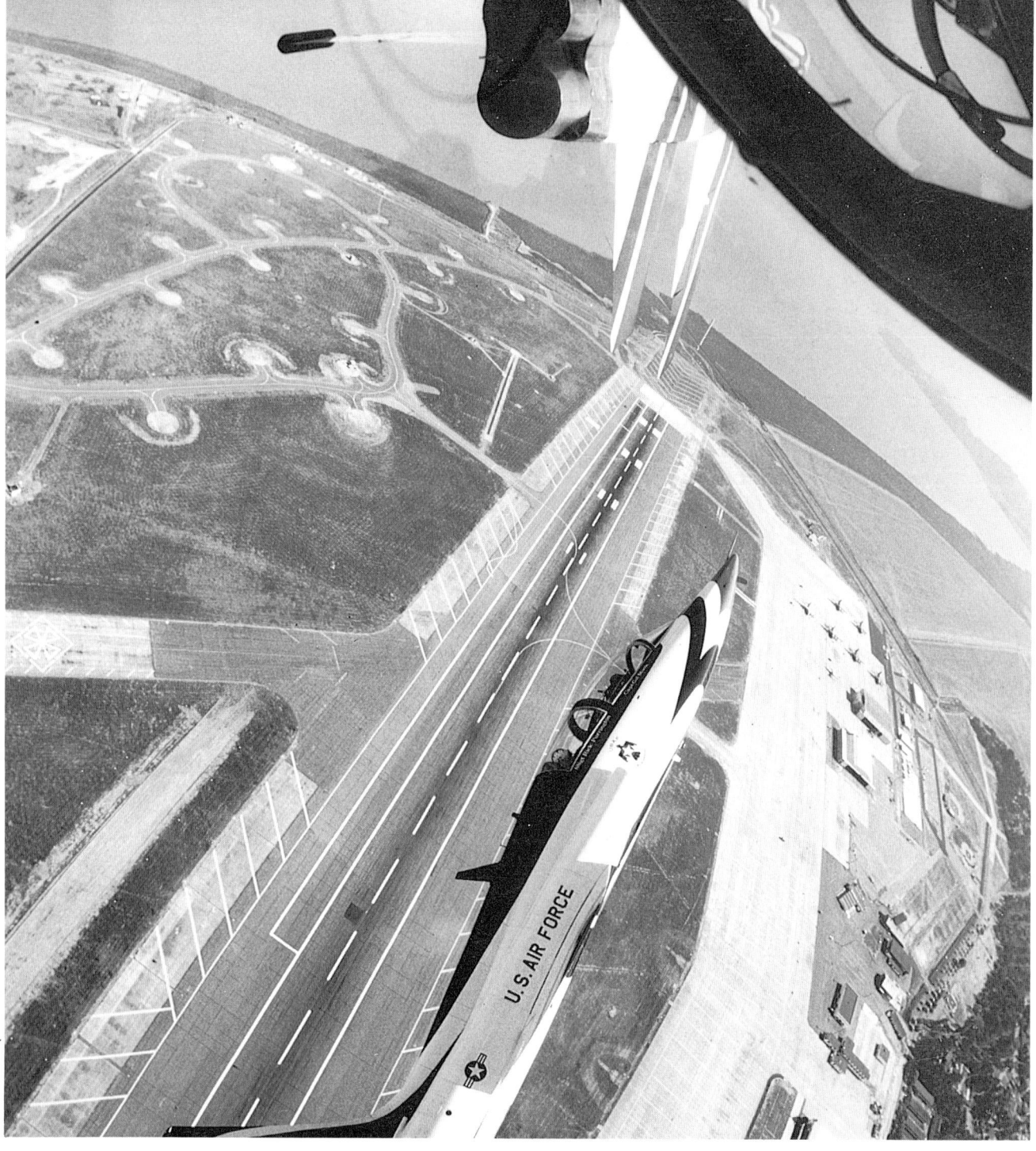

Dramatic wide-angle view from within the formation, during a display by T-38A Talons of the USAF *Thunderbirds* in 1975. (US Air Force via S. Wolf)

The leader misjudged his height and flew into the ground, taking the three formating T-38As with him, whose pilots' eyes were firmly fixed on the leader! Following this accident, the rest of the *Thunderbirds* displays for 1982 were cancelled. With the loss of most of the team and the aircraft, the future of the *Thunderbirds* was in doubt. However, it was decided to continue the team and re-equip with a new type — the F-16A Fighting Falcon, once again reverting to a fighter type. New pilots were posted in, led by Major Jim Latham, the team giving their first demonstration with the type in October 1982. Major Latham led the team through a successful 1983 season and was replaced by Lieutenant-Colonel Larry Stellmon for the 1984 season. In 1984, *The Thunderbirds* made their first European Tour for 13 years during June/July of that year, visiting England, Belgium, France, Germany, Spain, Portugal, the Netherlands, Norway and Denmark. *The Thunderbirds* are current on the F-16A, which looks like being their mount for several years to come.

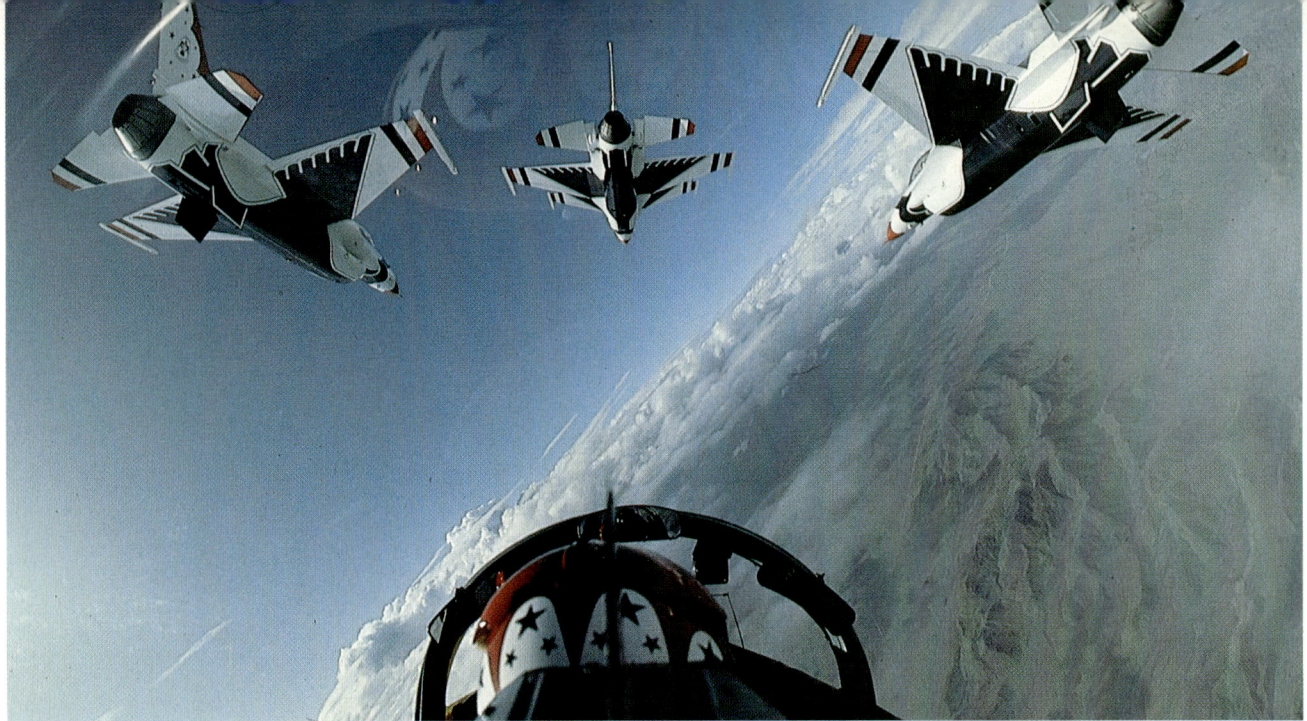

Above: Flying with the USAF *Thunderbirds* — a view from the 'slot' position during 1983. Note the paint scheme on the pilot's helmet and the *Thunderbird* motif under the other F-16s. (U.S. Air Force)

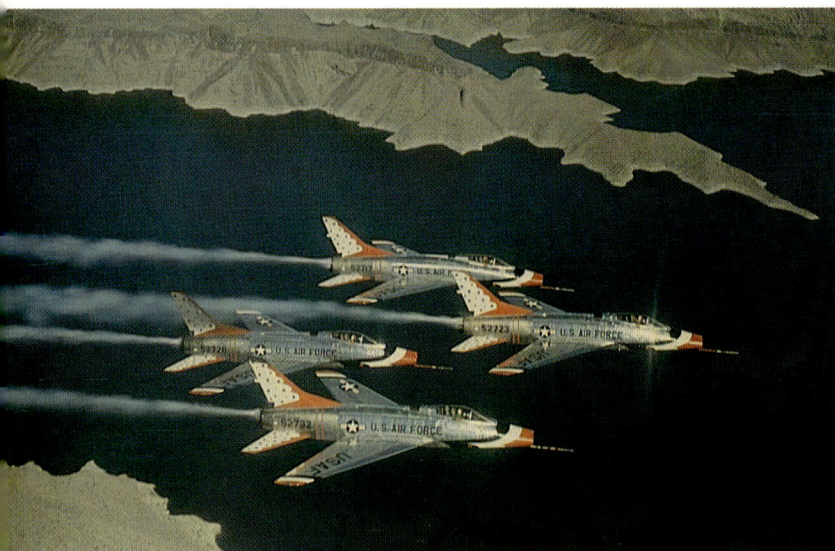

Above: F-100C Super Sabres of the USAF *Thunderbirds* in 1963. (US Air Force)

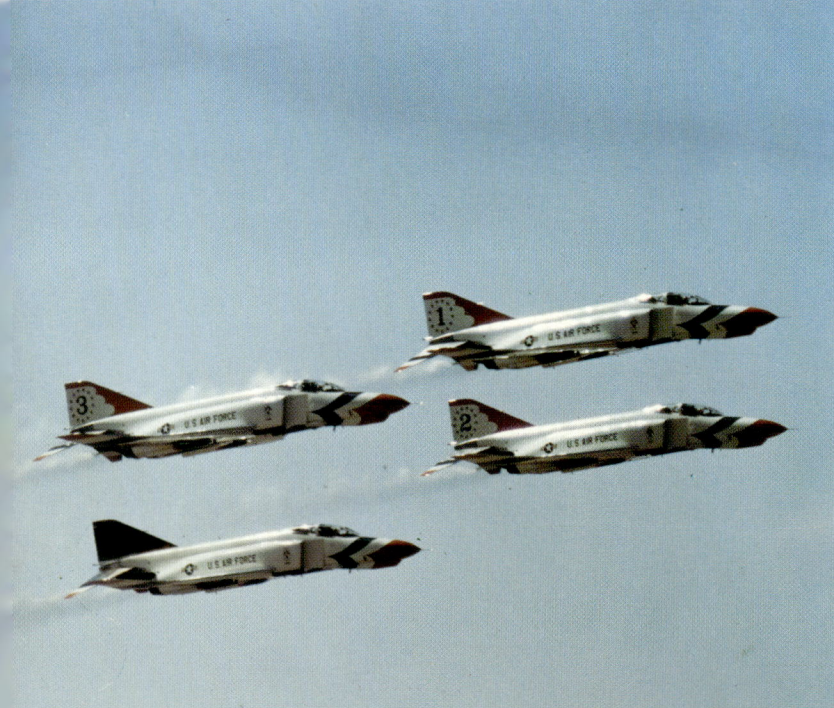

Left: Four F-4E Phantoms which equipped the *Thunderbirds* during 1969-73. Note No.4 has a blackened tail from the leader's smoke. (Harry Gann)

Aircraft used by *The Thunderbirds:*

1953-55: F-84G Thunderjet — 51-16714, 51-16719, 51-16720, 51-16722, 51-16723.
1955-56: F-84F Thunderstreak — 52-6732, 52-6735, 52-6751, 52-6770, 62-6771, 52-6779 and 52-6853.
1953-60: T-33A Support Aircraft — 51-4076, 52-9221, 53-5547, 53-6089.
1956-63: F-100C Super Sabre — 53-1718, 53-1740, 54-1860, 54-1882, 54-1969, 55-2717, 55-2723, 55-2724, 55-2725, 55-2727, 55-2728, 55-2729, 55-2730, 55-2732, 55-2733.
1960-68: F-100F Super Sabre — 56-3875, 56-3924, 56-3927.
1964: F-105B Thunderchief — 57-5782, 57-5787, 57-5790, 57-5793, 57-5797, 57-5798, 57-5801, 57-5814.
1964-68: F-100D Super Sabre — 55-3506, 55-3507, 55-3520, 55-3560*, 55-3561, 55-3582, 55-3606, 55-3708, 55-3737, 55-3754, 55-3776, 55-3779, 55-3791.
*This aircraft is currently preserved in the Air Force Museum, Dayton, Ohio.
1968-73: F-4E Phantom — 66-0286'3', 66-0289 '8', 66-0290'3', 66-0291'4', 66-0294, 66-0296, 66-0302'1', 66-0315'5/7', 66-0319'2', 66-0321'5', 66-0329'6/7', 66-0377.
1974-81: T-38A Talon — 68-8100, 68-8106, 68-8131, 68-8137, 68-8156, 68-8174, 68-9175, 68-8176, 68-8177, 68-8182, 68-8184.
1982-to date: F-16A Fighting Falcon — 81-0663/1, 81-0667/2, 81-0670/4, 81-0676/3, 81-0677/5, 81-0678/7, 81-0679/6, 81-0687/8 and F-16B 80-0638.

Transport support aircraft:
1959-63: C-54D Skymaster — 42-72674
1958-61: C-123B Provider — 54-0671, 54-0672, 54-0683
1954-57, 1959: C-119F Boxcar — 51-8120, 51-8137, 51-8146
1962-to date: C-130E/H Hercules — 73-1588 (one of many used by the team, but the only one known to have carried a Thunderbirds badge and code '14' on the nose.)

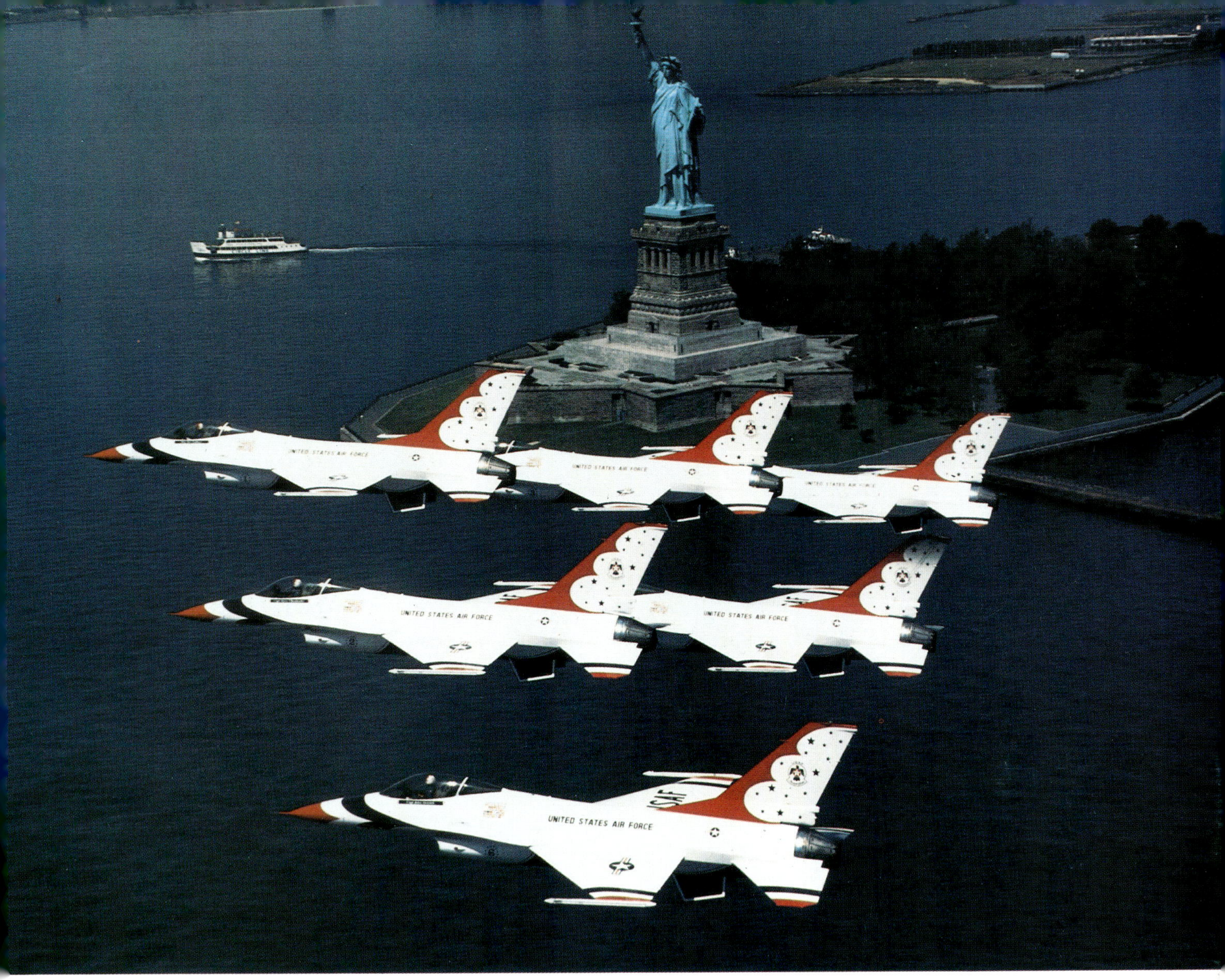

1947-59: Colorado Air National Guard, "Minute Men", Colorado Springs.

The *Minute Men* team was formed in 1947, when three Colorado Air National Guard pilots made up a trio of F-80C Shooting Stars to put on exhibitions at local fairs, rodeos and air shows. Led by Colonel Walter Williams, the team became more proficient and was called on for more and more demonstrations around Colorado and in neighbouring States. The team was about to move out on the national scene, when the Korean War broke out and the team's pilots were called overseas. After that war, the team reformed with an additional fourth aircraft to complete the diamond formation. In 1956, the *Minute Men* added a fifth pilot, Major Wynn Coomer, to perform solo manoeuvres to supplement the four-ship team's demonstration. At the end of 1956, it was almost decided to disband the team due to costs. However, the team went on to become the official jet precision demonstration team of all the USAF Air National Guard units. In 1957 the *Minute Men* changed to the F-86F Sabre, some of which were converted F-86E models. There were several changes of team members, but Colonel Williams continued to lead the team. Coming from an Air National Guard unit, the pilots were all part-time, having civilian jobs during the week. The team staged the first jet precision demonstration ever held in Hawaii, in April 1957.

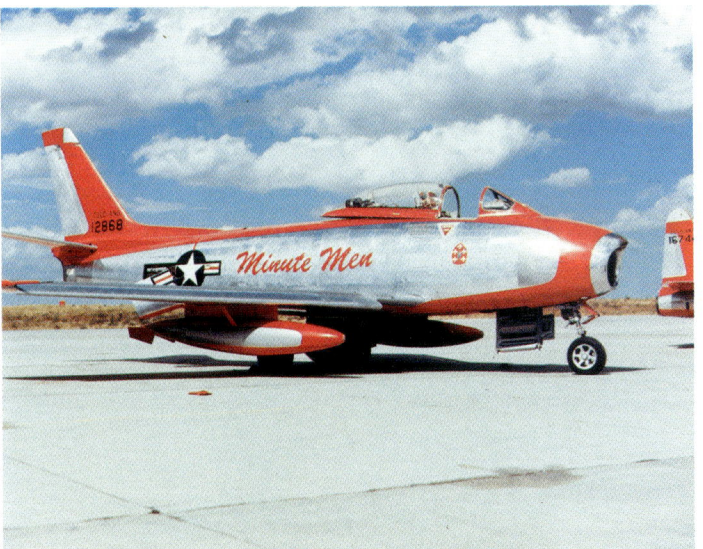

N.A. F-86F Sabre, 51-2868, of the USAF Colorado Air National Guard *Minute Men* team at Colorado Springs in 1958. (Colo. ANG)

Top: The USAF *Thunderbirds* with their F-16As fly past The Statue of Liberty in New York harbour during 1983. (USAF)

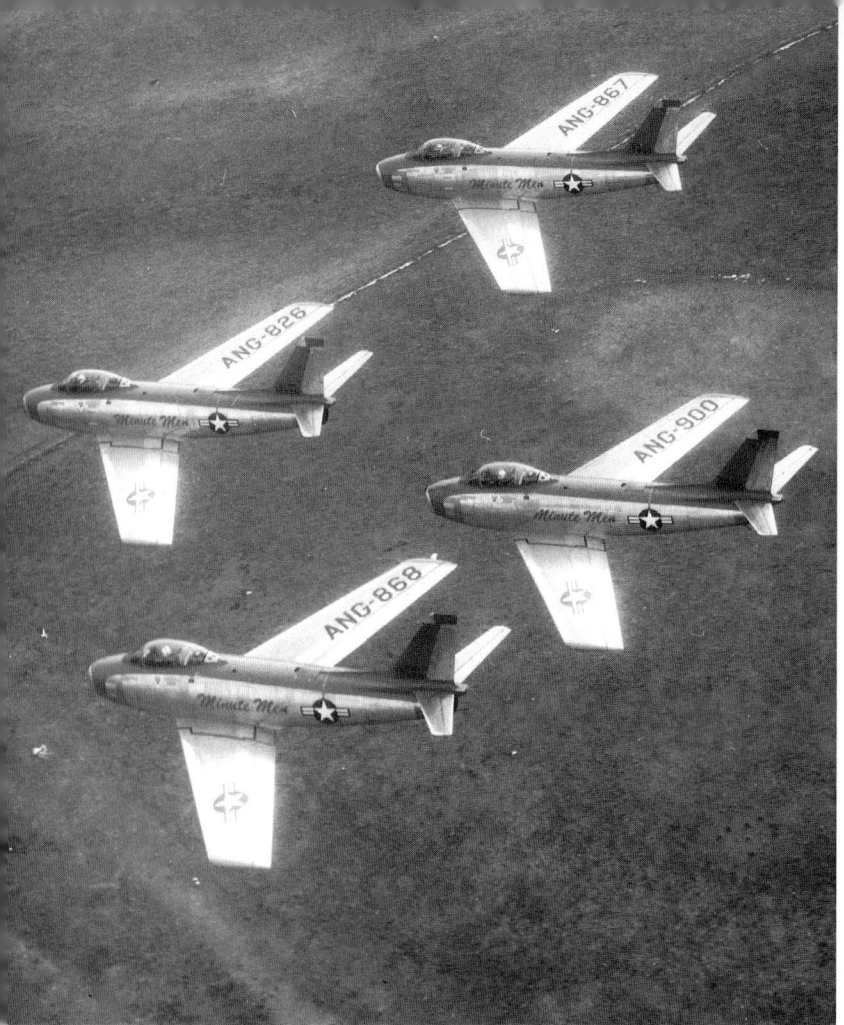

Left: F-86F Sabres of the Colorado ANG *Minute Men* team in 1957. Colour scheme is red on natural metal.
(USAF via Walter Williams)

The *Minute Men* gave a 25-minute display, highlighted by 20 minutes of smoke trails. It was the first team to carry enough smoke so that it could be used throughout the show. Other jet aerobatic teams carried only about three minutes' supply. Apparently, the team claimed they could lay a trail of smoke from Montreal to Miami! During 1958, the team claimed to be the first to do 5-ship loops and rolls in the U.S.A. It was also the first team to do the low-altitude 'corkscrew' manoeuvre, in which the two wing aircraft simultaneously did rolls around the leader and tail aircraft, forming spiral smoke-trails in the air.

During their period of operation, the *Minute Men* only had one accident. This was on 7 June 1958, when Captain John T. Ferrier was killed during an air show at Patterson Air Force Base, Ohio. Rather than eject from his Sabre, Captain Ferrier guided his ill-fated aircraft away from a densely-populated area and crashed on open ground. Captain Bob Cherry, who started with the team in the slot position in the autumn of 1955 and later moved to the left-wing position, replaced Colonel Walter Williams as team leader in March 1959. The team took six F-86F Sabres, including a spare, around to air shows, accompanied by a T-33 support aircraft. They continued until the end of the 1959 season, then disbanded.

Colour scheme of both the F-80C and F-86F aircraft was natural metal with red fuselage top, fin, undersides of the fuselage, wings and tailplanes. *Minute Men* in red script appeared on the fuselage sides and all other lettering was in black. The F-80C Shooting Stars included 45-8675, 45-8673 and 45-8583. Serial numbers of the F-86F Sabres were: 51-2826, 51-2867, 51-2868, 51-2855, 51-2884 and 51-2900 with supporting T-33 51-6744.

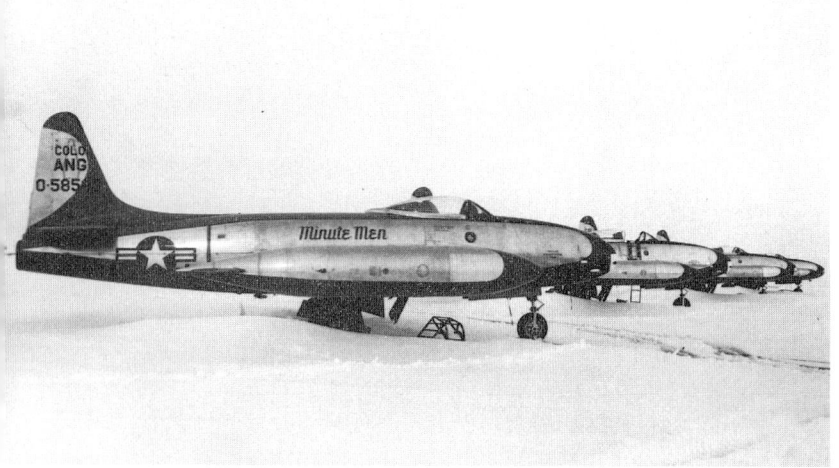

Above: 55-8583 heads a line-up of Lockheed F-80C Shooting Stars of the Colorado ANG *Minute Men* team in a wintery setting 1955/56. (Colo ANG via R. Ward)

1950-62: USAFE "Skyblazers". Fürstenfeldbruck/Neubiberg/Chaumont/Bitburg

When the 36th Fighter Bomber Group, with three squadrons of F-80Bs, moved from Panama to Fürstenfeldbruck, Germany, during 1948, the *Skyblazers* were formed. They were led by Captain Vince Gordon, flying four F-80 Shooting Stars until late 1950, when the 36th FBG began to re-equip with the F-84E Thunderjet. In 1951, the 22 FBS, 36FBG re-equipped the *Skyblazers* team with four F-84E Thunderjets, painted in standard squadron colours comprising blue and white diagonal stripes on all tail surfaces. The nose and tip tanks were painted in the squadron's red colour, including the front of the nose-wheel doors. Major Harry ('The Horse') Evans became the leader and took the team all over Europe and to North Africa, until the 36th FBG returned to the USA in 1952, where the *Skyblazers* gave their last display with F-84Es at Detroit in August 1952. F-84E Thunderjets operated by the team included: 49-2162, 49-2225, 49-2229, 49-2230, 49-2233, 49-2234 and 49-2249.

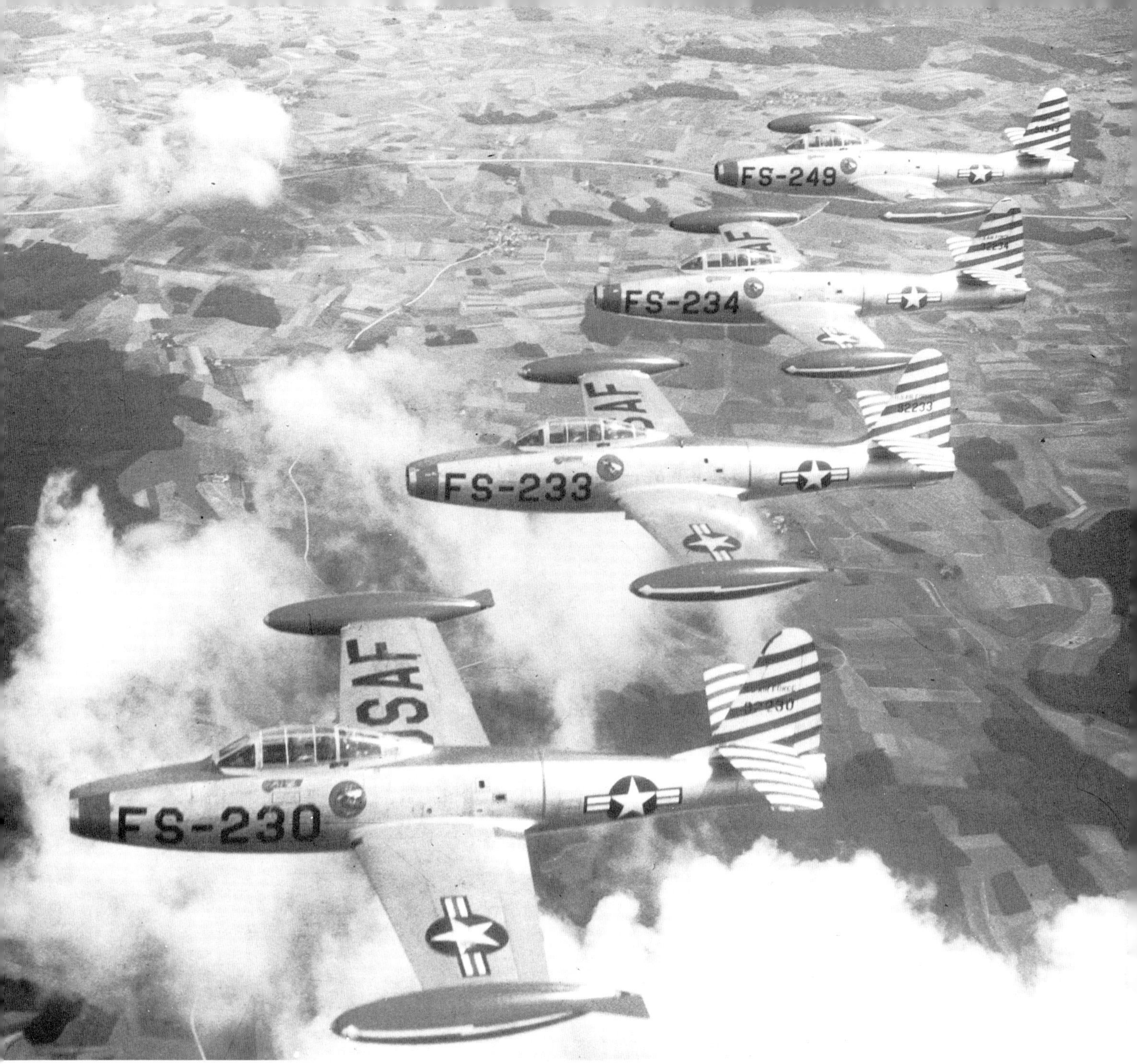

The USAF *Skyblazers* in 1951, flying F-84E Thunderjets from 22 FBS, 36 FBG. All tail surfaces were painted in light blue and white stripes. Nose and tip tanks were red. (USAF via David W. Menard)

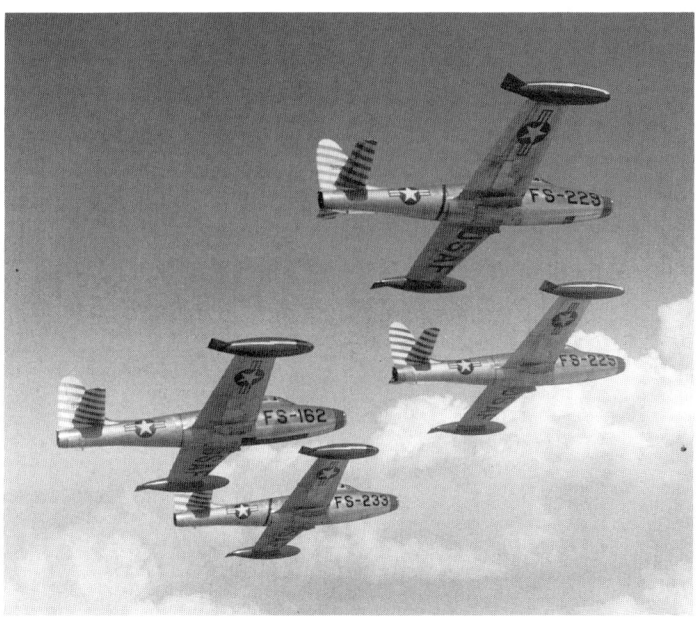

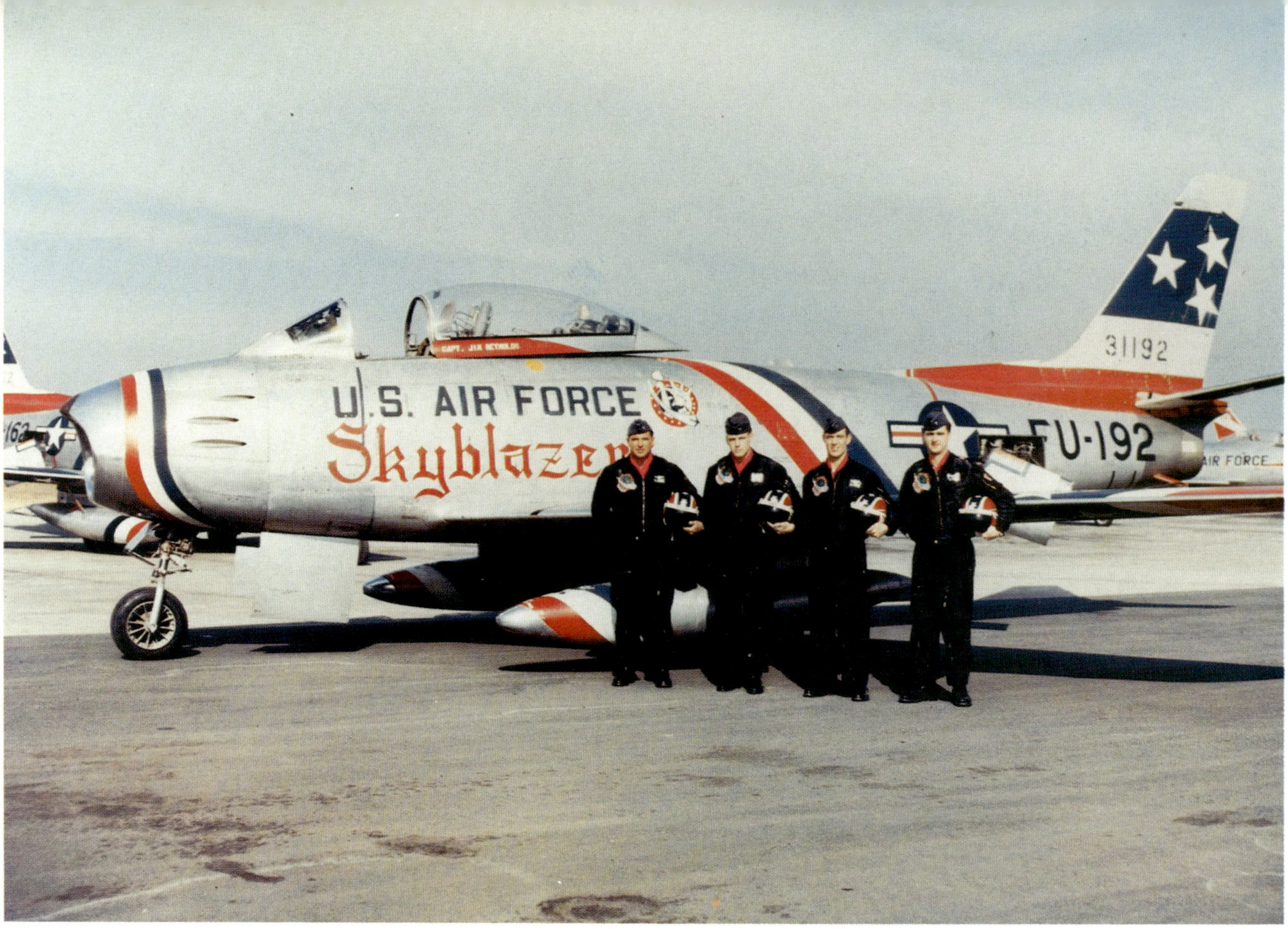

Above: Members of the *Skyblazers* aerial demonstration team stand in front of one of their F-86F aircraft at Chaumont Air Base, France. March 1956 (US Air Force)

Opposite: Good plan view of the *Skyblazers* F-100C Super Sabres, showing the wing markings to advantage during 1960. Note fuselage sash on lead aircraft. (US Air Force via R. Ward)

Below: Living up to their name, the 36 TFW *Skyblazers* F-100C Super Sabres are seen burning off fuel to dramatic effect in 1961. (US Air Force via D. W. Menard).

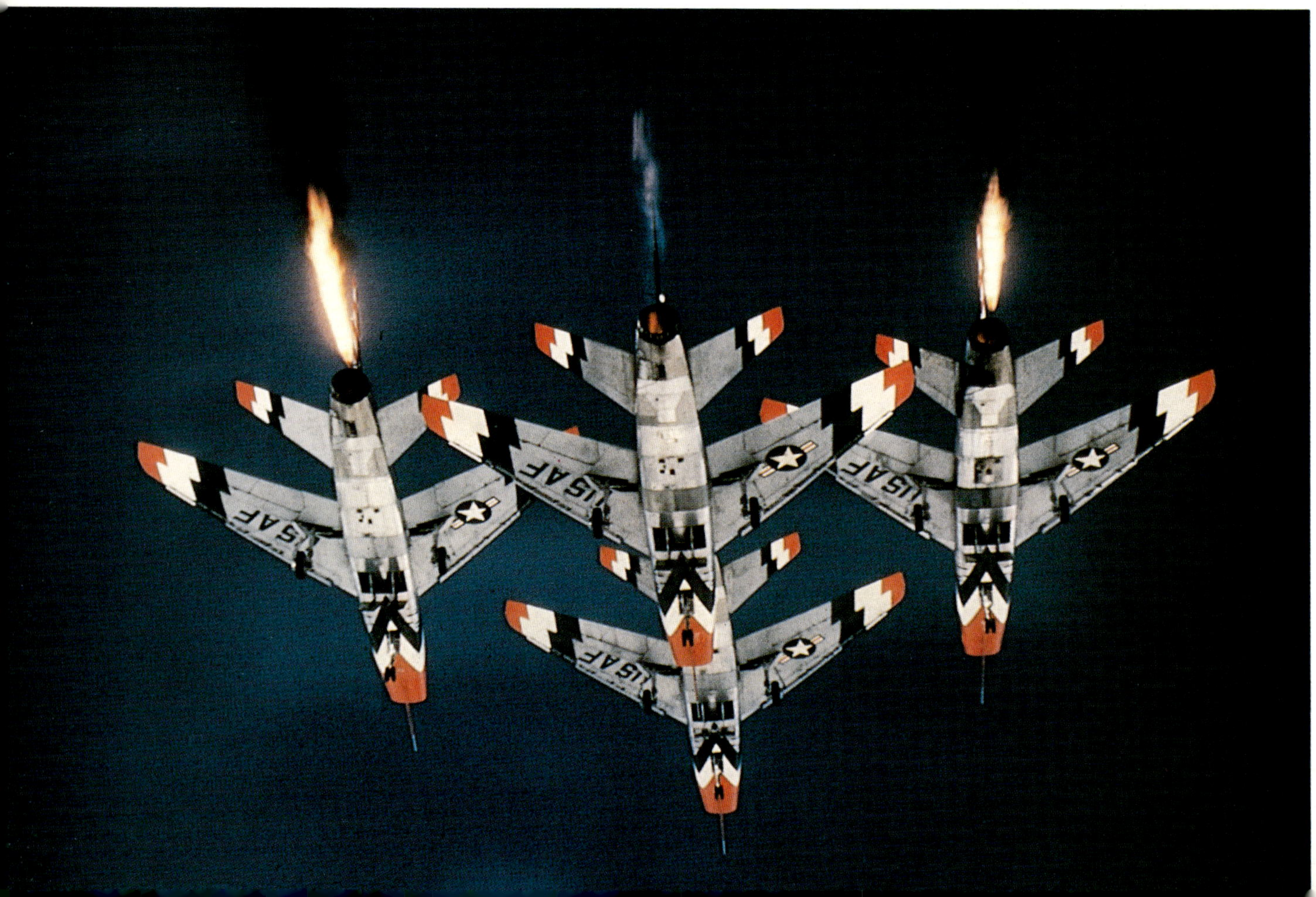

USAFE was eager to continue the *Skyblazers* team, so the 86th Fighter Wing at Neubiberg, Germany, was ordered to continue the team. Major Robert 'Tommy' Tomlinson was chosen as leader and practice with four F-84E Thunderjets began in July 1952. In early 1953, the 86th FW began to convert to the F-86F Sabre. At this time, USAFE decided the 48th Fighter Wing at Chaumont, France, would be responsible for continuing the *Skyblazers* team. So, the 86th FW gave their last *Skyblazers* display with F-84Es in July 1953.

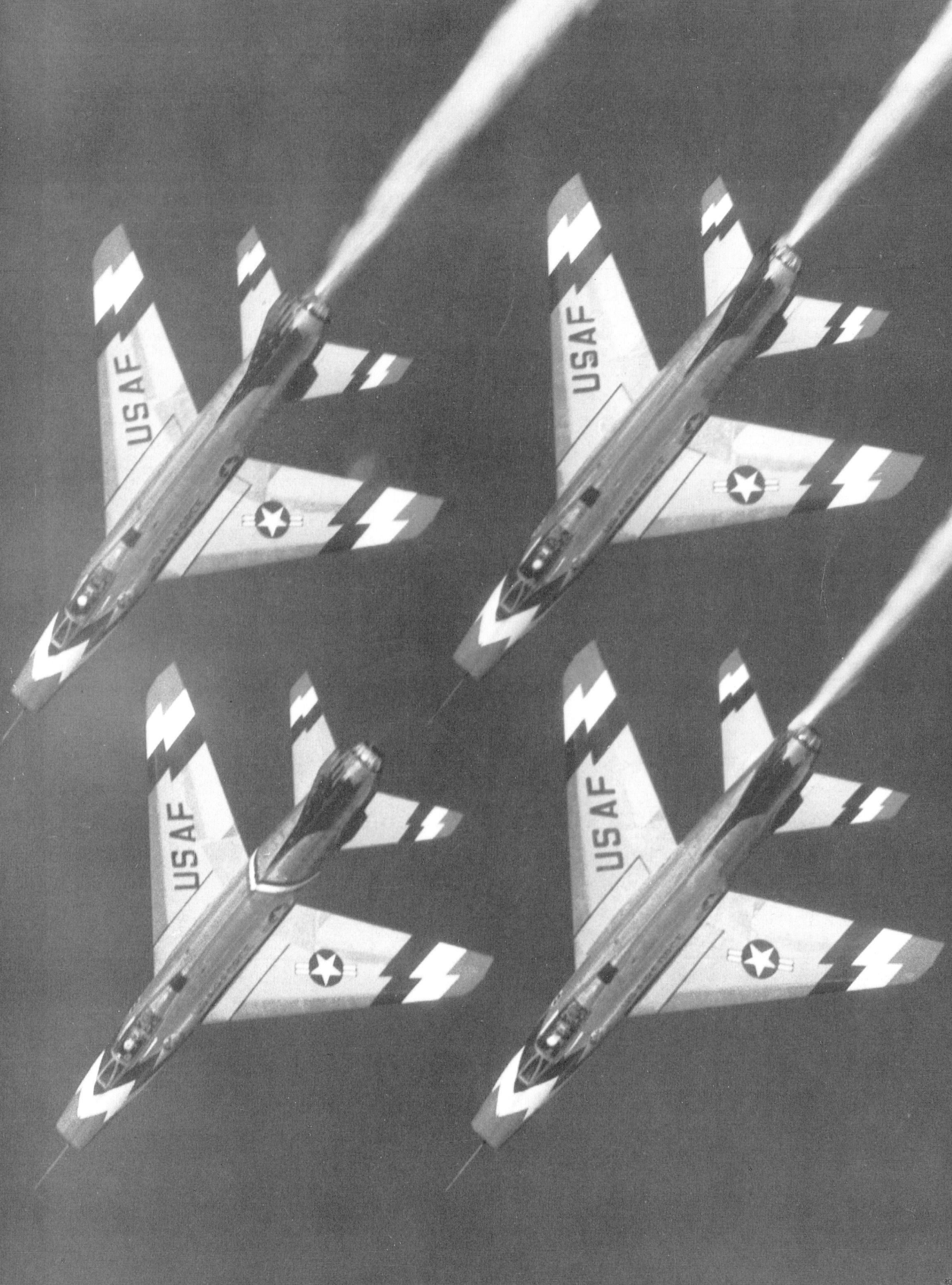

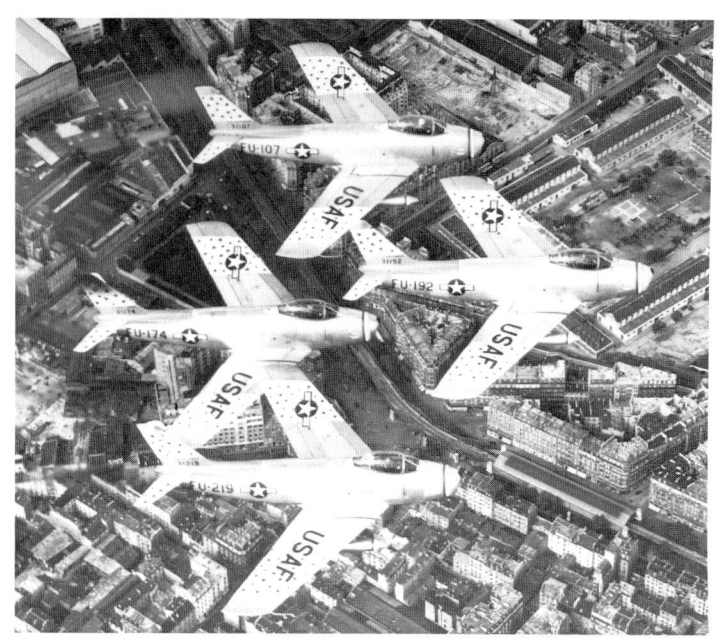

In July 1954, the team reformed under the 48th FW, with four F-86F Sabres painted with red, white and blue trim. The first colour scheme included the tail surfaces and outer wing panels being painted with large areas of red and white, with various-sized medium blue stars in the white areas. Led by Major William N. Dillard, the *Skyblazers* continued in this form throughout 1955, then changed the colour scheme for the 1956 season to include white stars on blue tail surfaces and outer wing panels. The *Skyblazers* legend was painted in Old English Style red script on both fuselage sides. The Statue of Liberty badge also appeared on both sides of the fuselage. The *Skyblazers* gave their last display with F-86F Sabres in October 1956, the aircraft used including: 53-1192, 53-1162, 53-1186 and 53-1201.

Left: Tight 'diamond' formation by F-86F Sabres of the *Skyblazers* team from the 48th FW over Paris in 1955. (Col. W. Dillard via D. Menard)

Below: Flying F-86F Sabres, the USAFE aerobatic team, the *Skyblazers*, perform precision flying over France. They were stationed at Chaumont Air Force Base, France, in October 1955. (US Air Force)

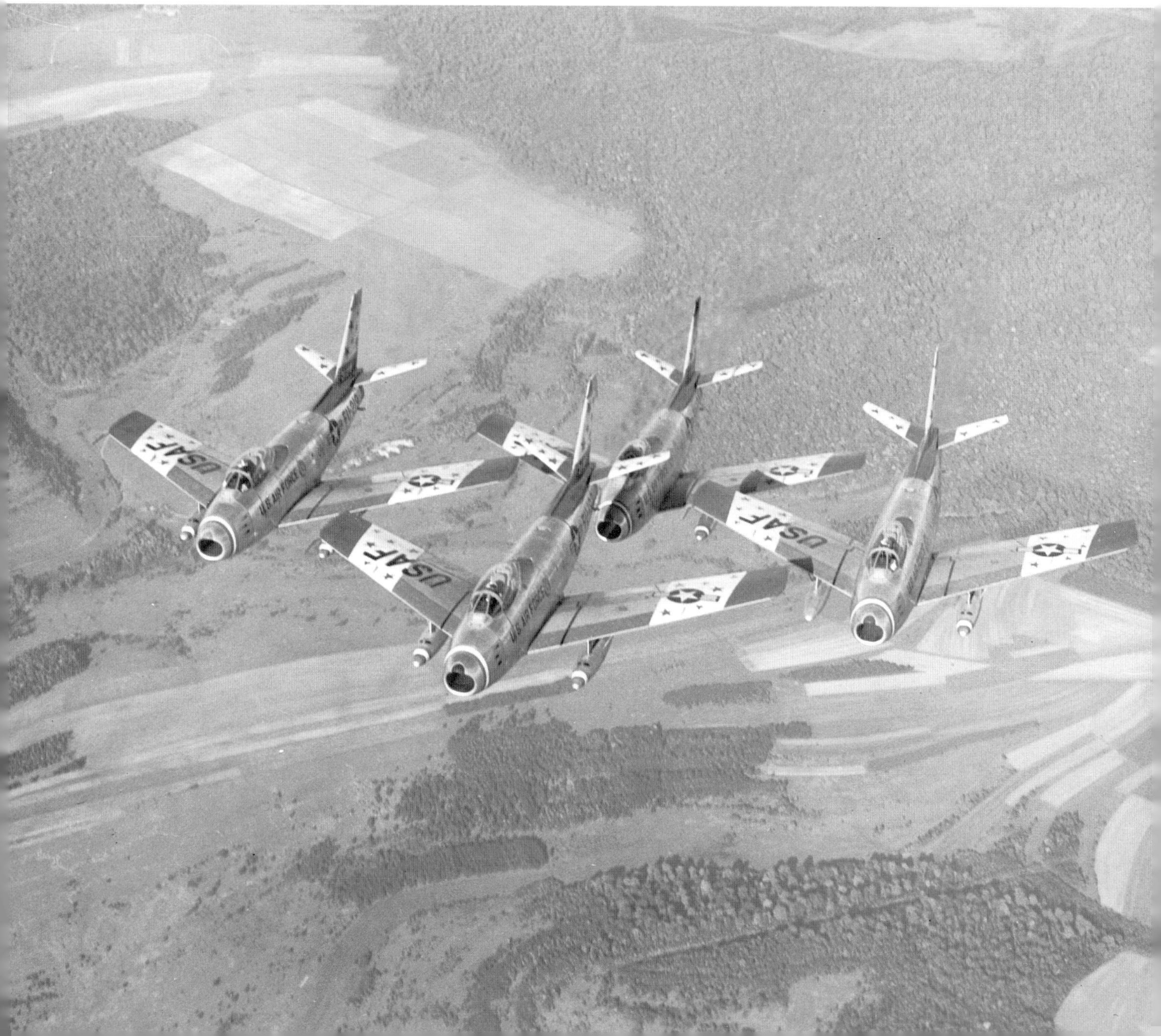

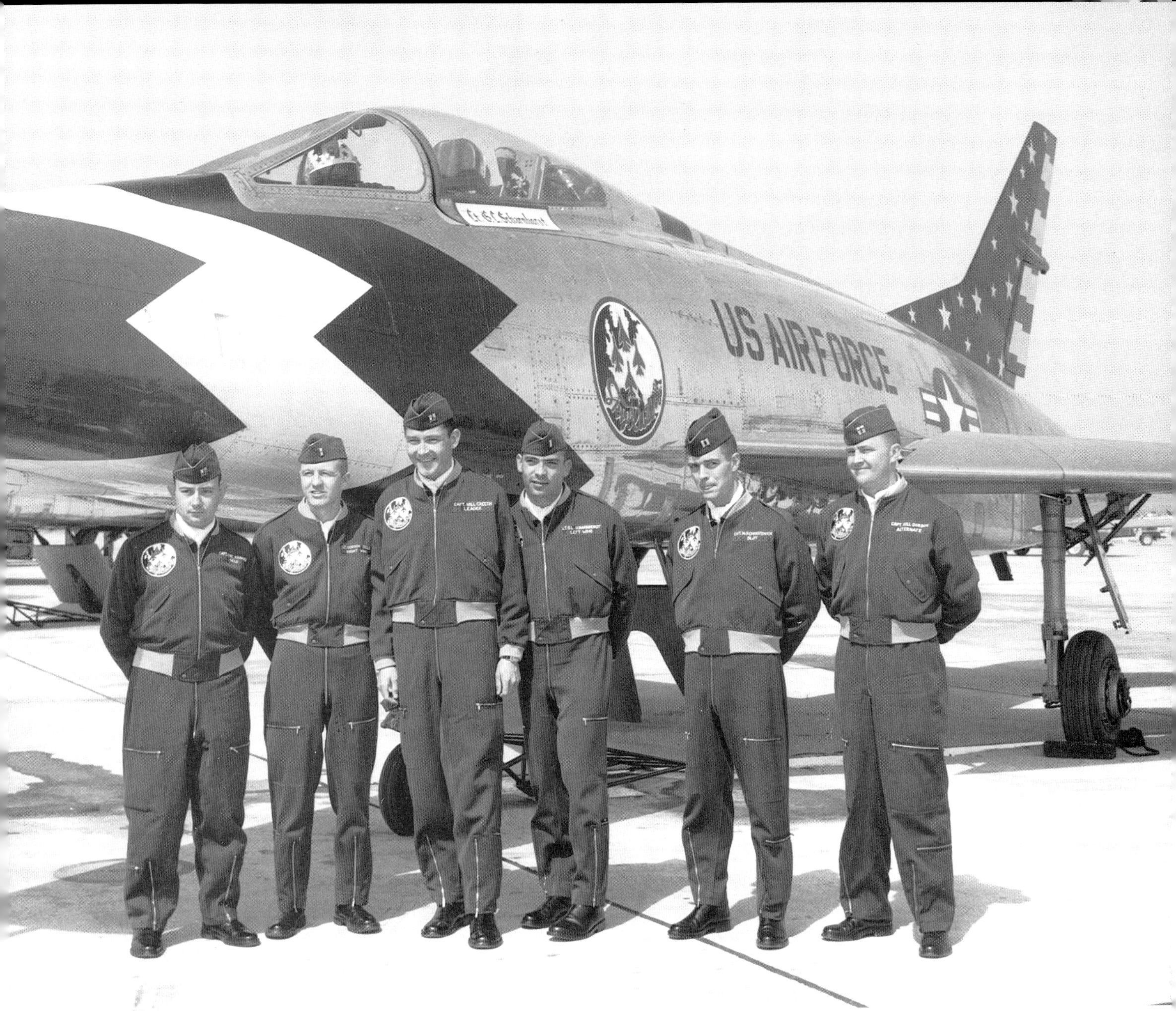

During the late 1950s, the 36th Tactical Fighter Wing at Bitburg Air Base, Germany, had re-equipped with the F-100C Super Sabre. Therefore, USAFE decided that this would be an ideal mount for the *Skyblazers* to continue with, complementing the *Thunderbirds* who were equipped with the type in the U.S.A. Captain Wilbur L. Creech was assigned the leader, who had previously flown F-84F Thunderstreaks with the Thunderbirds at Luke AFB, Arizona. The team's F-100cs were painted in a striking red, white and blue scheme and training began in 1958. They appeared in public for the 1959 season and displays took them all over Europe, as well as to Greece and Libya. Drop tanks were not normally carried during displays, but were added towards the end of the team's career. The *Skyblazers* emblem was carried on the left side of the fuselage and that of USAFE on the right. F-100C, 54-2009, was the lead aircraft and bore a sloping red, white and blue fuselage band just behind the national insignia on the rear fuselage. F-100C Super Sabres known to have flown in the team were 54-1959, 54-1980, 54-2002, 54-2010, 54-1992 and 54-1891. The *Skyblazers* last season was 1961, when Captain Pat Kramer became leader and the team's last display was in January 1962, when they disbanded.

Above: Capt. Bill Creech (3rd from left) poses with the rest of the *Skyblazers* team in front of one of their F-100C Super Sabres during a show at Athens, Greece in May 1959. (US Air Force)

Below: N.A. F-100C Super Sabres of the 36 TFW, *Skyblazers* team in their 1959 markings.
(USAF via Raymond F. Toliver)

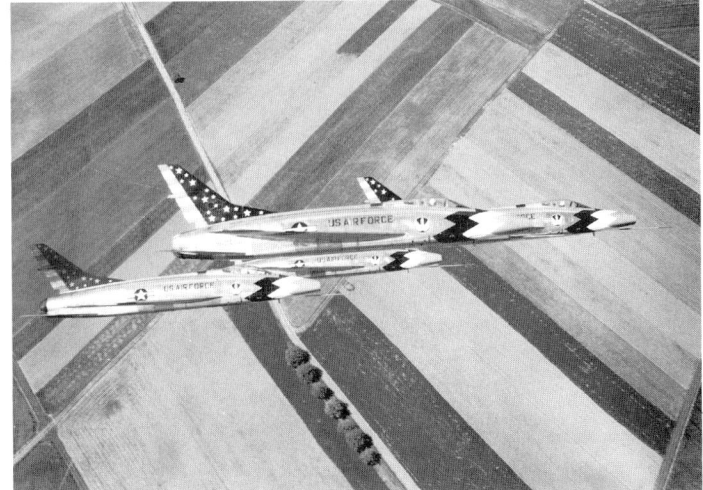

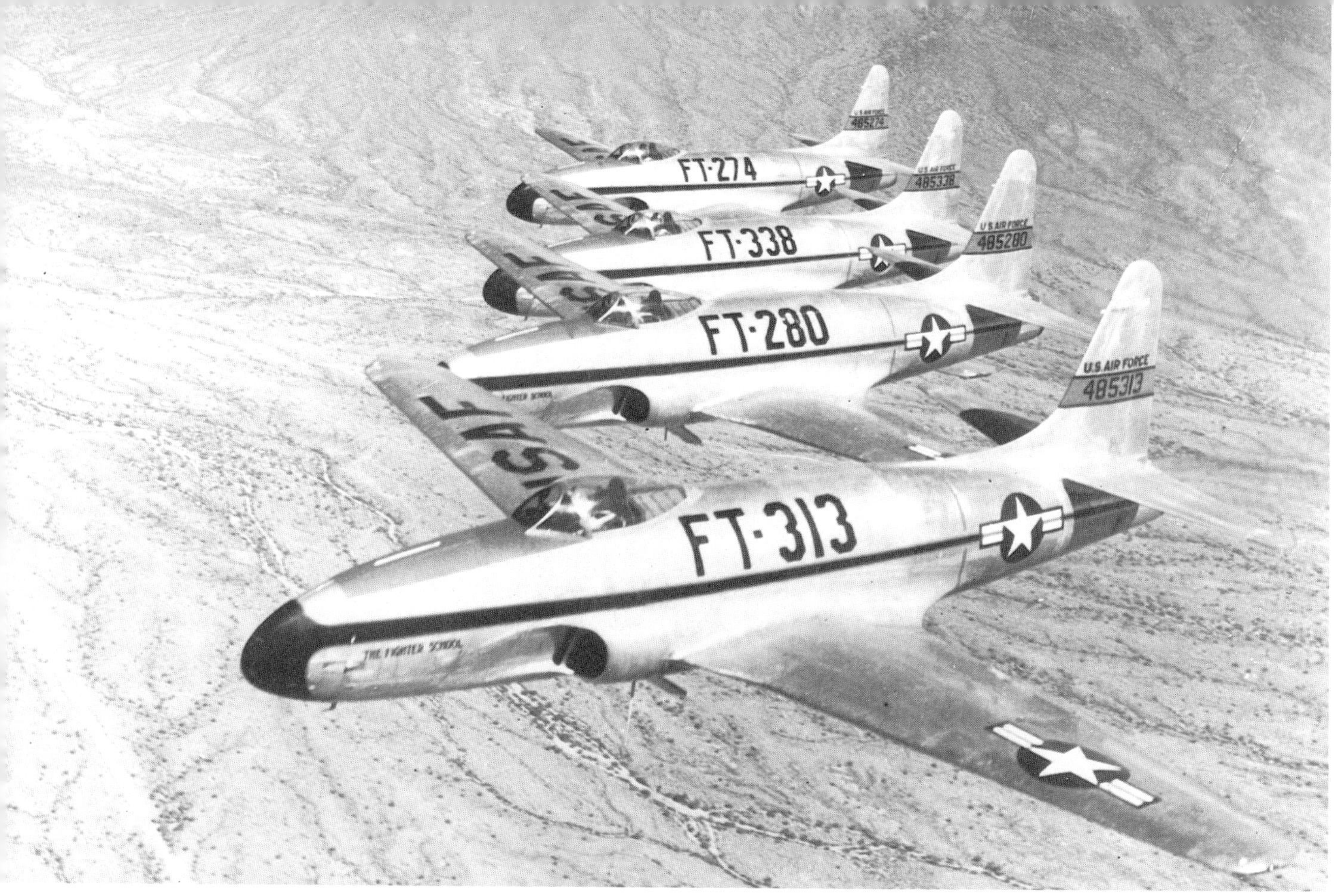

Above: The *Acrojets* from the USAF's Fighter School was one of the first jet teams, flying Lockheed F-80A Shooting Stars from Williams Air Force Base, Arizona, in 1949. (US Air Force)

Below: Worthy of inclusion are the world's first jet bomber aerobatic team, the USAFE *Black Knights* with four Martin B-57 Canberras. Operated by the 38th Bombardment Group (Tactical), this team was based at Laon, France in 1956. Colour scheme was overall gloss black with red scalloping on the nose, engine intakes and on all tail surfaces.
(USAFE via A. Pearcy).

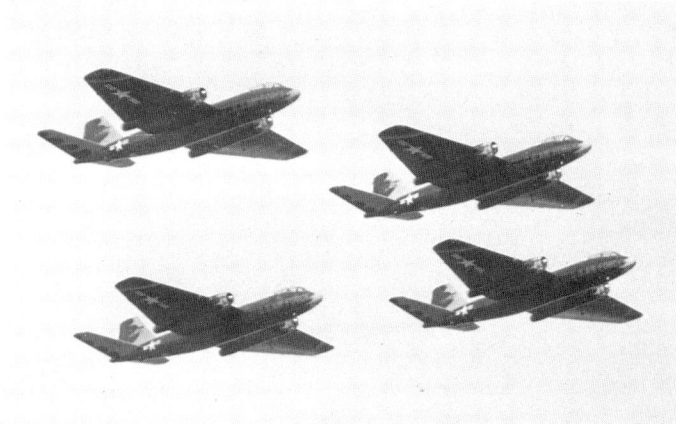

Other U.S.A.F. Aerobatic Teams

Following World War II, USAF squadrons found their aircraft were not in such great demand for operational tasks and time was found to form demonstration teams for the air displays which were being staged. One of the first post-war teams was the *Red Devils* with F-51D Mustangs, which was followed by the *Guardian Angels* with F-51H Mustangs from Maryland Air National Guard. Both teams were flying in 1949 and into the early 1950s before the Korean War disrupted such activities and crews.

One of the first jet teams to form were *The Acrojets*, flying Lockheed F-80A Shooting Stars. They formed in 1949 with four squadron commanders and instructors of the Air Force's Fighter School at Williams Air Force Base, Arizona. Major Howard W. Jensen look the team to the Cleveland National Air Races in Ohio during 1949 and the team of four continued through to the end of the 1951 season, when their displays included one at Detroit, Michigan. The aircraft were natural metal overall with a black cheatline outlined in red down the fuselage side. The fin bore a black-outlined yellow band upon which the serial was painted. F-80As operated by the *Acrojets* included 44-85313, '280, '338, '274, '510, '511, '481 and '508.

The aircraft that replaced the F-80 in squadron service was the F-86 Sabre and several teams formed on this type during the 1950s. The first Sabre team was *The Silver Sabres* which formed in 1949 with F-80s, but soon re-equipped with F-86A Sabres. Based at Langley Air Force Base, Virginia, the team comprised five aircraft from the 4th Fighter Interceptor Group, 335 F.S. and was led by Captain Vermont Garrison. As their name implies, the aircraft were natural metal overall. The fuselage had the badge of an Indian Chief's head mounted on a flaming arrow. *Silver Sabre* F-86As included 48-233, '244, '262, '273, '293 and '294. The team flew over the eastern and southern U.S. during 1949-50 and were disbanded when the Korean War broke out.

Several other squadrons flew Sabre aerobatic teams including the 94th F.S. which had a team of four F-86As called the *Sabre Dancers*, based at Oxnard A.F.B.

One of the more well-known teams flying Sabres was the *Sabre Knights* from 325 F.I.S. at Hamilton A.F.B., California. This team of four F-86F Sabres was formed in August 1952 by Major Vince Gordon, who previously led the *Skyblazers* in Europe. The aircraft wore red and yellow striped fins and nose trim. Serial numbers were 51-2751, '842, '806 and '805. In May 1954 the *Sabre Knights* changed from the F-86F model to the F-86D, their first display with the new variant being at Hamilton AFB on 15 May 1954. They flew a 20-minute show at venues in California and surrounding States until they disbanded at the end of the 1955 season. F-86Ds used by the team included: 52-3678, '730, '692 and '697.

While the USAFE *Skyblazers* were flying F-86F Sabres from Chaumont, France, a lesser-known team was formed in 1956 at nearby Laon Air Base. This team is worthy of mention, as it was the first jet bomber aerobatic team in the world, flying four Martin B-57 Canberras. Called the *Black Knights*, this team was operated by the 38th Bombardment Group (Tactical), the aircraft being gloss black overall with red lettering and scalloping round the nose, engine intakes and on all tail surfaces. Display venues and serial numbers of the B-57s flown by the team are unknown.

As mention has been made of the world's first jet bomber aerobatic team, then it would only be fair to include the world's first four-engine transport aerobatic team, although they were not really aerobatic in the strict sense of the word and were never made official. *The Four Horsemen* were a precision demonstration team, flying four Lockheed C-130A Hercules transport aircraft. In the early days of the C-130's career, four captains with the 463rd Troop Carrier Wing at Ardmore AFB decided to put together a Thunderbird-type demonstration. The four pilots were Capts. Hubert (Gene) Chaney, James Akin, David Moore and William Hatfield. The Herk quartet originally called themselves the *Thunderweasels*, but soon changed to *The Four Horsemen*, giving demonstrations in the U.S.A., Denmark and Japan. With aircraft each weighing 100,000 pounds, the team performed a series of elaborate and precisely-executed manoeuvres that left veteran transport pilots shaking their head in wonder! There were four basic formations for the quartet — 'Diamond', 'Arrowhead', 'Arrow' (line-astern) and 'Echelon', the display culminating in a 'bomb-burst', which was actually a horizontal break rather than a loop and break! While the wingmen broke sharply to left and right, the 'slot' position pulled up steeply at 45 degrees. When the 463rd Wing moved to Sewart AFB, Tennessee, in late 1959, the team continued performing. However, in the Spring of 1960, due to pressure of airlift duties, the USAF denied permission for the team to become official and they disbanded.

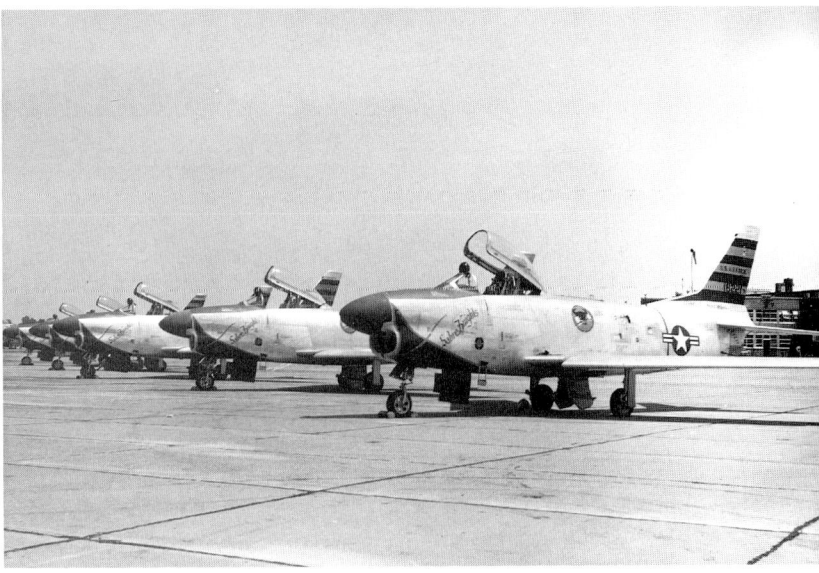

Above: N.A. F-86D Sabres of the 325 FIS *Sabre Knights* team in 1954. (David W. Menard)

Below: A quartet of F-86A Sabres of the *Sabre Dancers* team from 94 FS, Oxnard Air Force Base, California in 1954. (US Air Force)

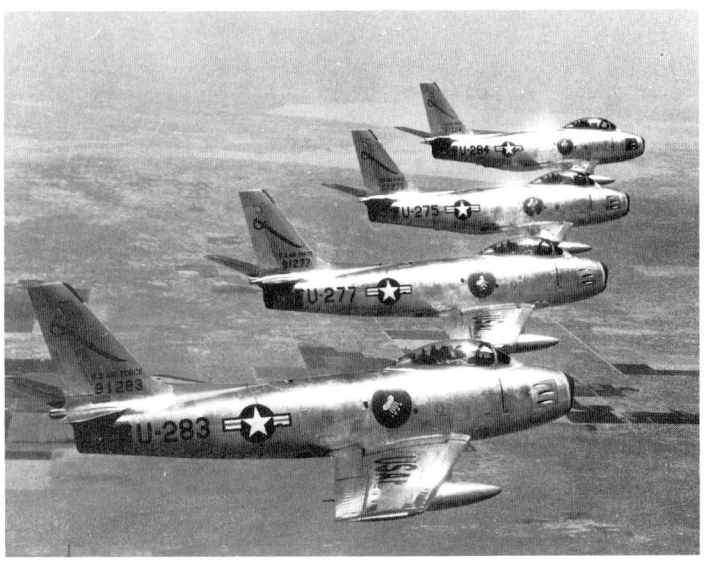

UNITED STATES NAVY
The First Display Teams

1928: VB-2B Squadron, "Three Sea Hawks", NAS North Island

The *Three Sea Hawks* were the first U.S. Navy demonstration team and were formed early in 1928 at NAS North Island, San Diego, California. Lieutenant D. W. Tomlinson, then Commanding VB-2B squadron, saw the need for a team for public relations and recruiting. Flying Boeing F2Bs-2s, the *Three Sea Hawks* gave their first public performance at Mines Field (now Los Angeles International Airport) during the National Air Races, 8-16 September 1928. Like the R.A.F., they flew many tied-together manoeuvres and performed before 100,000 spectators. In order to permit the Boeing F2B-1 to fly inverted without the engine cutting out, the carburettors were modified, so they could fly inverted indefinitely or until the oil pressure started dropping. The team participated in shows primarily along the west coast, including Seattle and San Francisco. The *Three Sea Hawks* represented the Navy until late in 1929, when all three pilots were posted to other units.

Below: The first *Blue Angels* flying Grumman F-6F Hellcats in 1946 and led by Lt. Cdr. R. 'Butch' Voris. (US Navy)

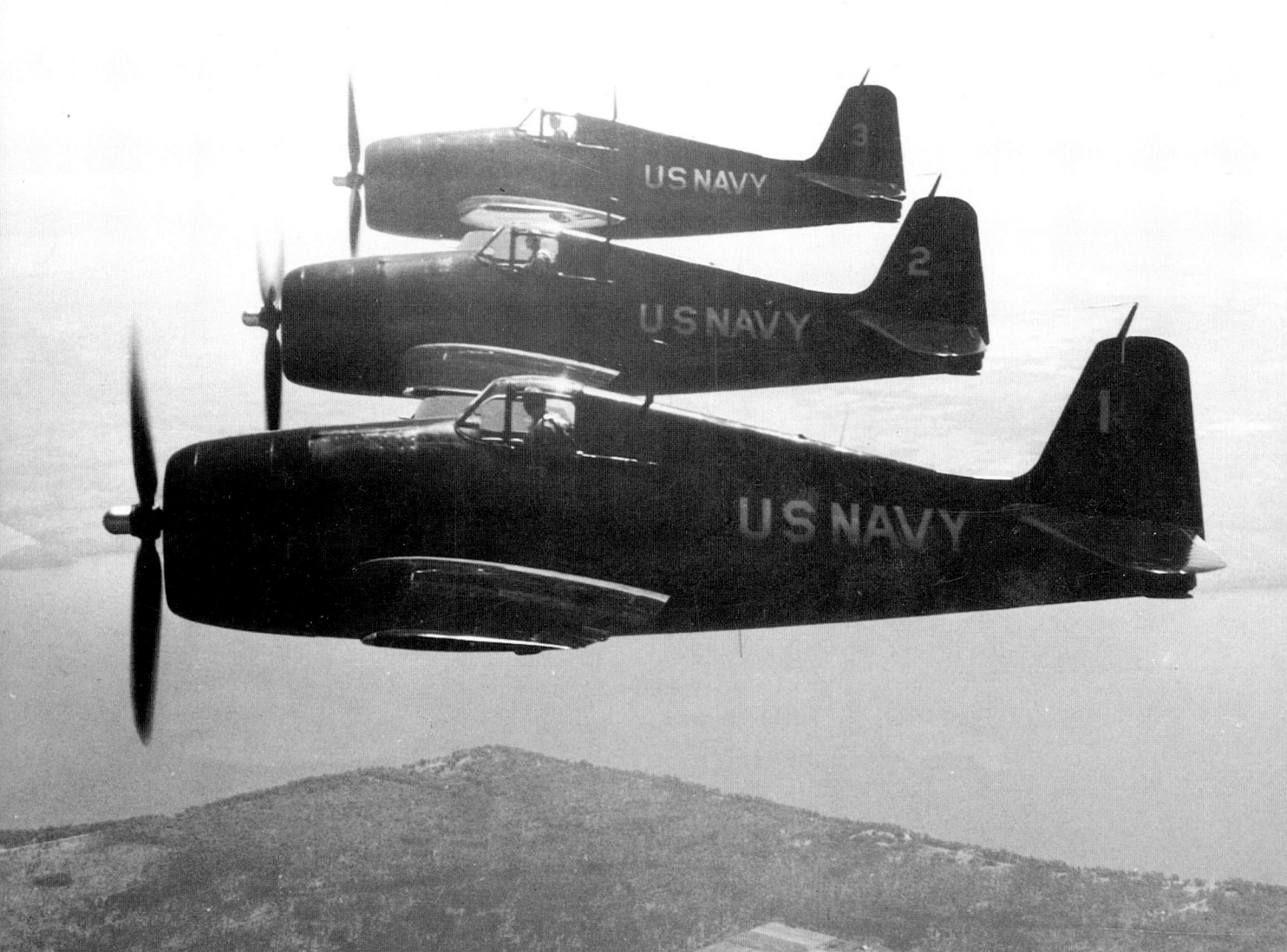

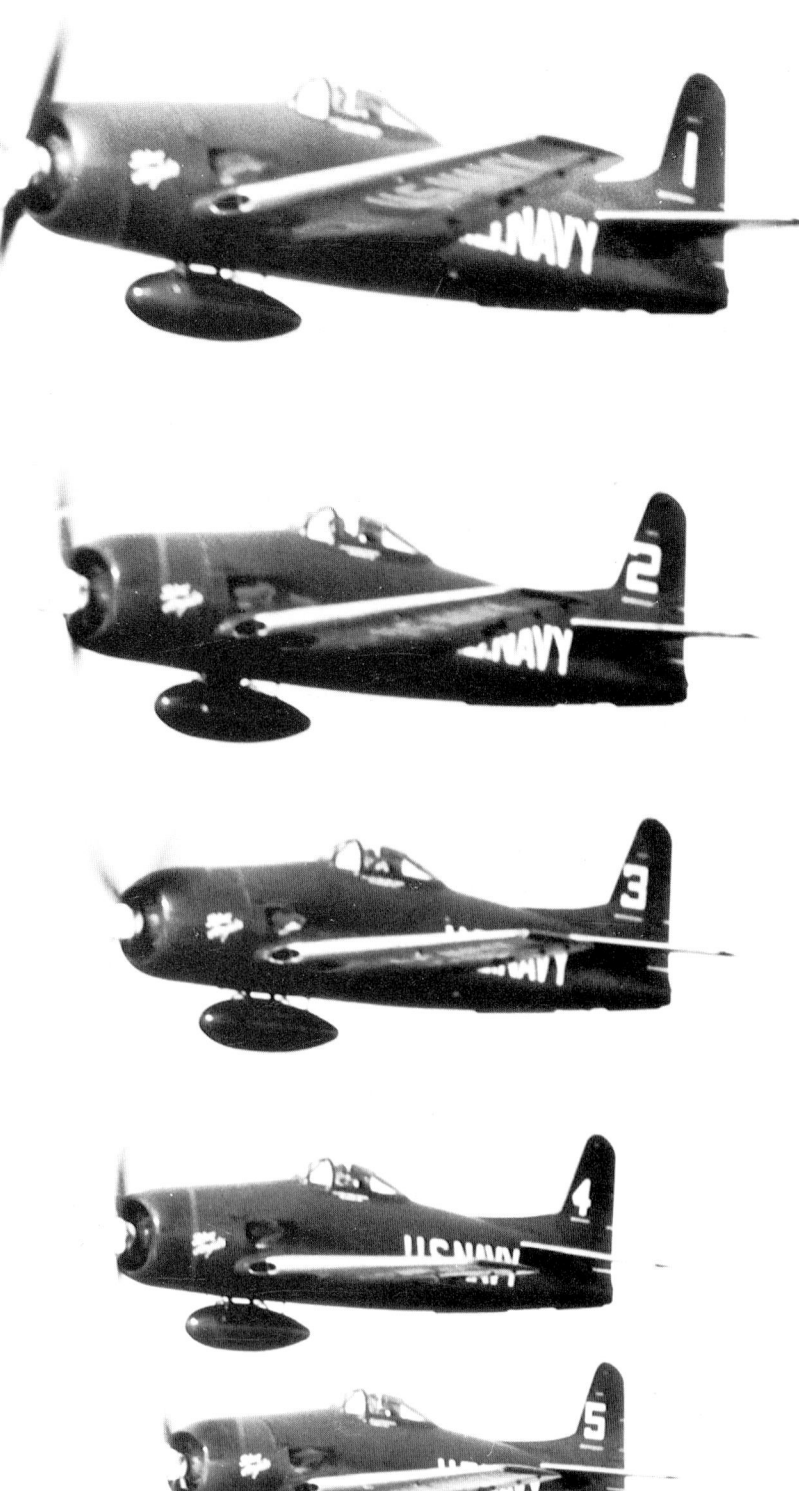

1929: VF-18 Squadron, the "High Hatters", USS "Saratoga"

This team existed briefly during the late 1920s and early 1930s and was formed within VF-1B squadron aboard USS *Saratoga*. Again the Boeing F2B-1 was used, of which three were led by Lieutenant L. E. Gehres. Different sections within the squadron were given the task of providing demonstrations by the *High Hatters*, so several pilots and aircraft were used during their display. The team also carried out tied-together demonstrations with nine aircraft, three flights of three being linked together with thirty feet of cord. The *High Hatters* were disbanded in the early 1930s, when the fleet squadrons underwent a major reorganisation.

Above: The second type used by the *Blue Angels* was the F-8F Bearcat during 1947-48. (US Navy)

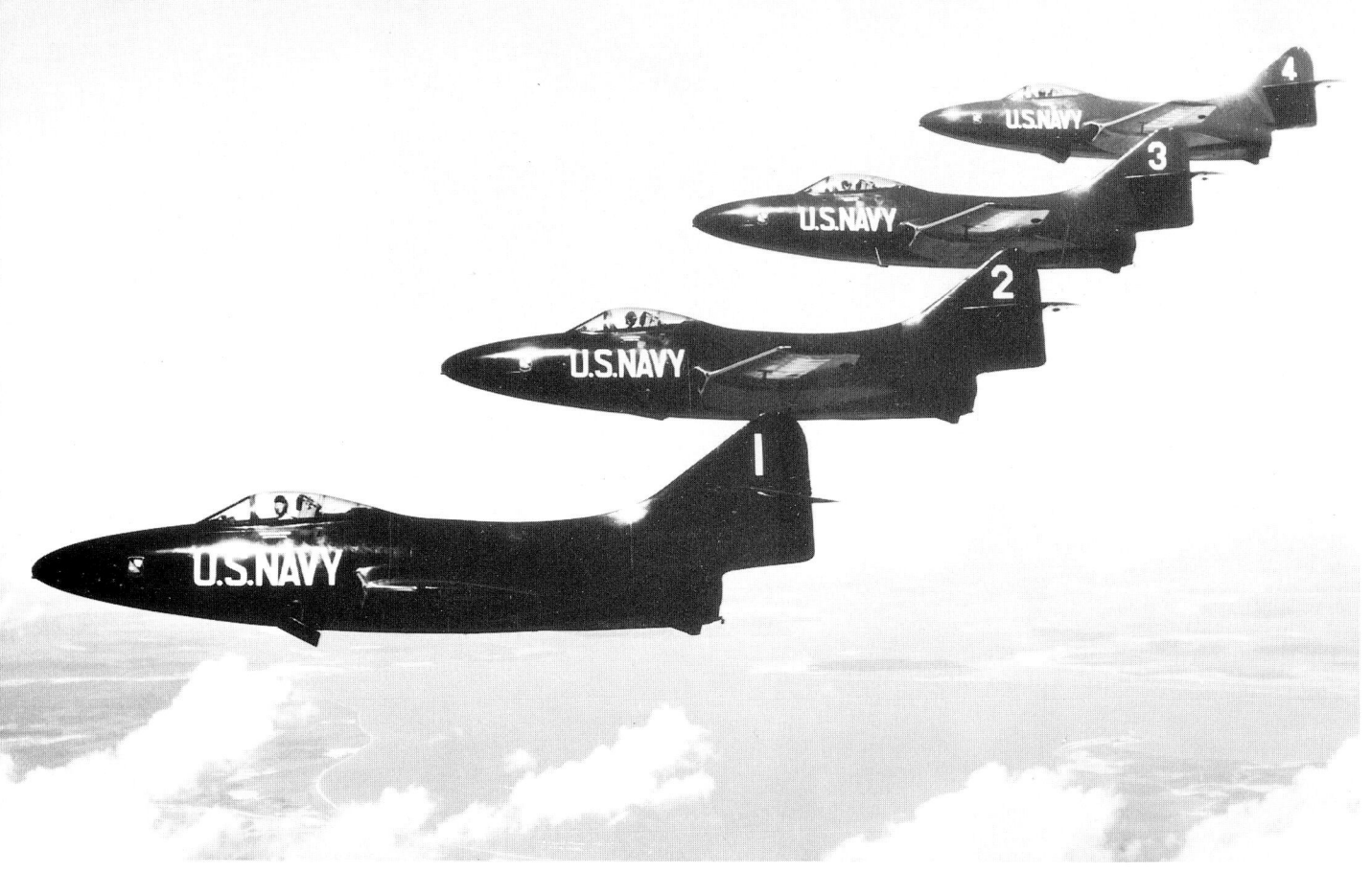

Above: Grumman F9F-2 Panthers were operated by the *Blue Angels* during 1949-50. (Grumman Aerospace Corp.)

1930: Naval Flight Test Group, "Three Flying Fish", NAS Anacosta

This team was formed in the spring of 1930 at NAS Anacosta, on the east coast. The Tactical Section of the Naval Flight Test Group provided this team, which flew three Curtiss F6C-4s, being flown by Lieutentants Gardner, Storrs and Trapnell. The aircraft also had to have their engines modified to allow extended inverted flight. This team participated in many displays including the Cleveland Air Races in August 1930 and disbanded in April 1931.

Early 1930s: Training Squadron 5 (VN-5D8) "Three T'Gallant'ls", NAS Pensacola

Yet another team which only existed for a brief period were the *Three T'Gallant'ls* flying Curtiss F6C-4s again. They were formed during the early 1930s within Training Squadron 5 (VN-5D8) at NAS Pensacola, Florida. The pilots were squadron instructors and the team flew demonstrations mainly at naval establishments until 1931 when they converted to the Boeing F4B-1. After another two years on this type, the team disbanded. These are the only known teams of the 1930s, which usually only flew for special ceremonies and naval occasions, but kept the early age of aerobatic teams alive. There were several un-named teams around this period, including a flight of six Curtiss F7C-1s flown by Marine pilots in August 1930. After the war, another U.S. Navy flight demonstration team appeared in 1946 — the famous *Blue Angels*. However, during the early years of this team, there were two other teams formed.

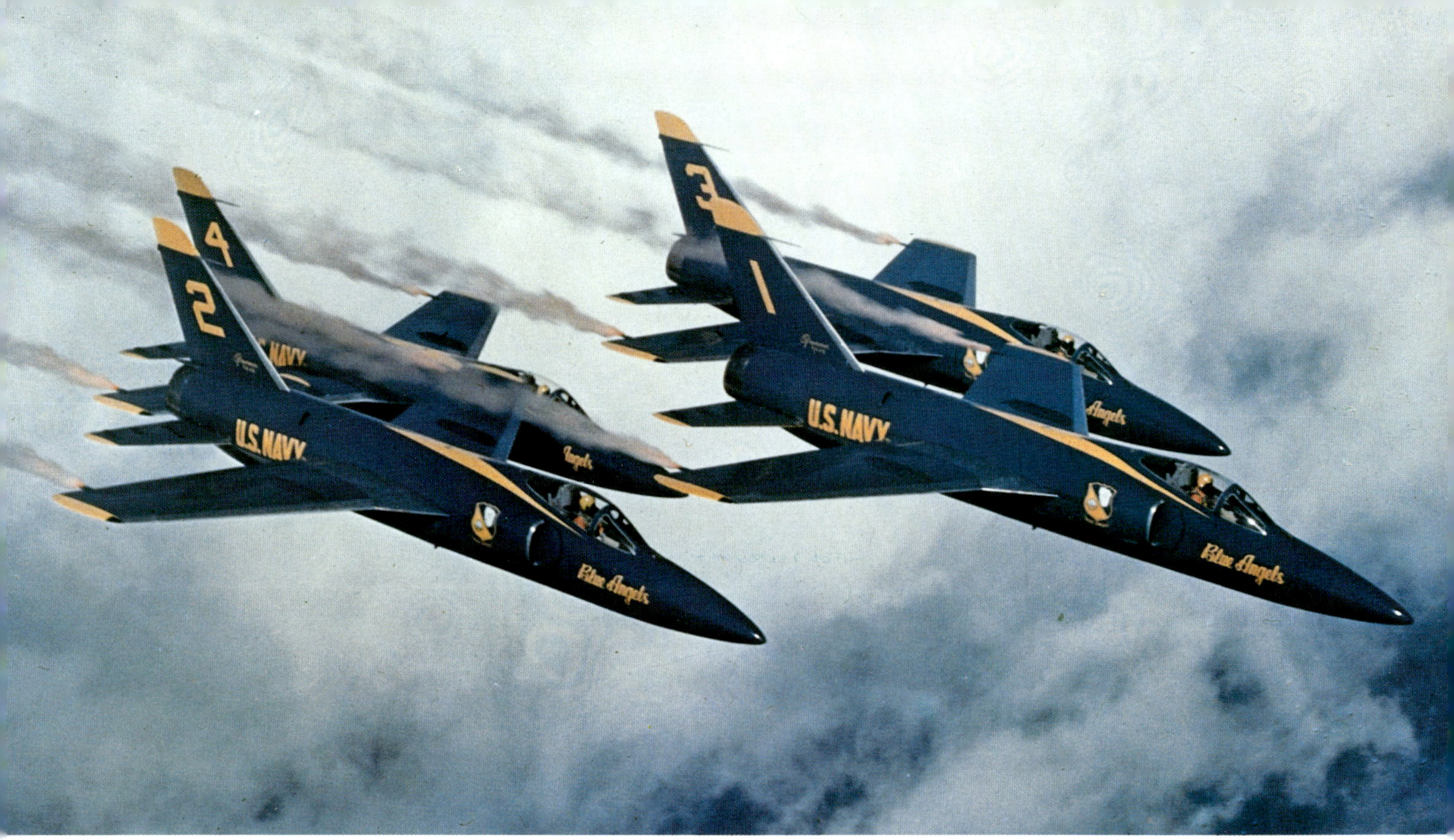

1948: The "Gray Angels"
This team only existed for the one season during 1948 and was set up to demonstrate the Navy's latest jet, the FH-1 Phantom, of which the team comprised three. The pilots were all Rear Admirals on active duty at the time, being Rear Admirals Dan V. Gallery, Edgar A. Cruise and Apollo Soucek. The first display was at Idlewild Airport, New York on 31 July 1948. Due to their popularity, the team continued to appear at numerous air shows, primarily in the mid-west and east. For many spectators, this was their first sight of a jet aircraft, so caused a lot of attention after the years of piston-engined aircraft. The team was never made official and was disbanded towards the end of 1948.

1949: U.S. Marine Corps, "Marine Phantoms", Cherry Point MCAS
This team was formed within VMF-122 Marine Corps Squadron at Cherry Point, North Carolina, early in 1949. It was organised and led by Lieutenant-Colonel Marion E. Carl, who was later relieved by Major Loren 'Doc' Everton. VMF-122 was the first Marine Squadron to be equipped with jet aircraft, the McDonnell FH-1 Phantom, of which 12 were assigned. However, the aerobatic team only comprised five of these aircraft at any one show. During 1949, the team took part in a major tour, which included the Cleveland National Air Races. One of their last official shows was on 15 May 1950 for the Aviation Writers Association. The team was disbanded mid-1950, when VMF-122 converted to the McDonnell F2H-1 Banshee and were involved in the war in Korea. Colour scheme was overall midnite blue with white 'LC' codes on the fin and large position numbers under the cockpit. These markings were replaced during the 1949 season, with an overall midnite scheme again, but with yellow nose, wingtips and tail trim. No codes were carried, one of the aircraft in this scheme being serial number '111785'. 'U.S. Marines' in white appeared on the nose in fairly small lettering.

Above: The long-nosed Grumman F-11A Tigers, which served with the *Blue Angels* from 1959 to 1968.
(Grumman Aerospace Corp.)

The current mount of the *Blue Angels* is the A-4F Skyhawk, which has served with the team since 1974.
(US Navy)

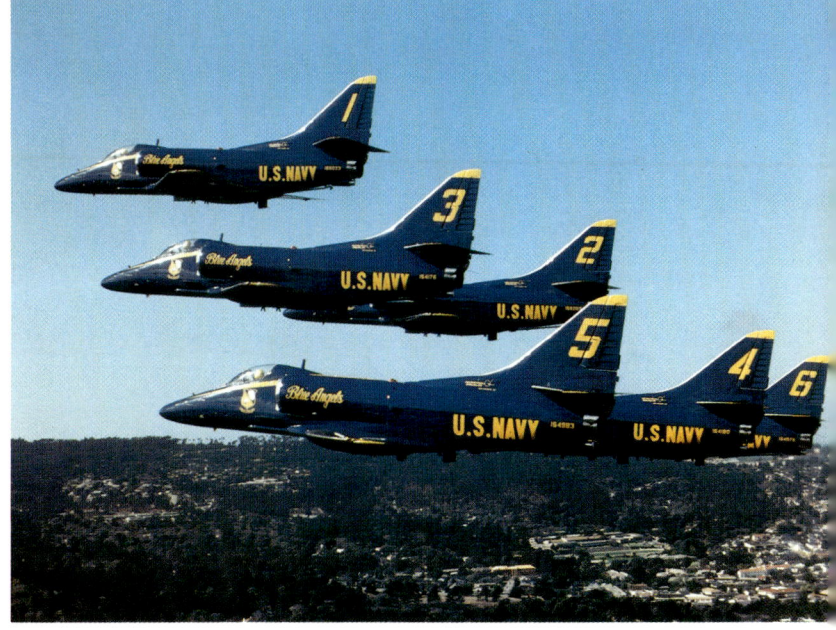

125

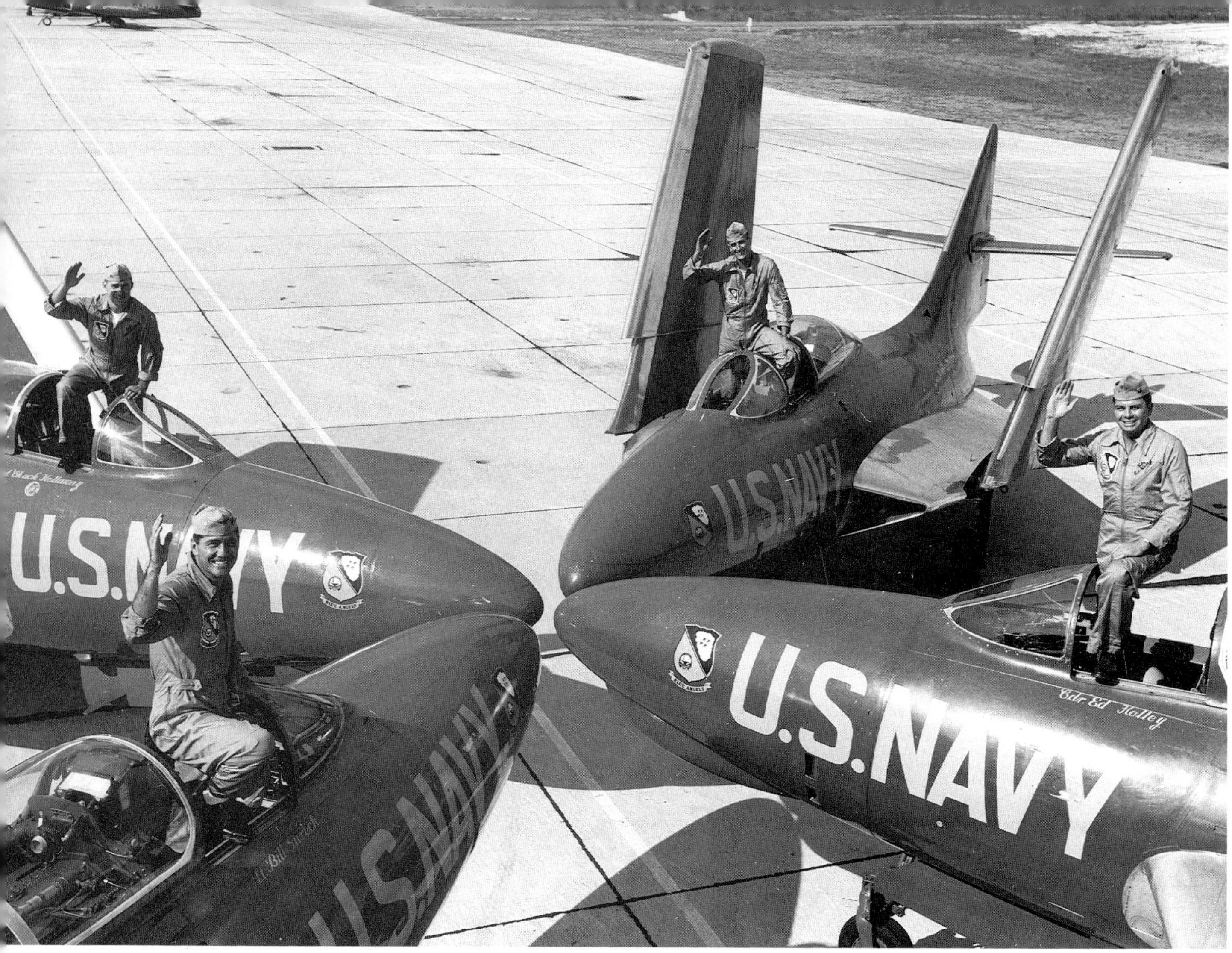

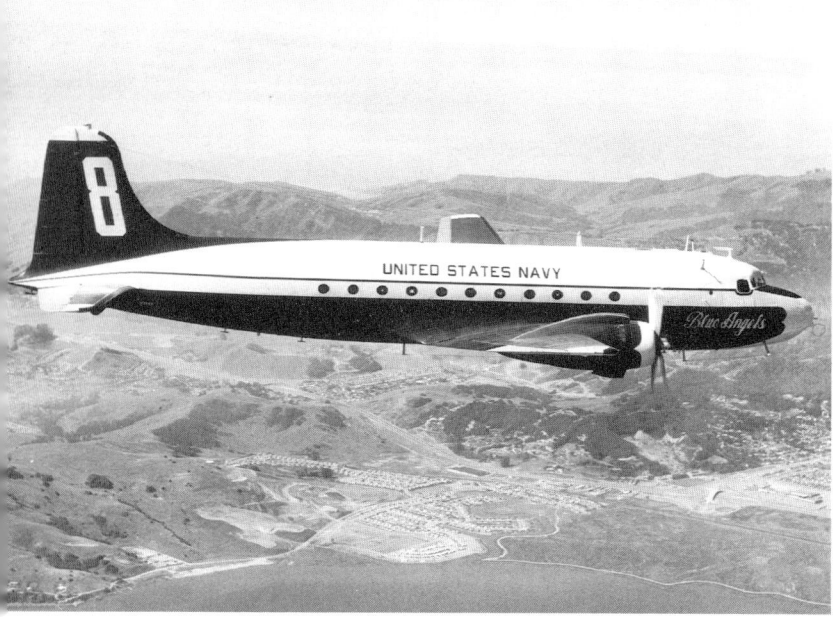

1946-to date: U.S. Navy Flight Demonstration Team, "The Blue Angels", Pensacola NAS, Florida.
The *Blue Angels*, officially known as the U.S. Navy Flight Demonstration Team, have over the thirty-five years since their organisation, earned world-wide fame.

In June 1946, a Flight Exhibition Team within the Naval Air Advanced Training Command was organised and directed by the Chief of Naval Operations. Lieutenant Commander Roy M. "Butch" Voris was selected to organise and lead the Team, which completed its first public performance flying Grumman F6F Hellcats at the Southeastern Air Show on 15 and 16 June. Their routine was most enthusiastically received by the public. There were four Hellcats on the original team, doing a very warlike routine. They would 'shoot down' an SNJ Texan painted as a Mitsubishi Zero, which descended trailing smoke and parachuted a dummy pilot who was promptly captured by a detachment of Marines. Most of these manoeuvres were done in tight formation, which became the basis for the present team's performance of aerial manoeuvres in thrilling combinations of high speed and close formation. They also evolved the *Blue Angels* famous 'Diamond' formation which is now their trademark. Operating from Jacksonville, Florida the *Blue Angels* would take a fourth Hellcat to shows, as a spare. It was not long before this aircraft started being used for solo performances. When they were first formed, the team didn't have a name, but by late July 1946, they became known as the *Lancers*. Within a month, a new name — the *Blue Angels* — had replaced it.

Above: Douglas C-54Q, 50868, was used by the *Blue Angels* from 1957 to '65. It carried the full team colours of blue, yellow and white. (Grumman Aerospace Corp.)

Top: Cmdr. Cormier and team pose with their Grumman F9F-8 Cougars during 1956-57 winter training. Note the narrator's TV-2 in the background. (Grumman Aerospace Corp.)

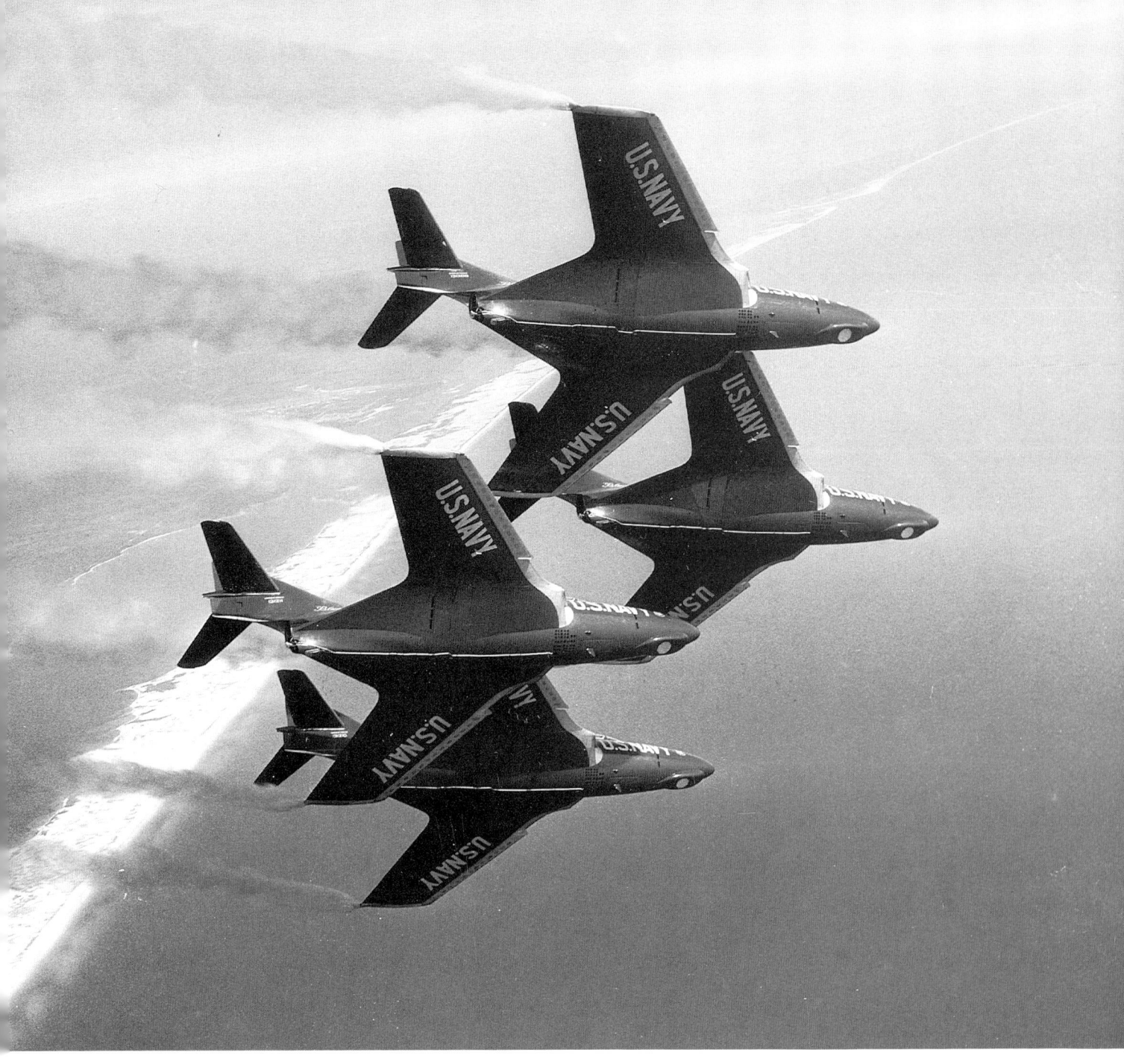

The *Blue Angels* operated Grumman F9F-8B Cougars during 1955-57. These aircraft are seen making smoke from wingtip generators. (Grumman Aerospace Corp)

In August 1946, a newer, faster machine was assigned to the *Blue Angels*, the F8F-1 Bearcat. Also manufactured by Grumman, it had a four-bladed prop and produced a 2,100 hp thrust which allowed speeds in excess of 450 mph. By mid-1947, there were changes in personnel and procedures, which produced an air show different from those in the first year. Lieutenant Commander Robert Clarke took over as leader in 1947 and he was relieved by Lieutenant Commander 'Dusty' Rhodes in January 1948, who led the team through the transition into jet aircraft in the summer of 1949. November 1948 saw the team move from NAS Jacksonville to NAS Corpus Christi, Texas.

In August 1949, the F8F Bearcats were replaced by the team's first jet aircraft, the Grumman F9F-2 Panther. Various adjustments in the type, timing and sequence were required. With the introduction of the jet, the *Blue Angels* association with the piston-engined plane was over, but never to be forgotten. The F6Fs and F8Fs had recorded more than 300 shows before some 12 million spectators.

127

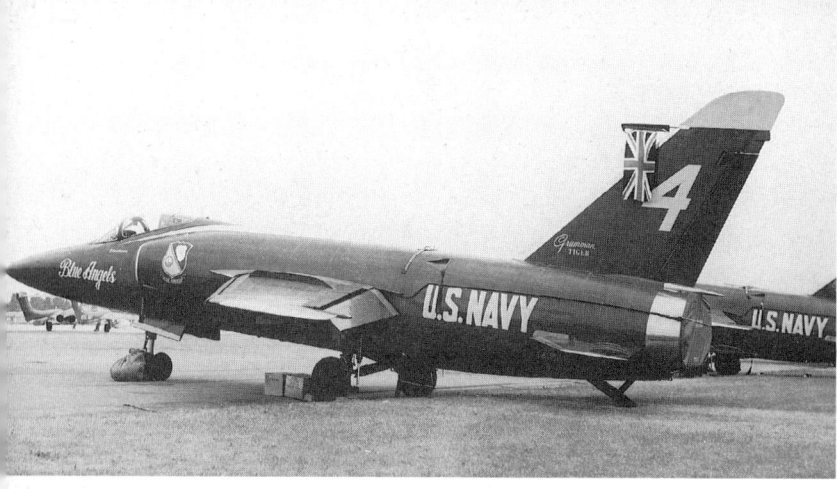

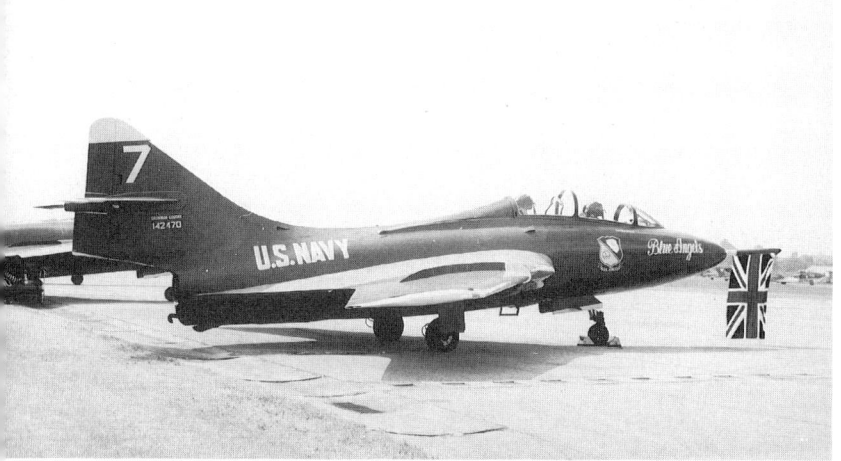

The US Navy's *Blue Angels* during their 1965 European Tour. Seen at RNAS Yeovilton in July 1965 are (top to bottom):

Grumman F-11A Tiger, 141849 '4'. Note smoke-making pipe down rear fuselage. (Peter R. March).

Grumman F9F-8T Cougar, 142470 '7', used by the narrator. It was the policy of the team to decorate their aircraft with the flag of the country visited. (Peter R. March)

The second Douglas C-54Q support aircraft used by the *Blue Angels* was serialled 91996. Note the huge flagpole on the roof, behind the cockpit. (Peter R. March)

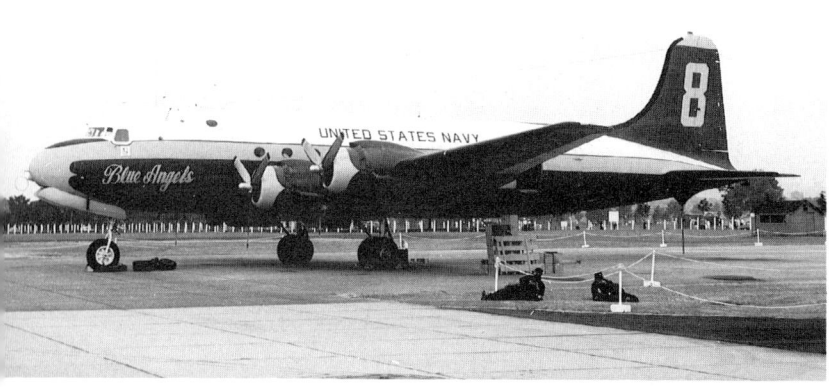

The Panthers were painted a special *Blue Angels* blue colour with polished metal wing leading edges and yellow lettering. *The Blues* introduced their new jets to the public for the first time at Beaumont, Texas, on 20 August 1949. The following month, the team changed its base again, moving to NAS Whiting Field near Pensacola, Florida. Lieutenant Commander Johnny Magda took over as leader early in 1950. The Grumman Panthers took part in twenty-four more shows, after which they gave their last display on 30 July at NAS Dallas. The outbreak of war in Korea disrupted the team's formation and in June 1950 the *Blue Angels* were ordered to duty in a combat status aboard the Aircraft Carrier USS *Princeton* as the nucleus of Fighter Squadron 191. Lieutenant Commander Johnny Magda, then Commanding Officer of the squadron, was the only *Blue Angel* ever to lose his life in combat when he was shot down off Korea's northeast coast in March 1951. During the period 1946 to 1950, the team had been seen by more than 14 million people in some 380 demonstrations.

In late 1951, seeing a recurring need for a demonstration team, the Chief of Naval Operations ordered the *Blue Angels* reactivation and Lieutenant Commander "Butch" Voris was again given the job of organising the team at NAS Corpus Christi, Texas. With new aircraft, the Grumman F9F-5 Panther — a later and faster version — and a group of highly skilled enlisted personnel, the team underwent a strenuous practice period in readiness for the coming schedule. The first public showing by the new team took place at the Memphis Mid-South Navy Festival in May 1952. In addition to seven F9F-5 Panthers, the *Blue Angels* were also assigned two F7U-1 Cutlasses and one F8F Bearcat. The two Cutlasses were to be used as solo demonstrators, but only participated in two air shows as they proved to be an excessive maintenance problem and were dropped from the team. The F8F Bearcat was a support aircraft and painted yellow overall, being named 'Beetle Bomb'.

The 1953 season began with Commander Voris being replaced as leader by Lieutenant Commander Ray Hawkins. In mid 1956, the F9F-5 Panthers were replaced by the F9F-6 version. However, problems developed with this version, so the team reverted to the F9F-5. Lieutenant Commander Zeke Cormier took over as leader in February 1954 and the team continued flying the Panther until the end of the 1954 season.

The *Blue Angels* changed to the swept-wing Grumman F9F-8 Cougar in January 1955 and new manoeuvres were developed including tight formations with wings overlapped and the 'Fleur-de-lis' performed at the end of their 25-minute show. In June 1955 the team moved base again from Corpus Christi to Pensacola NAS, Florida, home of Naval Air Training Command. This was their last move to date, as they have been based there ever since. Commander Edward Holley took over as leader in 1956 and during the 1957-58 seasons 3½ million spectators saw the team at air shows across the nation, with many million more seeing them on films and television.

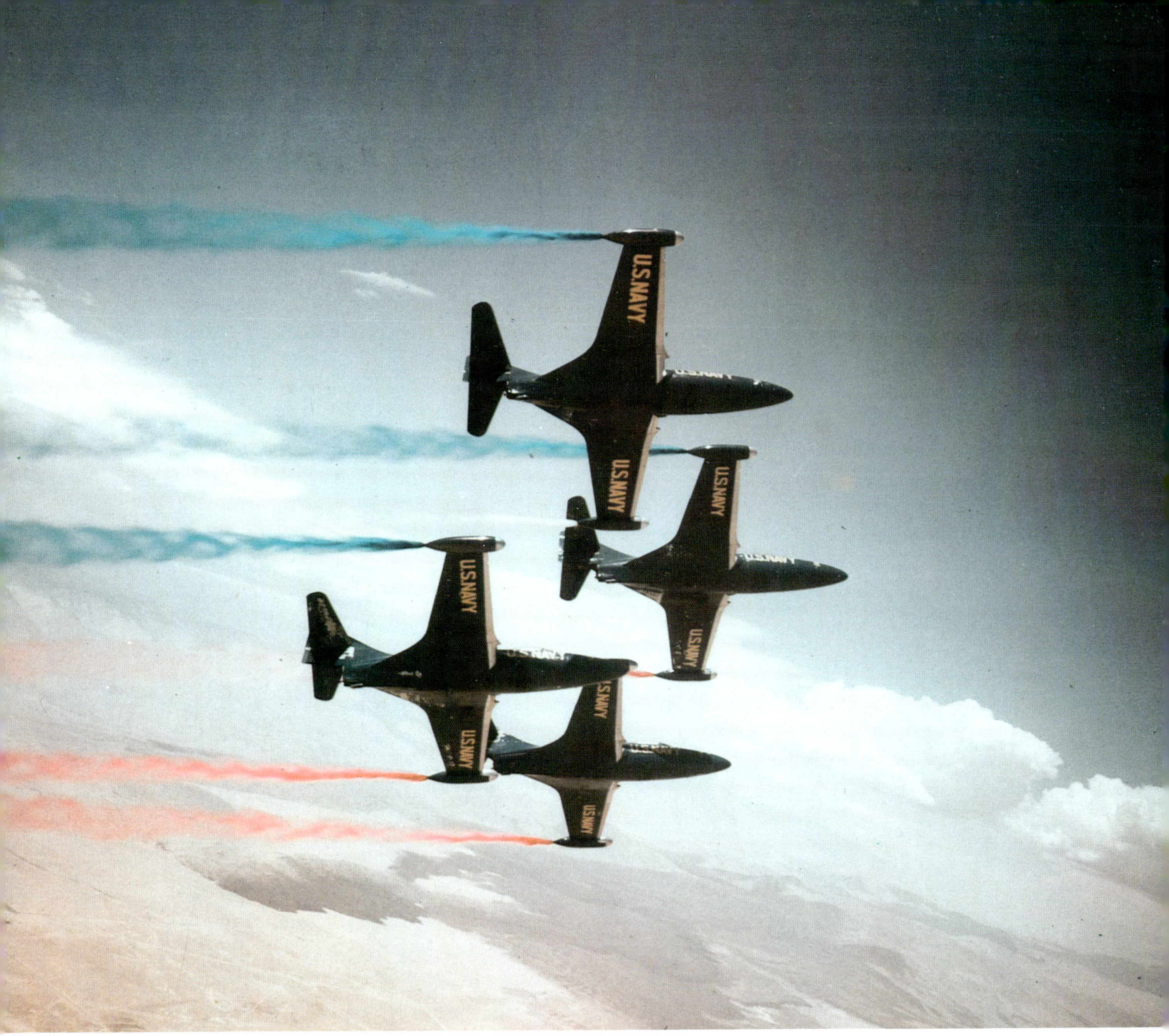

After 2½ years with the team, the F9F-8 Cougar was replaced by the F11F-1 Tiger, which came from the same Grumman stable. The change came in mid-1957 and this was the *Blue's* first supersonic jet aircraft. The first Tigers used by the team were the short-nosed version, which served from May 1957 until the end of the 1958 season. The long-nosed version served with the team from 1959 to the end of the 1968 season. In 1959 the team, now led by Commander Zeb Knott, added Bermuda to its overseas display sites as they performed there before 25,000 spectators, including the Duke of Edinburgh. Under the leadership of Commander Ken Wallace during the 1962-63 seasons, more intricate manoeuvres were added and the team made their 1000th performance at NAS Lemoore, California in 1963. On 3 January 1964, Commander Bob Aumack relieved Lieutenant Commander Ken Wallace as leader of the *Blue Angels* and went on to lead the team in 75 shows before 4½ million spectators, boosting the total attendance to an estimated 76½ million spectators since 1946. The *Blues* continued their overseas visits in 1965 with a spring Caribbean trip, followed by a 25-day European tour taking in displays at Paris, France and Yeovilton, England. In the autumn,

Above: Grumman F9F-5 Panthers of the 1952 *Blue Angels* trailing coloured smoke from their tip tanks. (Grumman Aerospace Corp.)

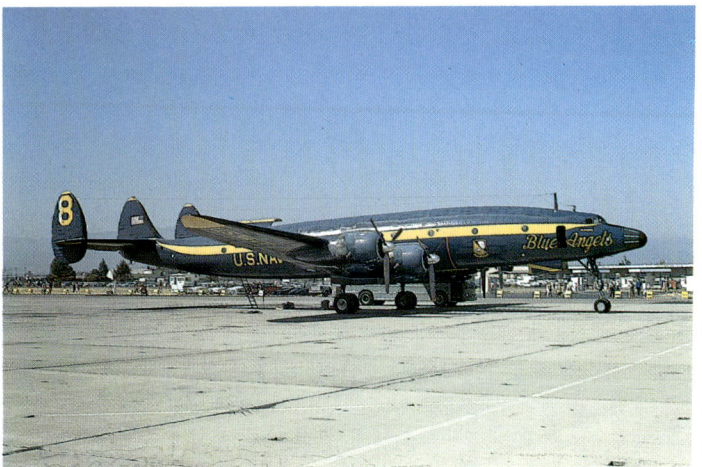

Lockheed C-121J Constellation, 131623, was used as support aircraft by the *Blue Angels* during 1968-70. It is seen here at Moffett Field, California in August 1969. (Author's collection).

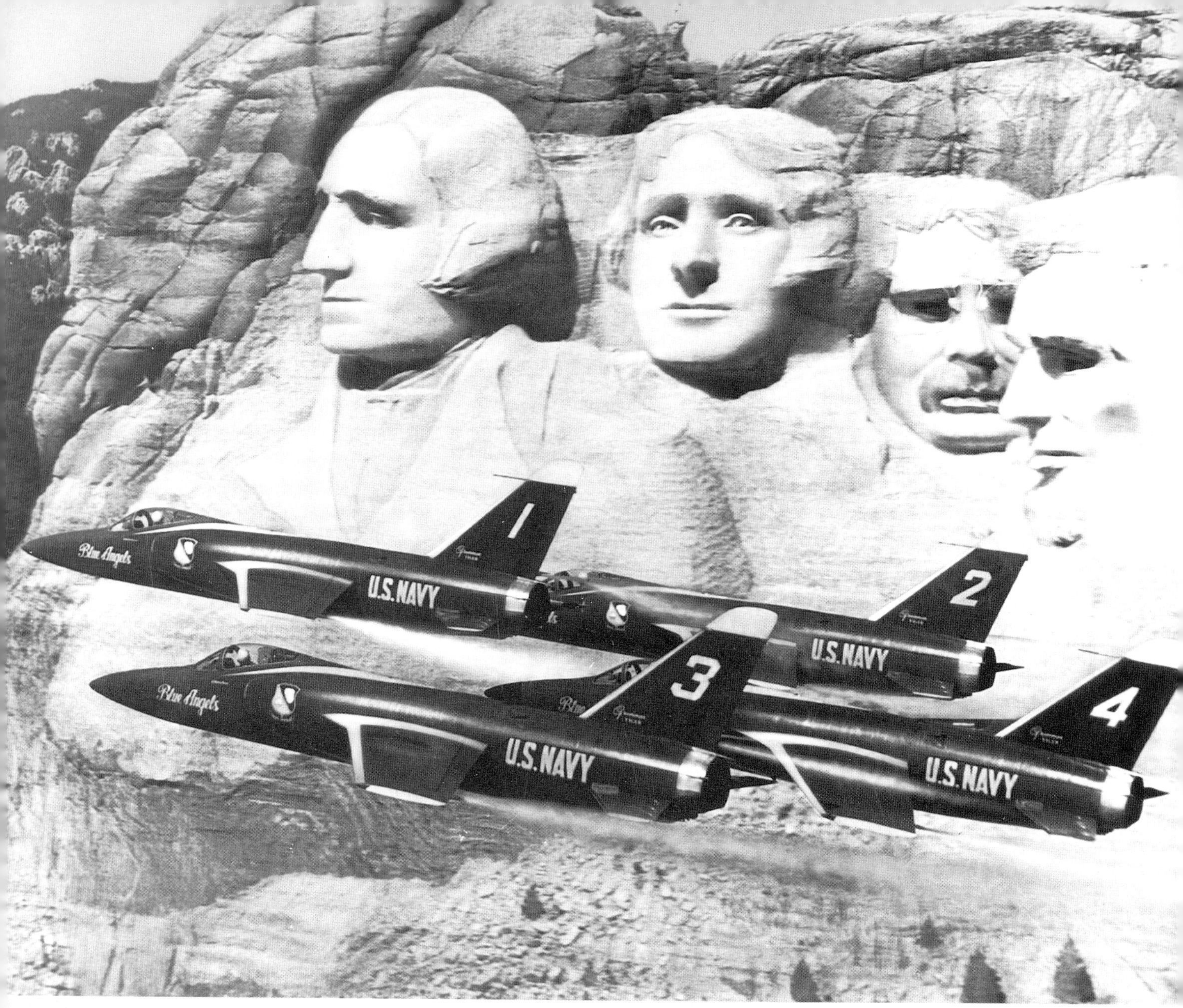

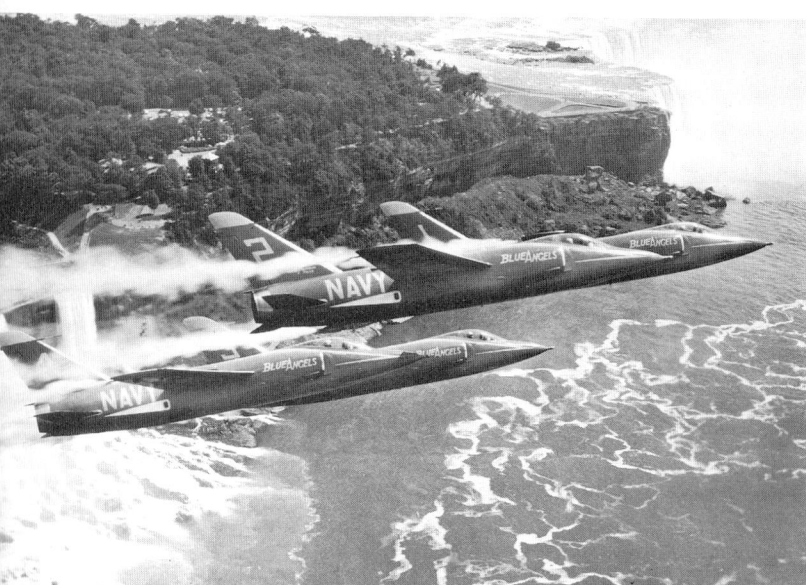

Above: The earlier short-nosed F-11F-1 Tigers seen over Niagara Falls in 1957. (Grumman Aerospace Corp)

Top: The *Blue Angels* F-11A Tigers flying by Mount Rushmore in 1964. (U.S. Navy)

they deployed to the Bahamas, where they flew two shows before 25,000 spectators. Commander Bill Wheat assumed command early in 1967 and took the team on another European tour in mid-May with shows in Italy, Tunisia, Turkey and France. In August of the same year, they flew three shows in Canada and continued flying the Grumman Tiger until the end of the 1968 season. This was the end of an era, as the next type of aircraft to be used was not a 'cat' from Grumman. Many were nostalgic about the long association with Grumman, but wouldn't stand in the way of progress.

In December 1968, the *Blue Angels* took delivery of their McDonnell F-4J Phantoms to replace the Tigers. Modifications had to be made to the Phantoms, which included ballast weight substituting the fire control system, VHF radio additions, afterburner modifications and the addition of dummy Sparrow missiles. The forward missiles carried oil and those in the rear were fitted with smoke dye. 1969 was the first season with the Phantom, with Commander Bill Wheat continuing to lead the team. Commander Harley Hall took over as leader in 1970 and the team participated in displays in Puerto Rico, Panama, Ecuador and Hawaii, as well as performances in the United States and Canada. The team celebrated their 25th anniversary the following year with 94 air shows.

From 21 October to 25 November, their first Far East tour took them to Korea, Japan, Taiwan, the Philippines and Guam. Commander Don Bently led the *Blues* through the 1972 season and into 1973, but a non-fatal accident caused him to relinquish his position to Lieutenant Commander Skip Umstead in April. The team made another European tour in 1973, which took in shows in England, France, Spain, Turkey, Iran and Italy. A tragic accident occurred at Lakehurst, New Jersey on July 26, when Lieutenant Commander Umstead, Captain Mike Murphy and his Crew Chief were all killed. The team immediately cancelled the rest of its shows for the season. The Phantom had been with the team for five years, but it was a thirsty aircraft and expensive to maintain, so it was decided to transition to a more economical aircraft for the 1974 season. The Phantom had been an impressive aircraft, but McDonnell-Douglas were to provide another fine and worthy successor — the A-4F Skyhawk.

Commander Tony Less took over as leader and the A-4F Skyhawks underwent several modifications in preparation for aerobatics. On 18 May, the *Blue Angels* made their first public appearance with their new planes at Omaha, Nebraska. They performed 52 displays during the 1974 season, with 69 the following year. 1976 was the bicentennial year and Commander Tony Less was replaced by Commander Casey Jones, who led the team through 80 displays. On 8 October 1977, the *Blue Angels* flew their 2,000th performance at NAS Atlanta, Georgia. Commander Bill Newman joined the team in 1978 as the *Blues* 17th Commander/leader and 75 shows were recorded in the U.S.A. and Canada. Tragedy struck again in 1978, when Lieutenant Mike Curtain, No.6 Solo, was making a high speed rolling pass down Miramar's runway, his aircraft struck the ground and disintegrated. This was the *Blues* first fatal accident with the Skyhawk. Commander Newman led the team through the 1979 season, but was relieved by Commander Denis Wisely in October. He took the *Blue Angels* through the 1980 and '81 seasons giving performances all over the United States and in Canada. A change of leader came once again in 1982, when Commander Dave Carroll led the *Blue Angels* through nearly 80 performances. Leaders and team members come and go, but the *Blue Angels* have now flown the Skyhawk for more than ten years, so must be due for an aircraft type change soon, although nothing has been announced.

The team leader for 1985 was Commander Larry 'Hoss' Pearson. A European tour had been planned for July-August 1985, but this had to be cancelled on economy grounds. It is hoped this can be arranged again soon, as a visit to Europe is long overdue.

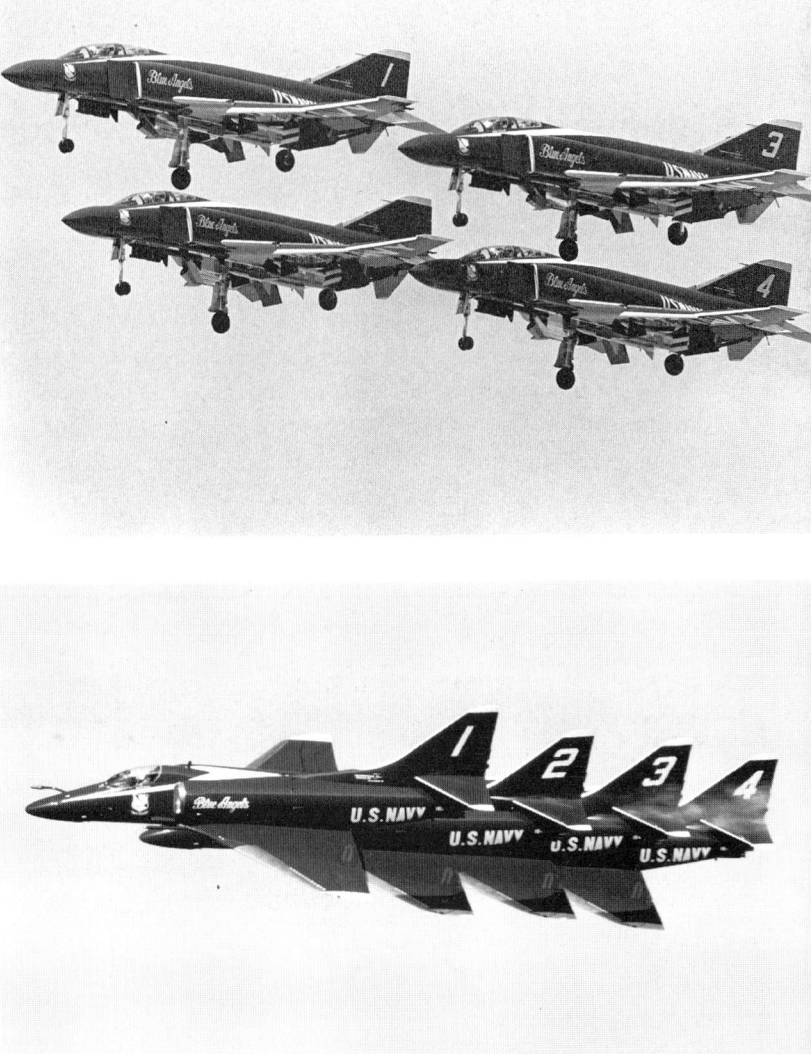

Top Right: McDonnell F-4J Phantoms of the *Blue Angels*, which equipped the team during 1969-73. They are seen here performing at Roosevelt Rhodes, Puerto Rico in March 1970. (U.S. Navy)

Right: No, it's not done with mirrors! This breathtaking shot shows just how close the *Blue Angels* fly with their A-4F Skyhawks on which they are current. (US Navy)

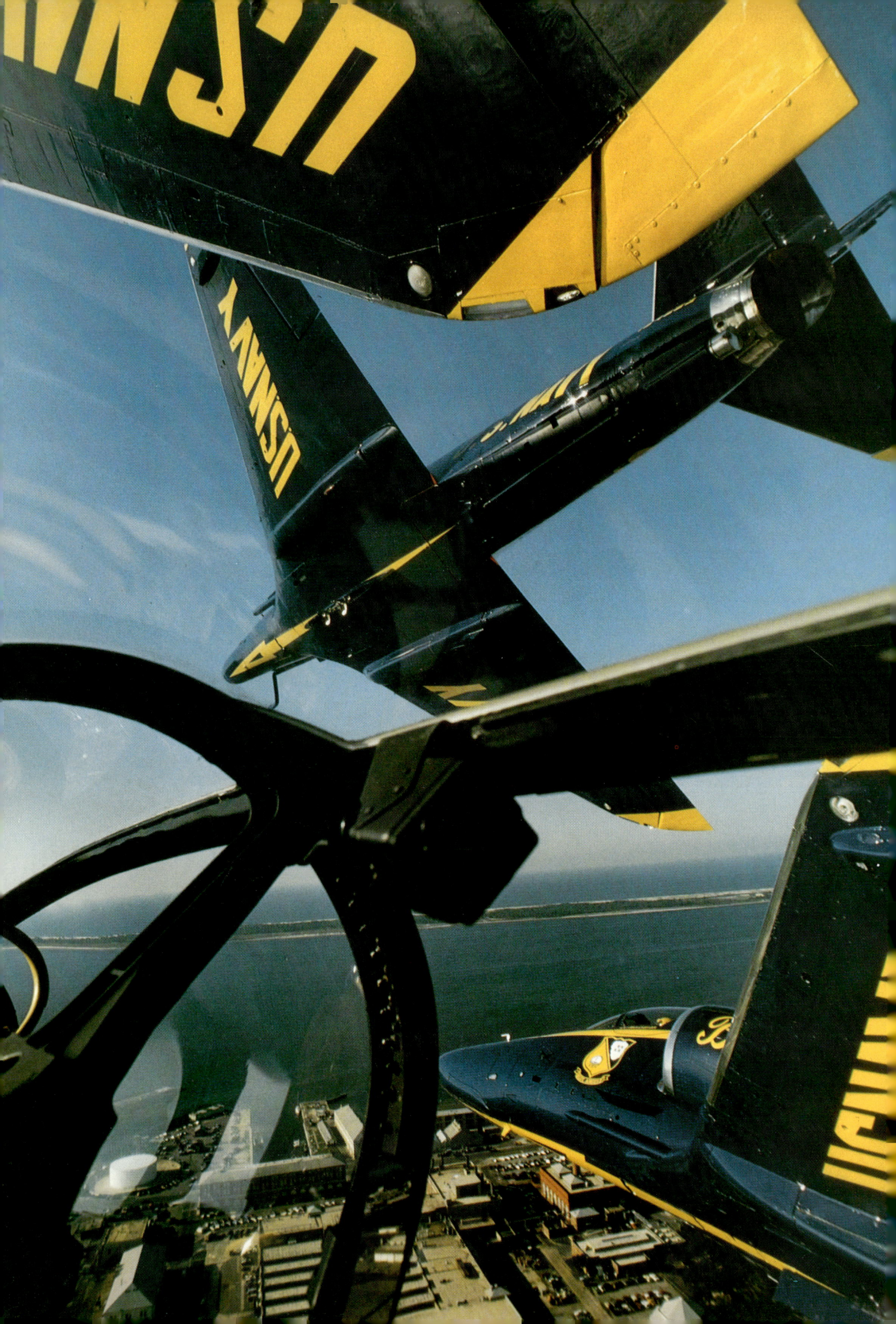

Aircraft used by the "Blue Angels"

1946: Grumman F6F-5 Hellcat — 79049, 79393, 79914, 80097.
1946-50/51/52: Grumman F8F-1C/D Bearcat — 94781, 94880, 94843, 94969, 94985, 94986, 94989, 94990, 94992, 94996, 95000, 95021, 95037, 95124, 95134, 95144 (Beetle Bomb) and 95187.
1949-50: Grumman F9F-2 Panther — 122585, 122587, 122588, 122589, 123016 and 123017.
1952: Chance Vought F7U-1 Cutlass — 124426, 124427.
1952-54: Grumman F9F-5 Panther — 125237, 125239, 125249, 125258, 125278, 125283, 125286, 125294, 125305, 125943, 125989, 125993, 126070, 126071, 126101.
1953: Grumman F9F-6 Cougar — 128080, 128116, 128128, 128129, 128152, 128446.
1955-57: Grumman F9F-8B Cougar — 131099, 131142, 131143, 131147, 131205, 131208, 131210, 131211, 131212, 131213, 138870.
1956: Grumman F9F-8 Cougar — 144279, 144368.
1957-68: Grumman F9F-8T (TF-9J) Cougar — 142470, 147404
1957-58: Grumman F-11F-1 Tiger (short nose) — 138633, 138639, 138640'6', 138641'5', 138642'4', 138643'3', 138644'2', 138645'1', 138647.
1959-68: Grumman F-11A Tiger (long nose) — 141738, 141764, 141765, 141775, 141777, 141790, 141797, 141802, 141811, 141812, 141816, 141823, 141829, 141831, 141837, 141847, 141849, 141850, 141851, 141853, 141859, 141863, 141867, 141868, 141869, 141870, 141871, 141872, 141873, 141874, 141876, 141882, 141883, 141884.
1969-73: McDonnell F-4J Phantom — 153072, 153075, 153076, 153077, 153078, 153079, 153080, 153081, 153082, 153083, 153084, 153085, 153086, 153839.
1974-to date: McDonnell-Douglas A-4F Skyhawk — 154175, 154176, 154177, 154179, 154383, 154904, 154975, 154983, 154984, 154985, 154986, 155029, 155033, 155056, 155502.
TA-4J Skyhawk — 158107, 158722 with 153477 temporarily assigned during 1981

Support Aircraft
1946-1949/54 — SNJ Texan 44008
AT-6 — 91047/112193
1953: Curtiss C-46A Commando, — 39507
1949: Douglas C-47A Skytrain — 17123, 17281
1953: Douglas TC-47K Skytrain — 99838
1953-55: Douglas C-117D — 12437
1957-65/68: Douglas C-54Q Skymaster — 50868/56508
1956: — 90407
1965-67: Douglas C-54Q Skymaster — 91996
1951-56: Lockheed TV-2 SeaStar — 128662, 128676, 137955
1968-70: Lockheed C-121J Constellation — 131623
1970-to date: Lockheed KC-130F Hercules — 149806, 150690

The four North American FJ-3 Furies used for evaluation by the team in 1956 were 141364, 141371, 141375 and 141379.

Opposite: Dramatic 'slot' position among the *Blue Angels'* Skyhawks, photographed from the team's two-seat TA-4J over Pensacola Naval Air Station, Florida in 1984. (US Navy)

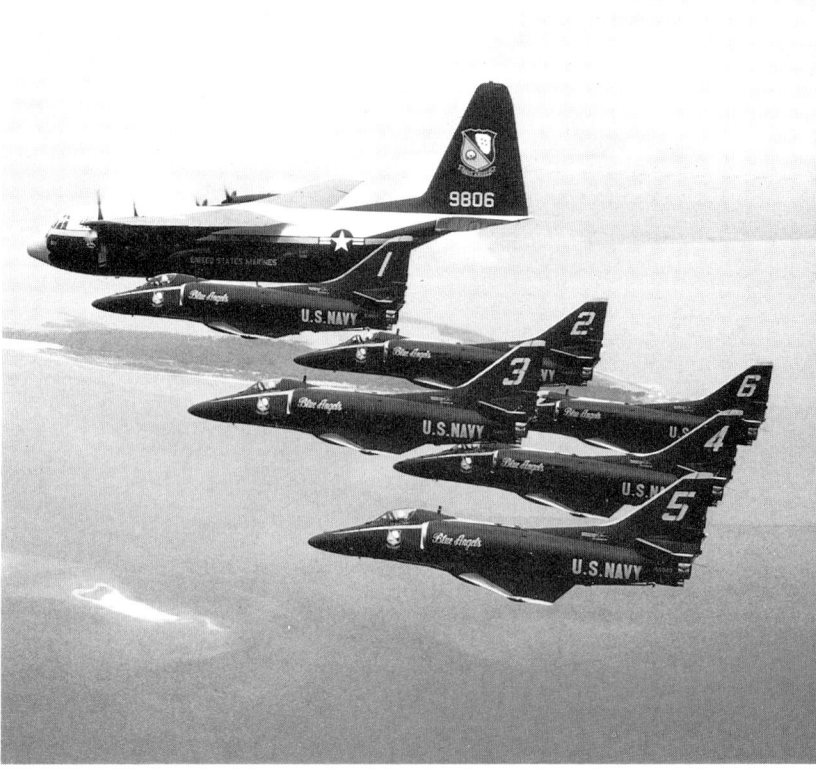

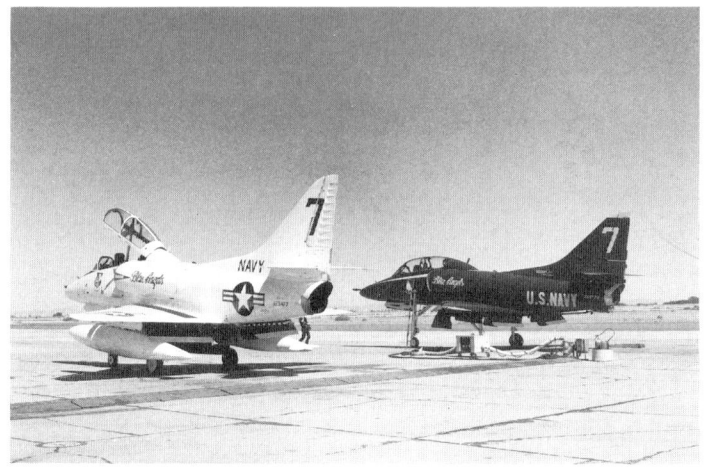

Above: Rare shot showing the *Blue Angels* two-seat TA-4J Skyhawk, 158722 '7', alongside all-white TA-4J 153477 '7' which was loaned to the team in 1981.
(Harry Gann/McDonnell-Douglas)

Top: Like a mother and chicks, the *Blue Angels* Skyhawks are seen here formating with their current support aircraft, KC-130F Hercules, 149806. (US Navy)

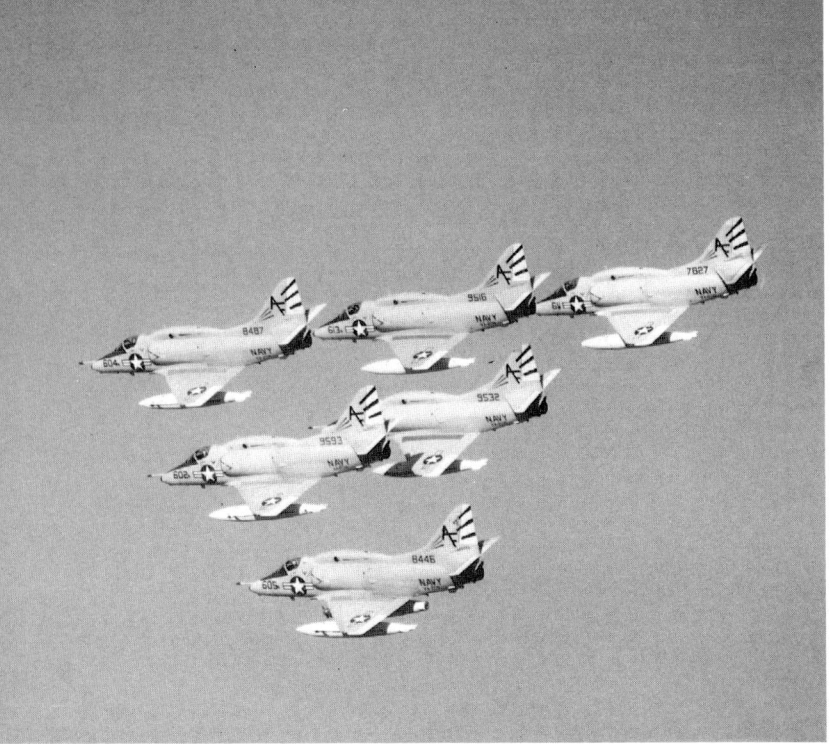

Above: Tight formation by six A-4L Skyhawks of the *Air Barons* team from VA-209 Squadron. (Harry Gann)

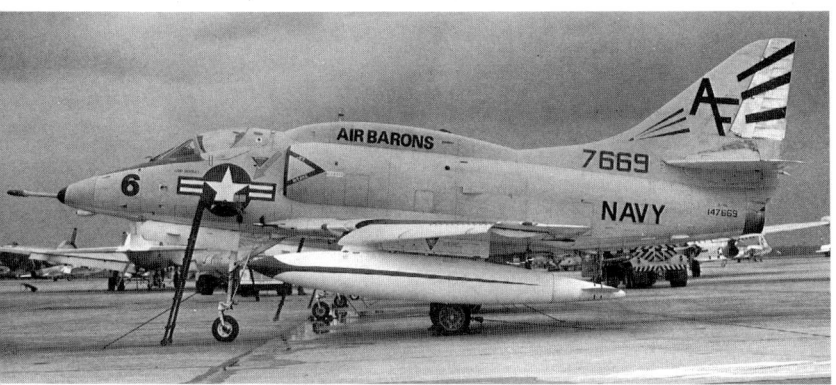

Above: Douglas A-4L Skyhawk, 147669, of VA-209 Squadron's *Air Barons* team, seen at Andrews Air Force Base in October 1971. All lettering, stripes on fin and underwing tanks were black.
(J. G. Handelman via R. Ward)

Below: Hughes OH-6A Cayuse, 12994, of the US Army *Silver Eagles* team dressed in full comic costume at Jacksonville, Florida in November 1973. (L. B. Sides)

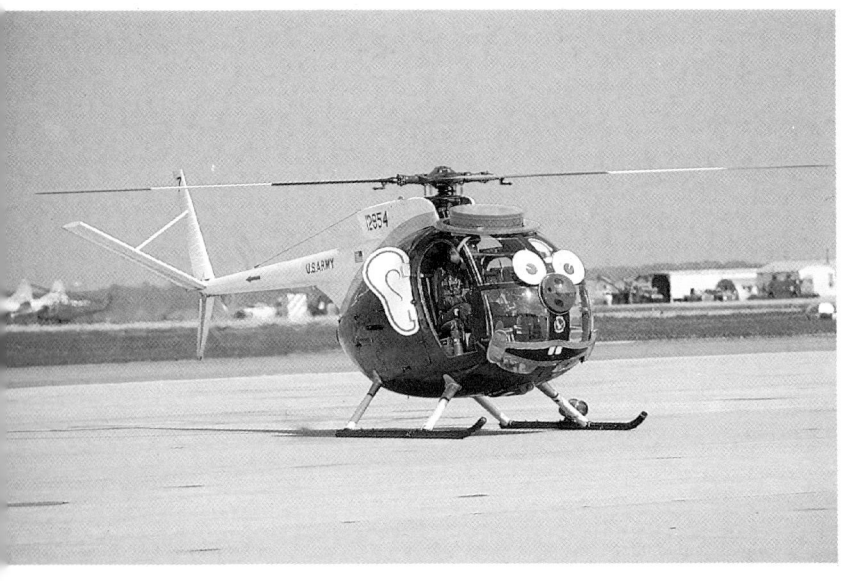

1967-71: U.S. Naval Air Reserve, the "Air Barons", NAS Glenview, Illinois

To recruit manpower for the Naval Reserve, a group of reserve pilots attached to VF-725 Squadron stationed at NAS Glenview, Illinois, organised a six-man flight demonstration team. It developed into a highly professional team and the Department of Defense nominated the team to officially represent the Naval Air Reserve at air displays and events. This team, the *Air Barons,* was the most important team to exist alongside the *Blue Angels*. The team was founded by Lieutenant Jim Mahoney, when he was posted to NAS Glenview in June 1958. At that time, VF-725 were operating Grumman F9F-6 Cougars, followed by FJ-4B Furies and A4B Skyhawks in July 1964, when the squadron was redesignated as an attack element of RAW-72.

On 1 September 1967, the *Air Barons* made their debut performance at Toronto, Canada. The team flew a 30-minute display which included a 'buddy-refuelling' demonstration.

In July 1968, VA-725 was re-designated VA-8 and, following his promotion to Commander, Jim Mahoney became the *Air Barons* commanding officer. The team participated in several displays during 1968-69, then in 1970 VA-8 was disestablished and VA-209 was formed. At this point, the team was operated independently and solely in the role of a flight demonstration team. On 15 May 1970, the team transitioned into the newer A-4L Skyhawk. In 1971, Commander Mahoney became the team's narrator, making way for Lieuteutant Commander Phil Lockard to become leader. On 26 March, VA-209 disbanded but the *Air Barons* were permitted to complete their show schedule up until their final performance on 4 November 1971 over Kissimmee, Florida for the opening of Disney World.

During their 5 years of operation, the *Air Barons* flew 66 demonstrations with no fatal accidents.

Their Skyhawks retained the standard light gull grey and white colour scheme with black lettering. The A-4Ls wore three dark green stripes on their fins, surmounted by the code 'AF' in black letters. On the avionics pack was a small black knight's helmet, which was replaced by 'AIR BARONS' titling by 1971. The teams' A-4Cs included 142101 and 142130, whilst examples of their A-4Ls were 147669 and 147706.

UNITED STATES ARMY

1973: "The Silver Eagles"

The Silver Eagles was a helicopter team comprising Hughes OH-6A Cayuses, which performed in the south-eastern U.S.A. during the early 1970s. Exact formation and disbandment dates are unknown, but the team were operational during 1973, the OH-6s being painted in a smart white and black colour scheme with a *Silver Eagle* badge on the door. One of the highlights of the performance was a solo routine by an OH-6 dressed up like a clown, with comic ears, nose, eyes, mouth and even hat! Cayuses operated by the team included 67-16060, 67-16066 and 65-12954.

LESSER-KNOWN AEROBATIC TEAMS

So little is known about the following teams, that they don't warrant a section in their own right. Many avenues of research have produced very little, however all deserve a mention to complete the world scene.

ARGENTINA
1962-63: "Escuadrilla Acrobatica Cruz del Sur" (Southern Cross Aerobatic Flight)
Six N.A. F-86F Sabres were operated by this team in a distinctive silver/blue/red/yellow colour scheme. The only known serial number is 'C-113' and the team disbanded at the end of 1963.

BOLIVIA
1984; The Bolivian Air force is reported to operate a team of Pilatus PC-7 Turbo-Trainers, painted with sharkmouth markings on the nose. Based at Santa Rosa Air Base, serials of team aircraft include: FAB 451, 454, 456 and 461.

CHILE
1981-to date: Chilean Air Force "Falcons" Aerobatic Flight
The only known aerobatic team operated by the Fuerza Aerea de Chile is the *Falcons* Aerobatic Flight with four Pitts Special bi-planes. Although four were delivered for the aerobatic team, two were written-off on 21st December 1981 in a mid-air collision, but may have been replaced.

PEOPLES' REPUBLIC OF CHINA
Air Force of the Peoples' Liberation Army, Yangtsuon
In 1982, the Chinese Air Force was reported as having an aerobatic team of fifteen MiG 15UTI trainers painted red and silver. The team is based at Yangtsuon and one of these machines is serialled '506'.

CZECHOSLOVAKIA
This Air Force operated a team of MiG 15s from 1953 throughout the 1950s. At some stage, they were supplemented or replaced by a team of MiG 17s. Both types were basically natural metal overall, although the MiG 15s sported a red stripe along the wings, which terminated in a large red arrowhead on the nose.

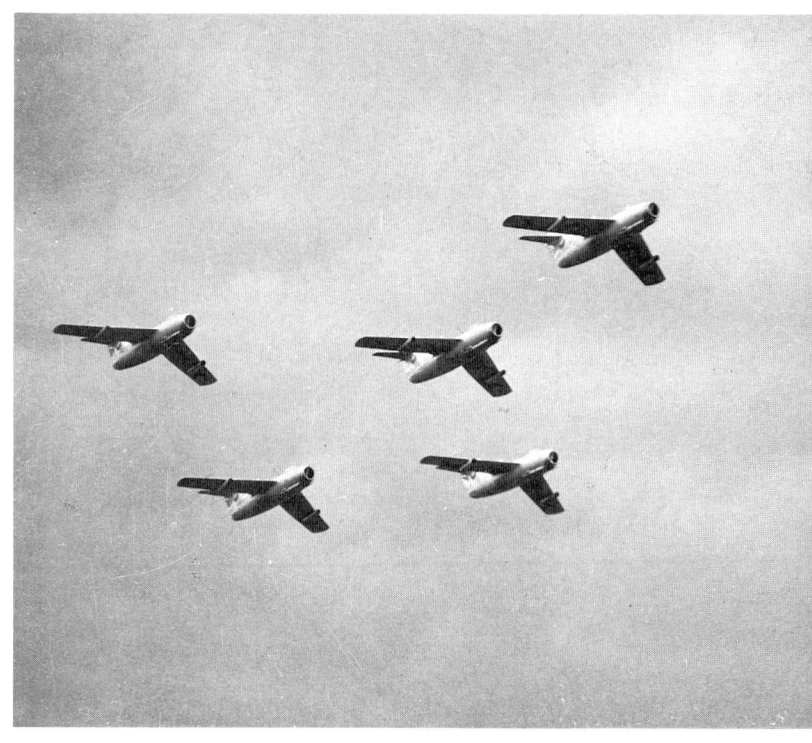

The Czechoslovakian Air Force aerobatic team of MiG-15s performing at Prague in September 1953.
(via R. Ward)

SOUTH KOREA
The Republic of Korea Air Force operated a team of Northrop F-5As during the late 1960s early 1970s in a smart colour scheme of white, orange, dark blue and red. (See page 98 for photo)

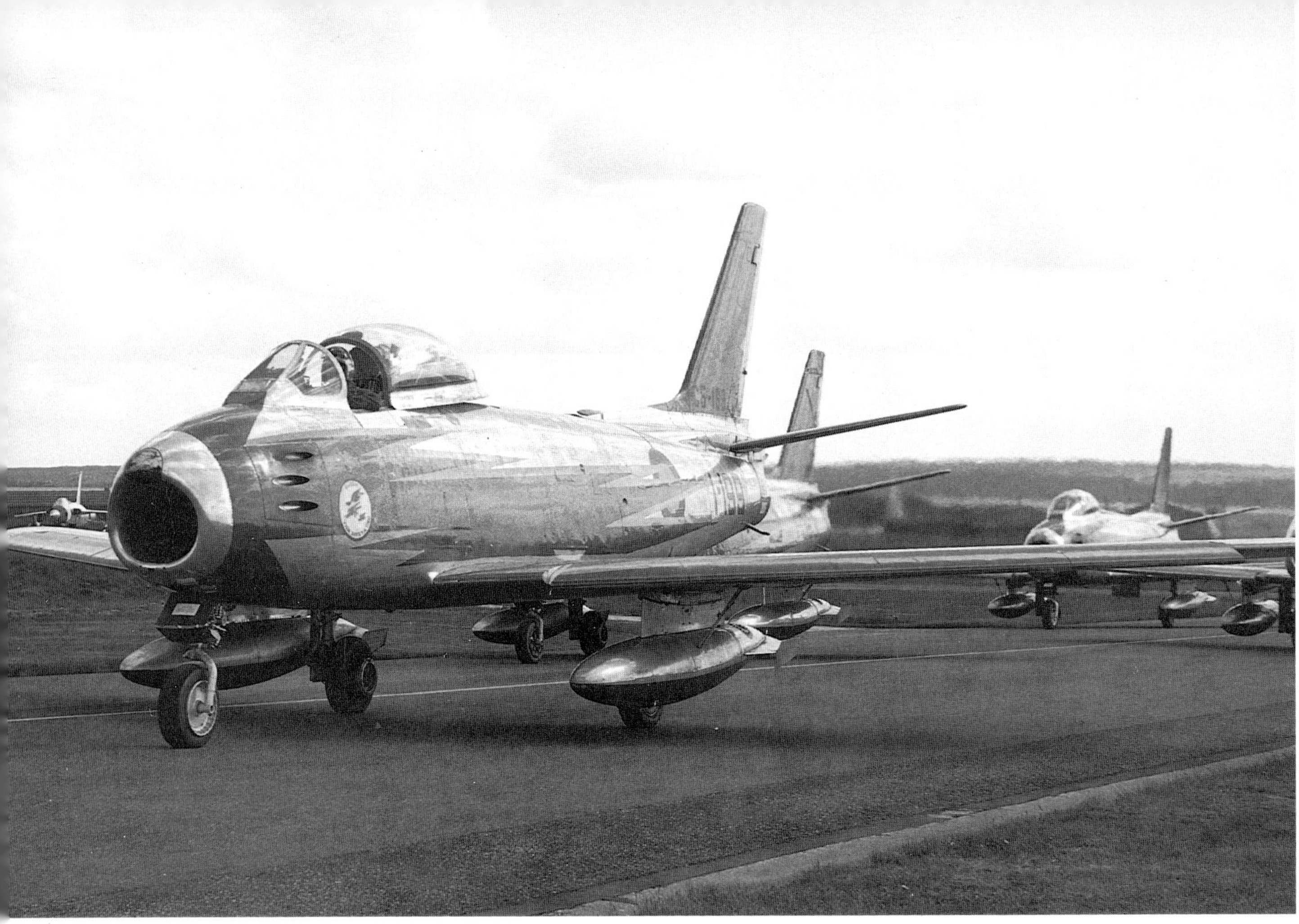

F-86F Sabre, C5-199, leads the Spanish Air Force *Arrowheads* team at Spangdahlem, Germany in May 1962. (Werner Gysin)

Canadair F-86E Sabres of the Turkish Air Force *White Swans* team. Trim is red on natural metal with white fin and swan.

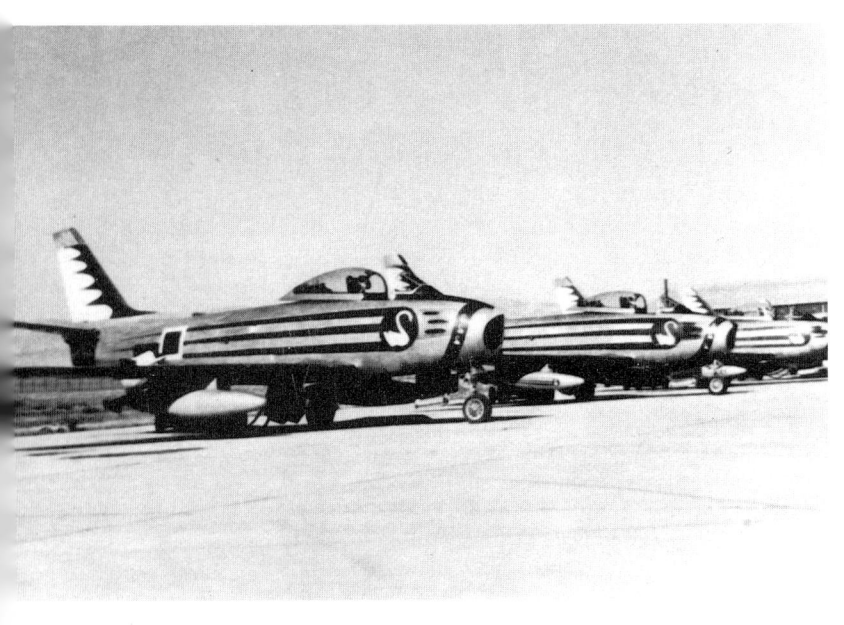

SOVIET UNION

The Soviet Air Force has had an aerobatic team since the mid-1950s. Starting with MiG 15s, the team progressed to MiG 17s, MiG 19s and the last known type was the MiG 21. With the latter mount, they performed at Domodedovo air display, Moscow, in 1967, but have not been reported since. All the types mentioned above have worn the same colour scheme of red on all upper surfaces and silver undersides. Two-figure codes are carried on the nose in white. No dates or other information is known.

SPAIN

The Spanish Air Force national aerobatic team was the *Ascuas* (Arrowheads) flying F-86F Sabres in a striking silver, yellow and red colour scheme. There were four aircraft in the team, which came from Ala de Caza 1, and the name *Ascuas* was chosen in memory of an Ala 1 pilot, killed in a crash, whose radio call sign was Ascua.

Known serial numbers of team aircraft were: C5-175, C5-199, C5-83, C5-104. No other Spanish Air Force teams are known and no others formed since *Ascuas* disbanded early in 1963.

TURKEY

The Turkish Air Force flew a team of Canadair F-86E Sabres called the *White Swans* during the early 1960s. Beautifully painted with red stripes down the fuselage and red scallops along the leading edges of all flying surfaces. A white swan insignia adorned the nose on a red disc. Serial numbers included '103' (19103) and '435' (19435). When the Northrop F-5A replaced the Sabre with the Turkish Air Force, a team of F-5As was formed during the mid-1960s.

Appendix I

AEROBATIC TEAM BADGES

AUSTRIA

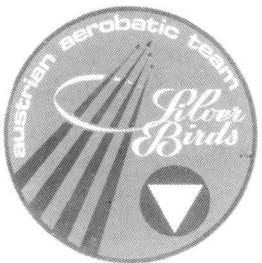

The Silver Birds

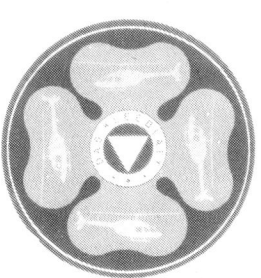

KARO AS
(Ace of Diamonds)

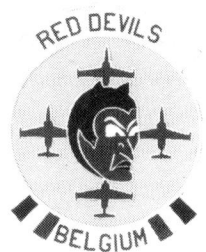

KLEEBLATT
Helicopter Team

BELGIUM

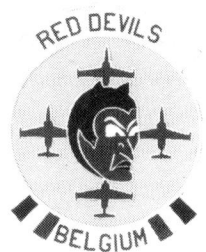

The Red Devils

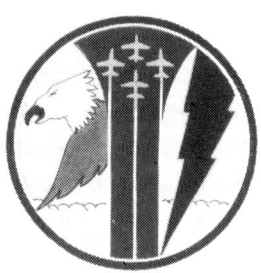

Esquadrilha da Fumaça
(Smoke Squadron)

BRAZIL

CANADA

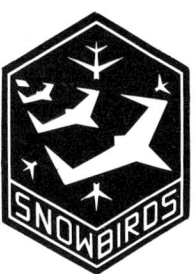

Snowbirds

FRANCE

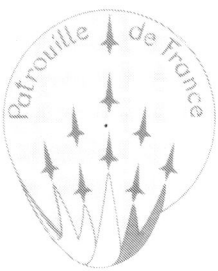

La Patrouille de France

GREAT BRITAIN

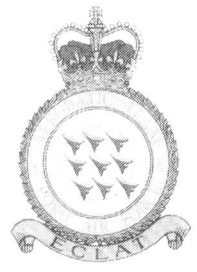

The Red Arrows

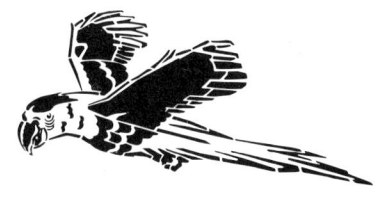

The Macaws

GREAT BRITAIN

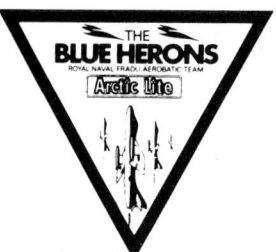

The Blue Herons

ITALY

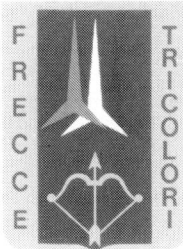

Frecce Tricolori
(Tricoloured Arrows)

SWITZERLAND

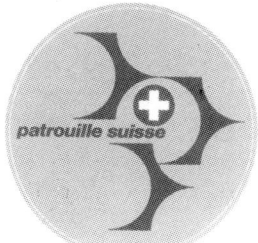

La Patrouille Suisse

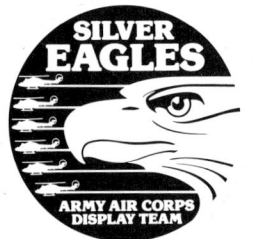

The Silver Eagles

NORWAY

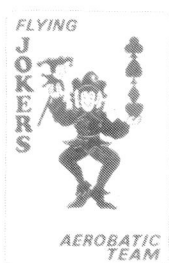

The Flying Jokers

UNITED STATES OF AMERICA

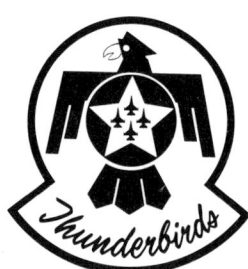

The Thunderbirds

INDIA

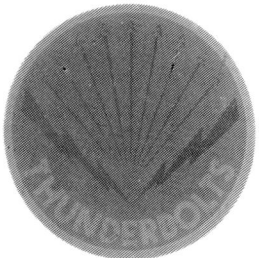

The Thunderbolts

PORTUGAL

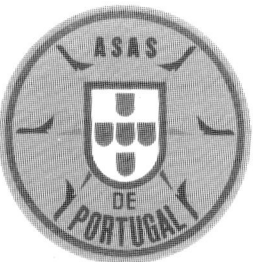

Asas de Portugal
(Wings of Portugal)

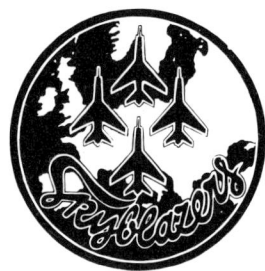

Skyblazers

ISRAEL

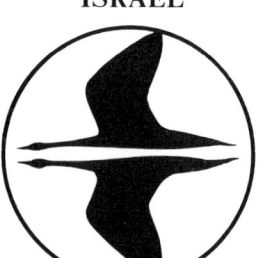

Israeli Airforce/
Defence Force
Aerobatic Team

SWEDEN

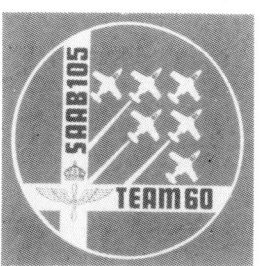

Team 60

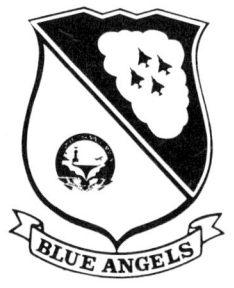

Blue Angels

Appendix II
AEROBATIC TEAM MANOEUVRES

THE RED ARROWS

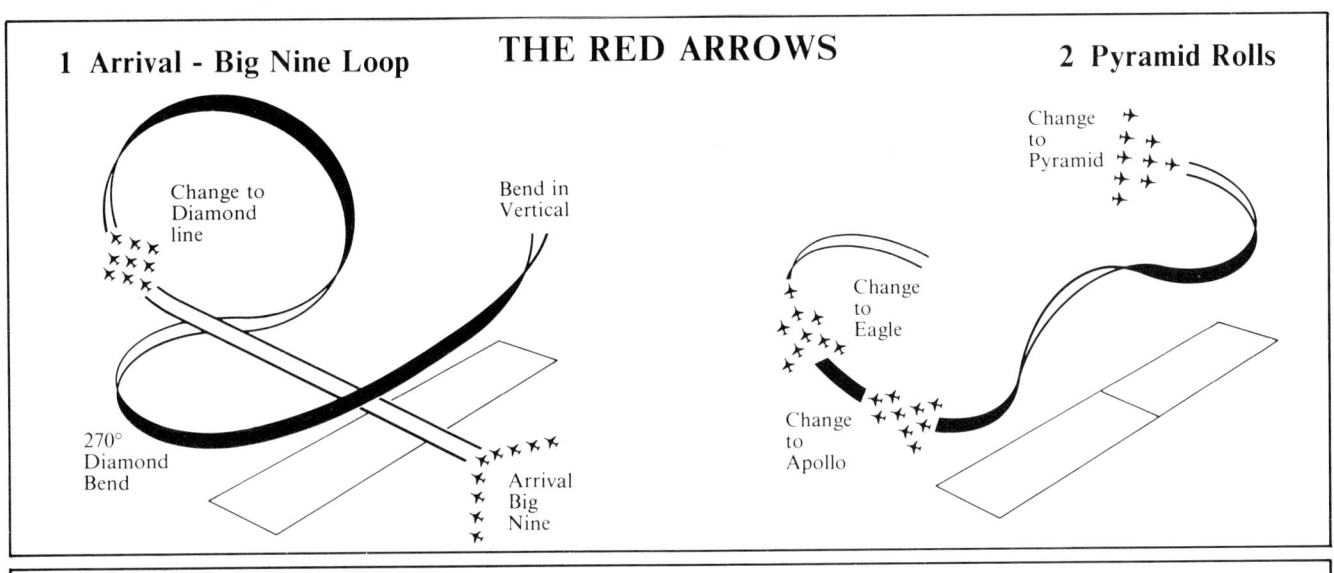

1 Arrival - Big Nine Loop

2 Pyramid Rolls

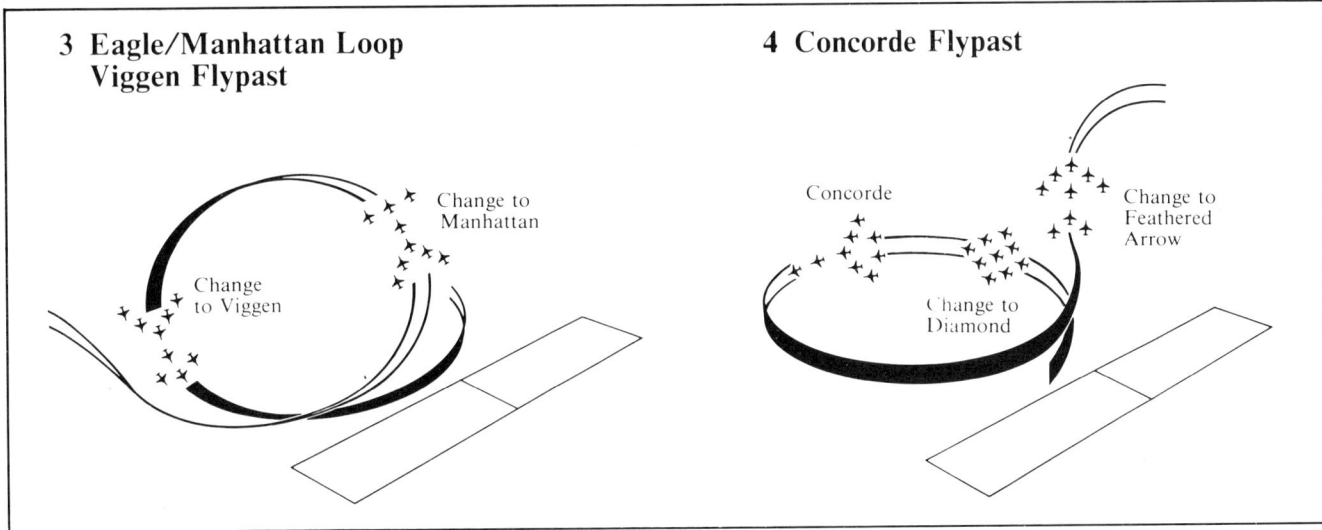

3 Eagle/Manhattan Loop Viggen Flypast

4 Concorde Flypast

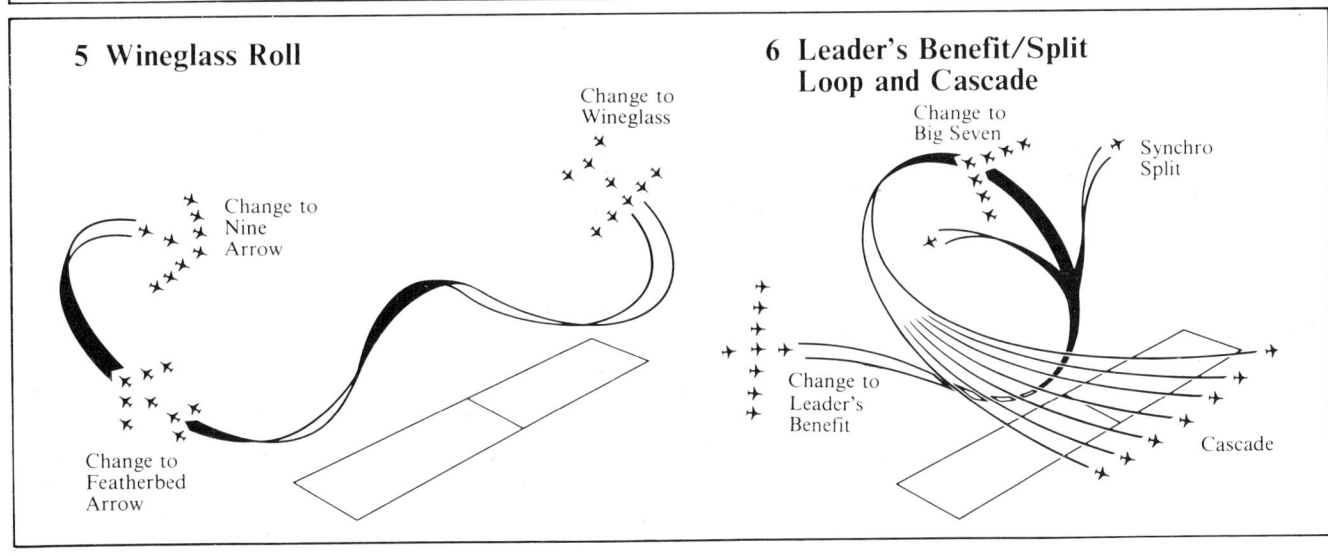

5 Wineglass Roll

6 Leader's Benefit/Split Loop and Cascade

7 Spectacles and Opposition Barrel Roll - Synchro Pair

8 Kings Cross

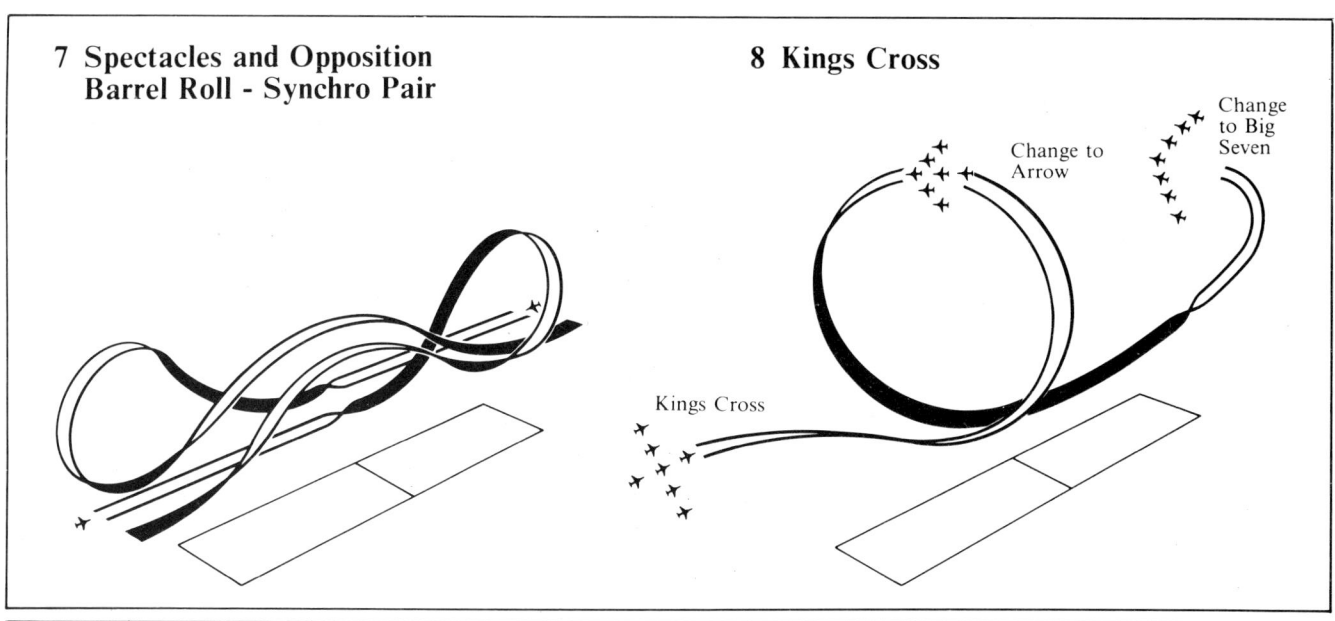

9 Boomerang - Synchro

10 Roll Backs

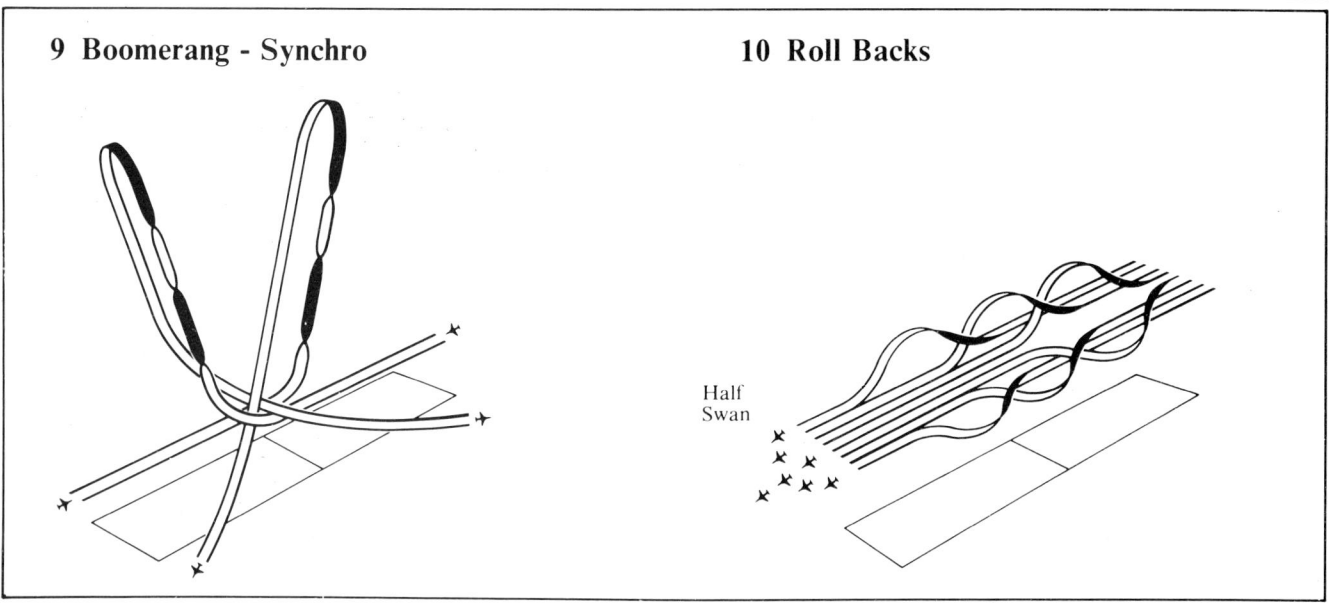

11 Looping Carousel - Synchro

12 Caterpillar Loop

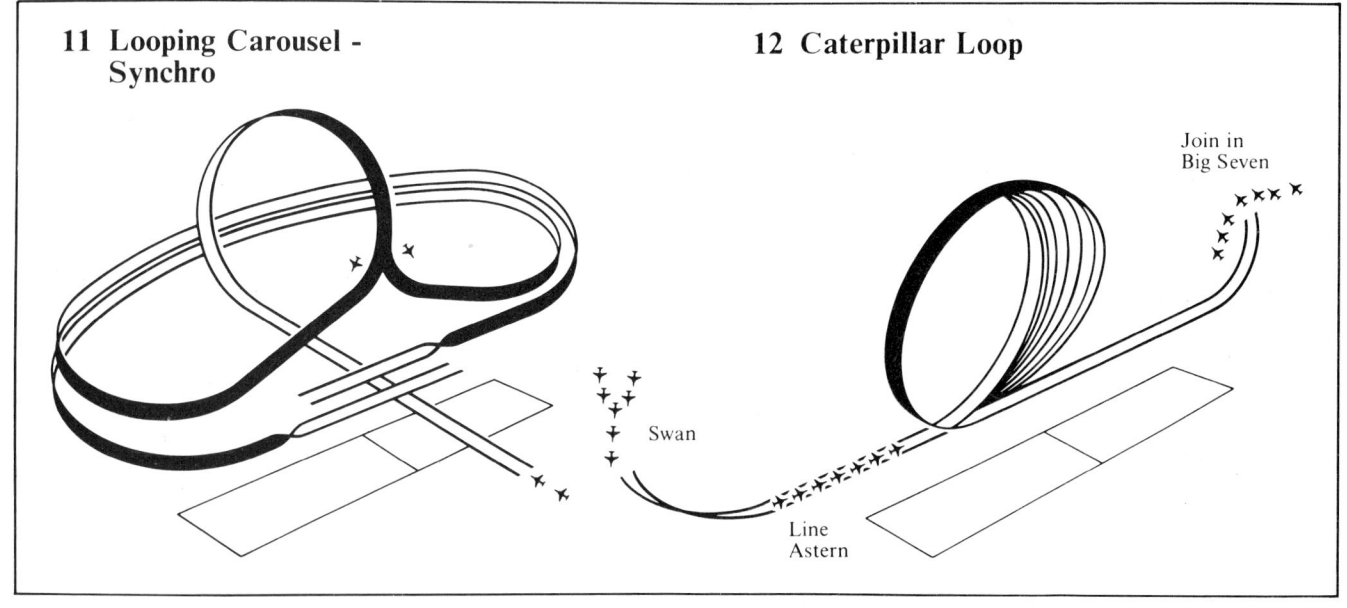

13 Double Rolls - Synchro

14 Synchro Southern Cross

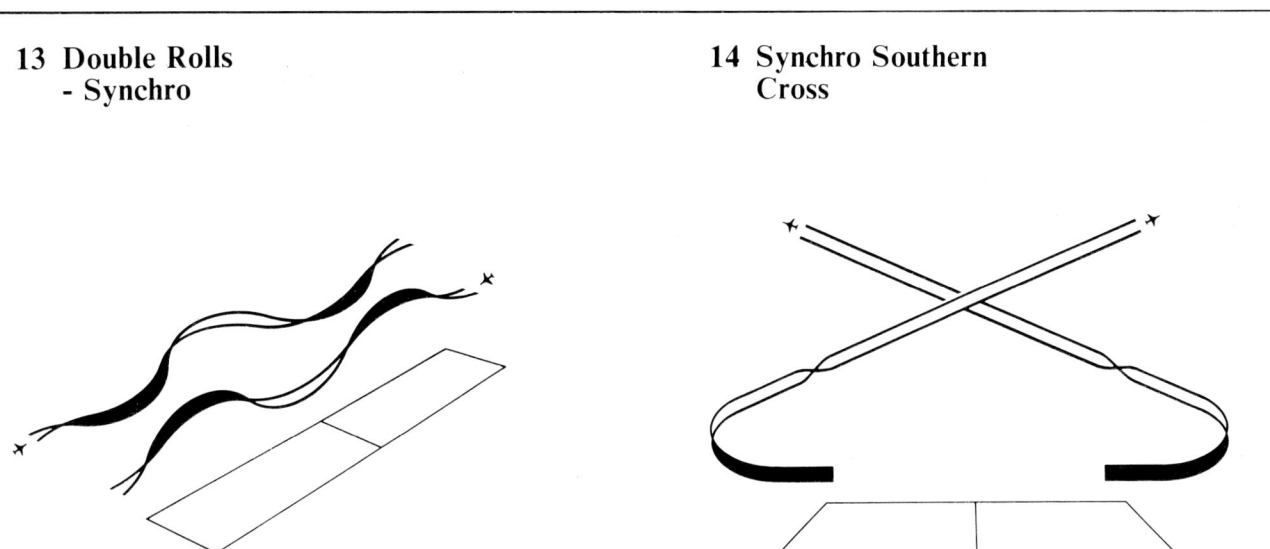

15 Box Loop - Vixen Break

16 Opposition Loop - Synchro

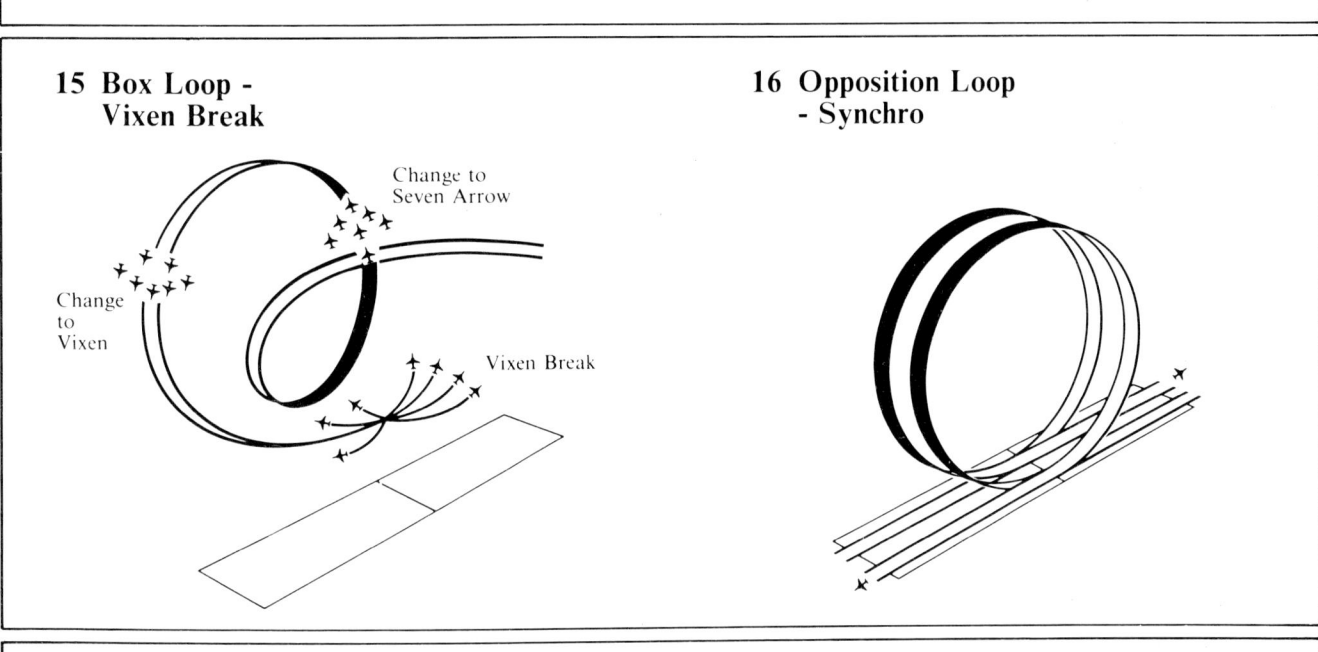

17 Parasol Break

18 Rocket Climb

Occasionally, if the site, weather, fuel, airspace and bird hazard permit, the team may finish with the Rocket Climb.
This manoeuvre is always preceded by the Parasol Break and headed by the team leader.
Aircraft are flown in echelon away from the crowd line and join in Loose Nine Arrow on completion.

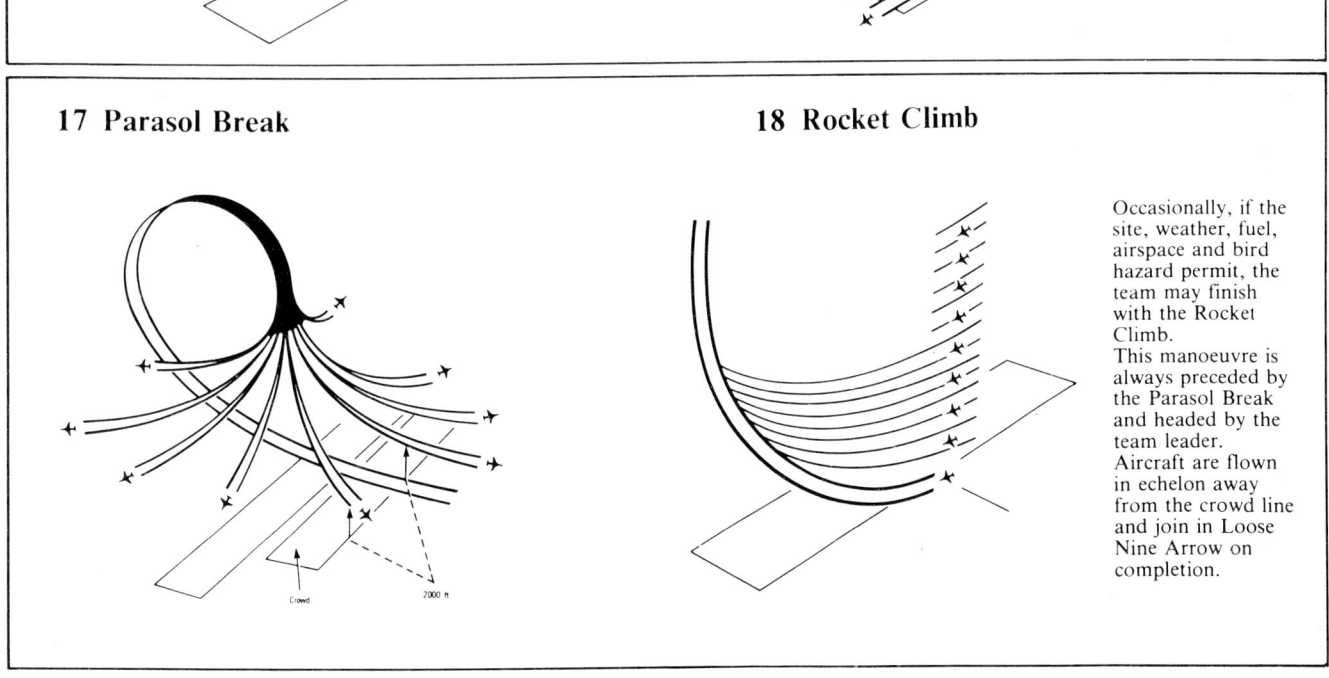

THUNDERBIRD MANOEUVRES

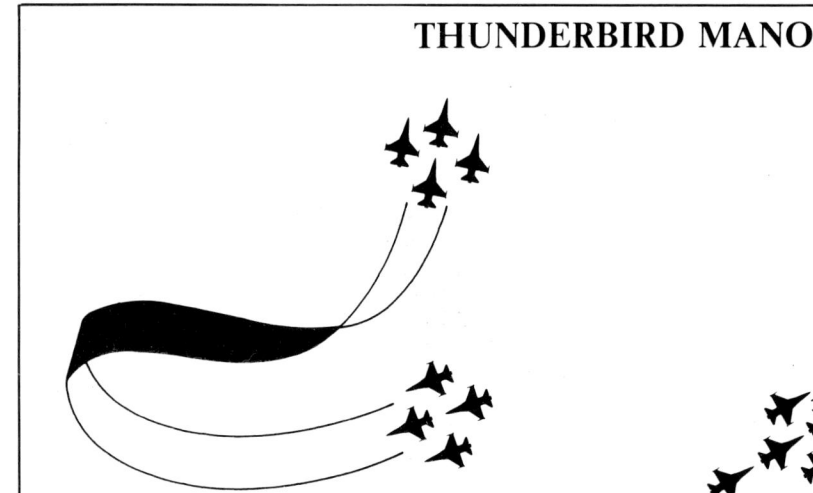

Diamond Cloverloop Opener

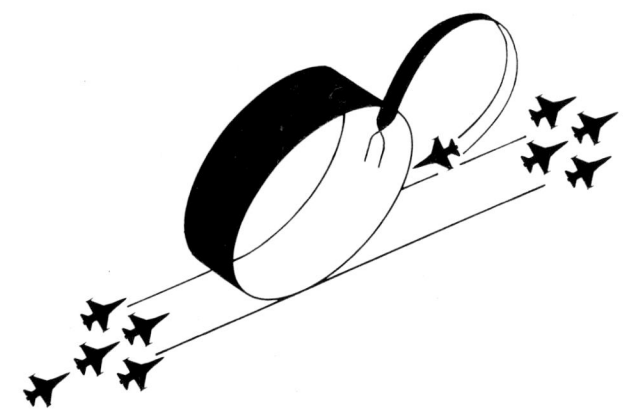

Stinger Loop Plus Solo Breakaway

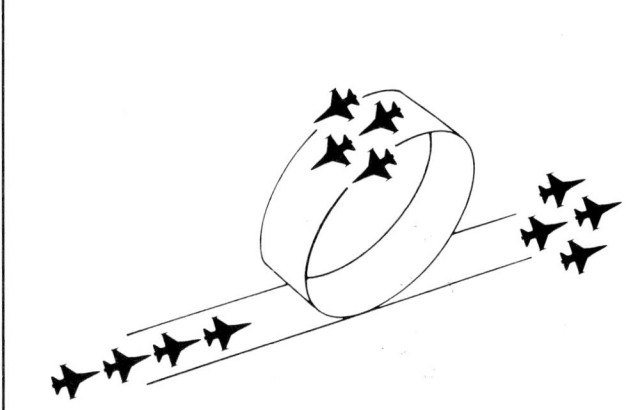

Trail to Diamond Loop

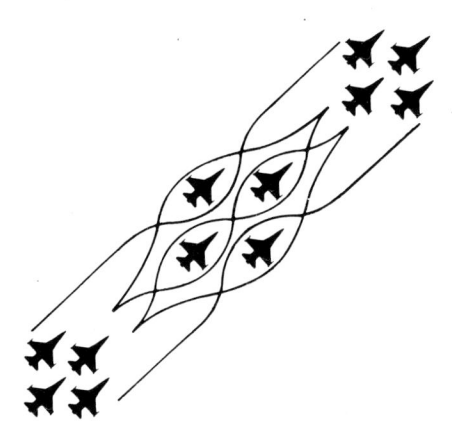

Bon Ton Roulle

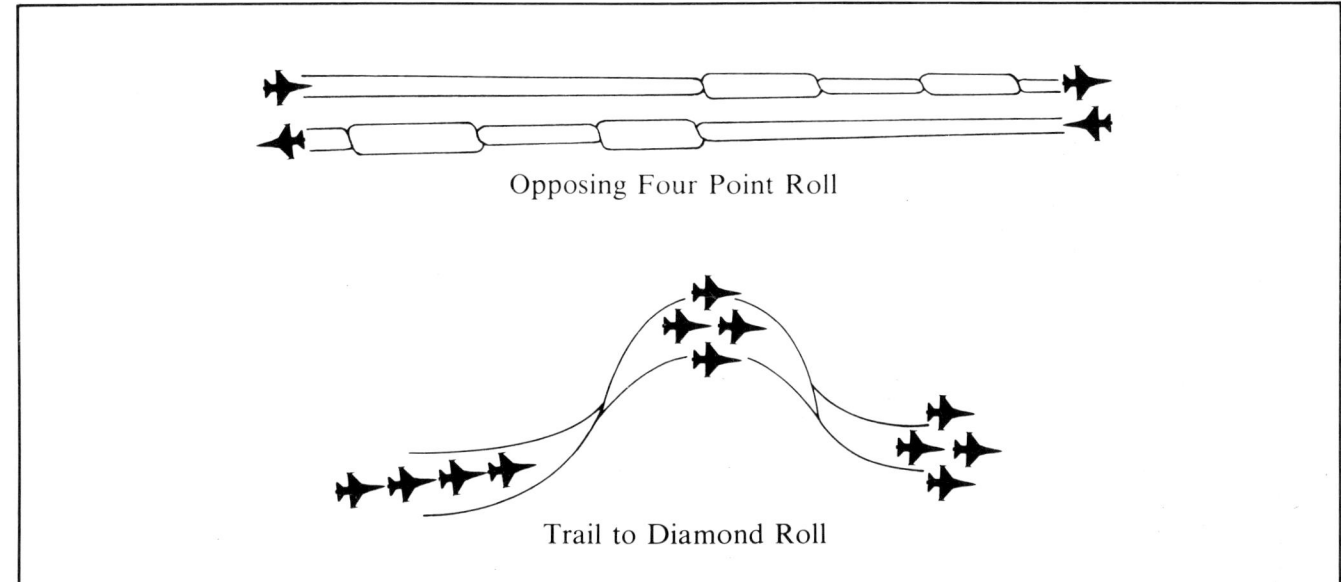

Opposing Four Point Roll

Trail to Diamond Roll

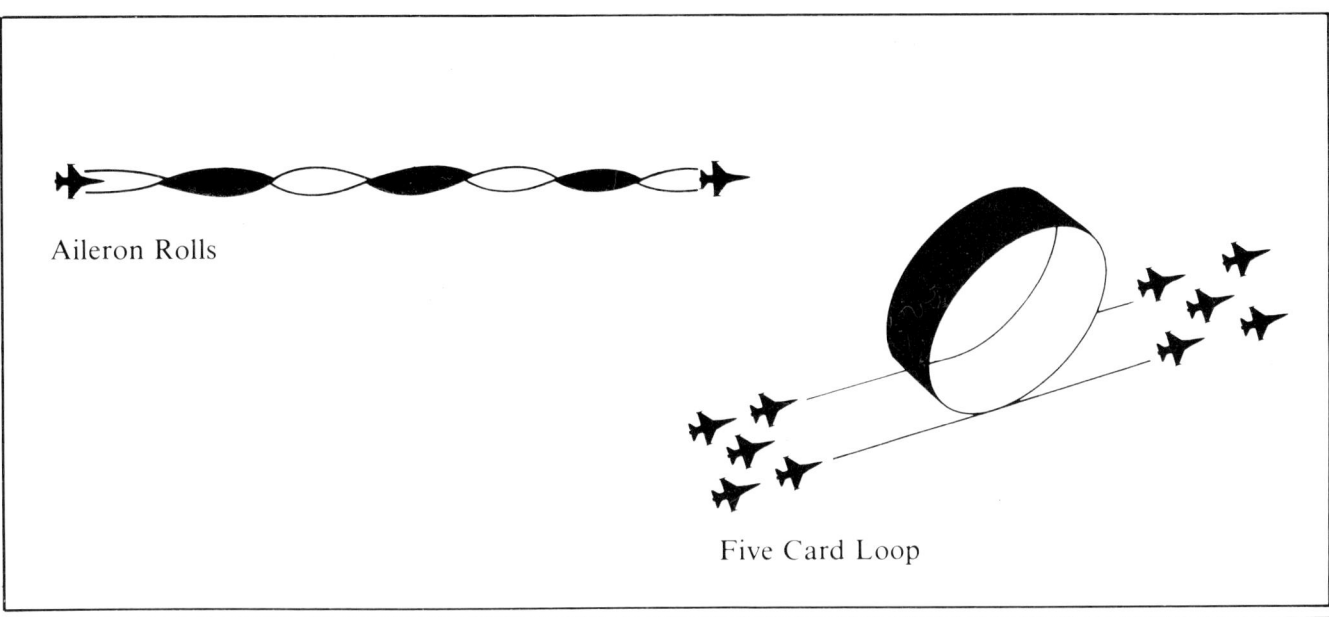
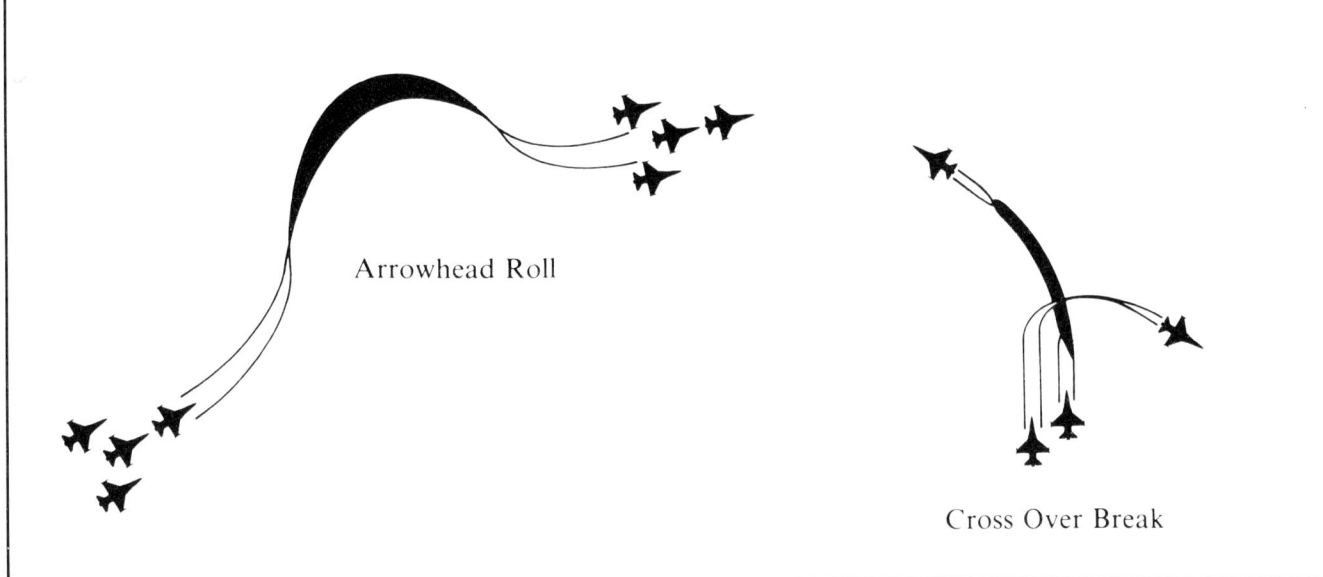
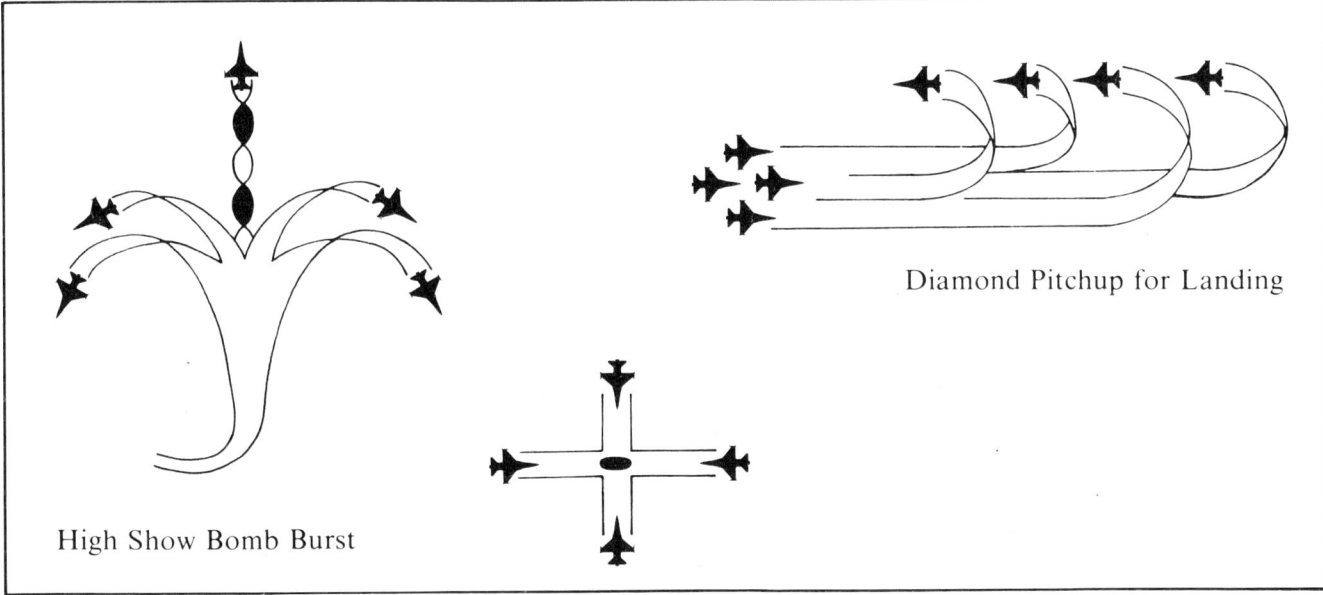

MINUTE MEN
Air National Guard Precision Team
Flying F-86 Supersonic Sabre jets

MANOEUVRES

Attention Pass	Solo Inverted Flight
Diamond Loop	Corkscrew
Change-Over Loop	Solo - Hawaiian "8"
Solo - 4-Point Roll	Bomb Burst
Diamond Roll	5-Ship Loop
Change-Over Roll	5-Ship Roll
Solo - 8-Point Roll	Echelon Roll
360° Low Turn	

Change-Over Loop

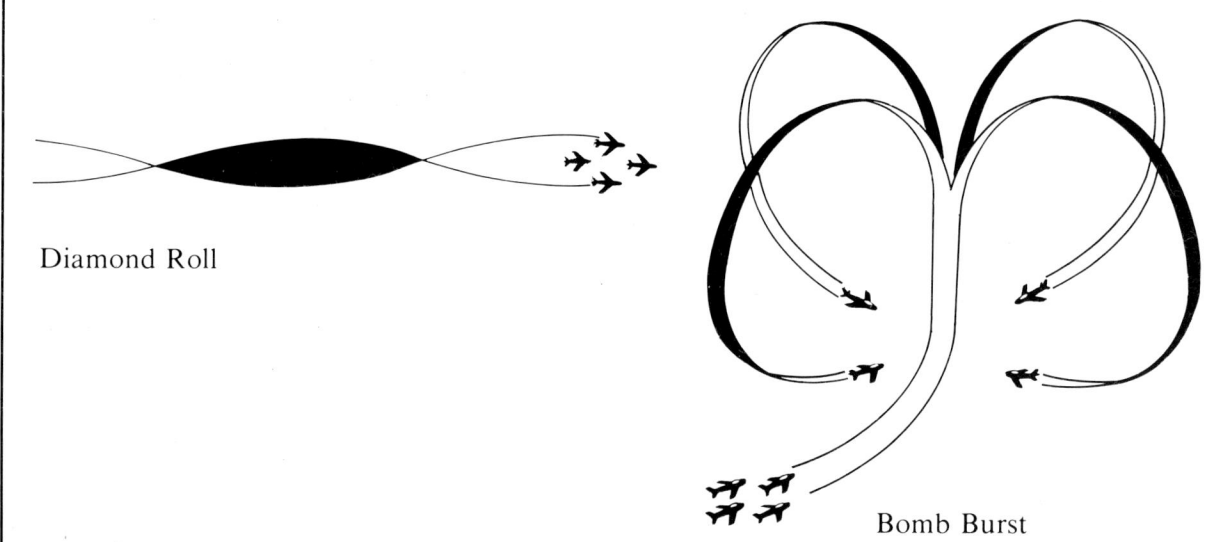

Diamond Roll

Bomb Burst

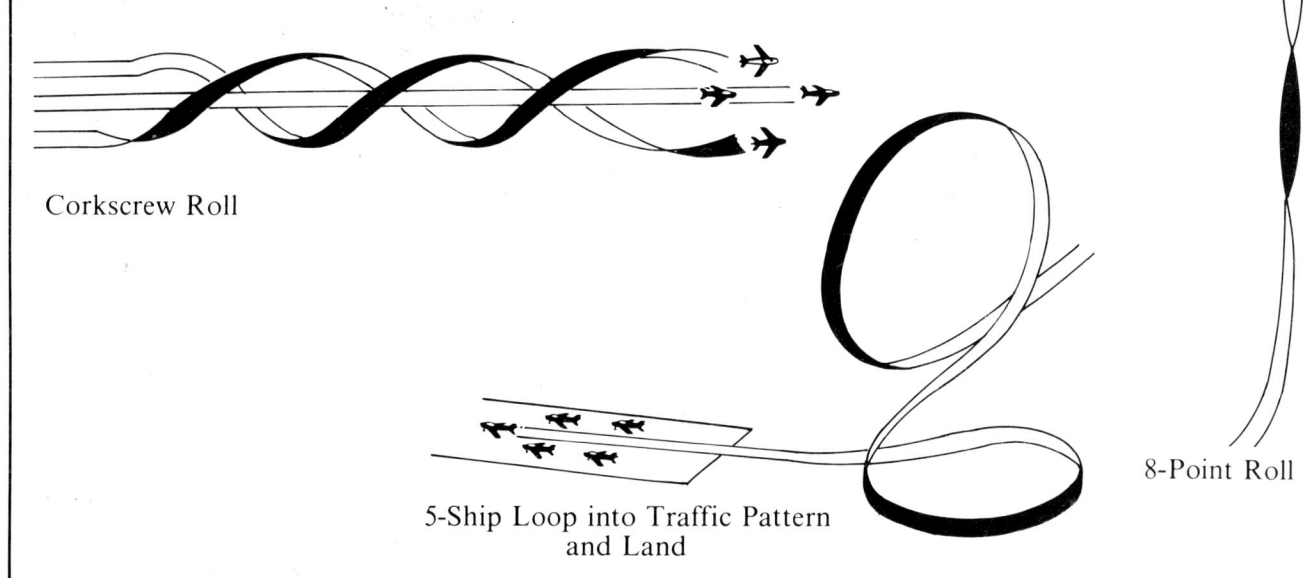

Corkscrew Roll

5-Ship Loop into Traffic Pattern and Land

8-Point Roll

Index

'P' after page numbers indicates a photograph of a particular aircraft type.

Ace of Diamonds (KARO AS), Austrian Air Force 12
Acrobobs, Belgian Air Force 13
Acro Deltas, Swedish Air Force 100
Acro Hunters, Swedish Air Force 100
Acrojets, USAF 120
Aermacchi MB-326 9P, 10P, 97P
Aermacchi MB-339 79P, 83
AESL CT-4 Airtrainer 90P(2)
Air Barons, US Navy 134
Argentine Air Force 135
Armstrong-Whitworth Siskin 19, 34
Army Air Corps 67
Asas de Portugal (Wings of Portugal) 96
Ascuas (Arrowheads), Spanish AF 136
Avro 504K 23, 34
Avro Tutor 35P, 36P
Austrian Air Force 11

BAC Jet Provost T.5 48P, 52P(2), 53P, 54P(2), 55P
Belgian Air Force 13
Belgian Army 15
Bell JetRanger/Kiowa 12P, 25P
Black Arrows, RAF 41
Black Diamonds, RAAF 9
Black Knights, RAF 38
Black Knights, USAFE 120, 121
Blackburn Buccaneer S.2 64P
Blades, RAF 54
Blue Angels, US Navy 126
Blue Bees, Belgian Army 15
Blue Chips, RAF 54
Blue Devils, RCAF 19
Blue Diamonds, RAF 45
Blue Diamonds, Philippine Air Force 94
Blue Eagles, Army Air Corps 67
Blue Herons, Royal Navy 66
Blue Impulse, Japan ASDF 84
Boeing F2B-1 122, 123
Boeing F4B-1 124
Bolivian Air Force 135
Brazilian Air Force 16
Bristol Bulldog 9, 35P, 36
British Aerospace Hawk 27, 58P(2), 59
Bulldogs, RAF 55

Campoformido Boys, Italian Air Force 80
Canadair CL-13 Sabre 19P, 20P(2), 21P, 72P(2), 73P, 80P, 81P, 82P, 136P
Canadair CT-114 Tutor 19P, 22P, 23P(2), 24P
Canadian Armed Forces 19.
CASA C-212 Aviocar 96
Cavallino Rampante, Italian Air Force 80
Cessna T-37C 93, 96P, 98P
Chance-Vought F7U Cutlass 128, 133
Chinese Nationalist Air Force 26
Chilean Air Force 135
Commonwealth CA-27 Sabre 9P, 10P(2)
Curtiss F6C-4 124
Curtiss C-46A Commando 133
Czechoslovakian Air Force 135

Dash-4, Royal Netherlands Air Force 87
Dassault Ouragan 29
Dassault Mystère IVA 30P
Dassault-Breguet/Dornier Alpha Jet 31P(2), 32P
de Havilland Genet Moth 34
de Havilland Gipsy Moth 9, 34P, 35
de Havilland Tiger Moth 34P, 35
de Havilland Sea Vixen 62P, 64P(2), 69P
de Havilland Vampire 10, 29, 37P, 89P, 97, 99
de Havilland Canada Chipmunk 49P, 68P, 69
Diavoli Rossi (Red Devils), Italian Air Force 81
Douglas C-47 Dakota 103, 133
Douglas C-54 Skymaster 105, 112, 126P, 128P, 133
Douglas A-4 Skyhawk 89, 125P, 131P, 132P, 133P(2), 134P(2)

Eagles, Army Air Corps 70
Embraer EMB-312 Tucano 17P, 18P(2)
English Electric Lightning F.1/1A 45, 46P, 47P(2)
Esquadrilha da Fumaça (Smoke Sqn) FAB 16, 17

Falcons, Chilean Air Force 135
Falcons, RAF 45
Falcons, Pakistan Air Force 93
Falcons, Philippine Air Force 94
Fairchild C-119 Flying Boxcar 83, 103P, 104P, 105, 112
Fairchild C-123 Provider 105, 107P, 112
Federal German Air Force 33
Fiat CR20 80
Fiat CR32 80P
Fiat G-91PAN 79P, 82, 83P
Fighting Cocks, RAF 40
Fireballs, RCAF 20
Firebirds, RAF 46
Finnish Air Force 27
Flying Jokers, R. Norwegian Air Force 92
Focke-Wulf FW-44 Steigliztz 99, 101P
Folland Gnat T.1 49P(2), 56P(2), 57P, 58P(3), 59P(3)
Fogde-Team, Royal Swedish Air Force 99
Fouga Magister 11, 12P(2), 13P, 15P, 17P(2), 18, 27P, 29P(2), 30P(2), 31P, 32P, 33, 77P, 78P(3)
Four Horseman, USAF 121
Fred's Five, Royal Navy 62
French Air Force 28
F-16 Team, Royal Swedish Air Force 101

Gazelles, RAF 56
Gemini Pair, RAF 54
General Dynamics F-16A Fighting Falcon 92, 111, 112P, 113P
Getti Tonanti, Italian Air Force 80
Gimli Smokers, RCAF 22
Gin Four, RAF 53
Gloster Gamecock 34
Gloster Gauntlet 36, 37
Gloster Gladiator 13, 36P, 37

Gloster Grebe 34
Gloster Meteor 9, 13, 38P, 43, 50P, 87P
Golden Centennaires, RCAF 23, 24
Golden Harvards, Israeli Air Force 78
Golden Hawks, RCAF 20
Goldilocks, RCAF 23
Grasshoppers, Royal Netherlands Air Force 88
Gray Angels, US Navy 125
Grey Owls, Army Air Corps 69
Grumman F6F Hellcat 122P, 126, 133
Grumman F8F Bearcat 123P, 127, 128, 133
Grumman F9F Panther 124P, 128, 129P, 133
Grumman F9F Cougar 126P, 127P, 128P, 129, 133
Grumman F-11A Tiger 125P, 128P, 129, 130P(2), 133
Guardian Angels, USAF 120

Haglind-Team, Royal Swedish Air Force 100
HAL Kiran 74
HAL Marut 74
Hawker Fury 35, 36, 37P
Hawker Hunter 13P, 38, 39P, 40P, 41, 42P, 43P(2), 45P(2), 45P(3), 46P, 62P, 66P, 74P, 100P(2), 102P(2)
Hawker Sea Hawk 60, 61P(2), 62P
Hellenic Flame, Greek Air Force 72
Hellenic Air Force 71
High Hatters, US Navy 123
Hunting Provost 40P
Hunting Jet Provost 40P, 41P(3), 44P(2), 48P, 51P(2)
Hughes OH-6A Cayuse 134P

Imperial Iranian Air Force 75
Indian Air Force 74
Israeli Defence Force/Air Force 77
Italian Air Force 79

Japanese Air Self-Defense Force 84
Jasska-Four, Finnish Air Force 27

KARO AS, Austrian Air Force 11, 12
Kleeblaat, Austrian Army 12

Lanceri Neri (Black Lancers), Italian Air Force 81
La Patrouille de France, French Air Force 28
La Patrouille d'Etampes, French Air Force 29
La Patrouille de Tours, French Air Force 29
La Patrouille Weiser, French Air Force 28
La Patrouille Suisse, Swiss Air Force 102
Larks, Belgian Army 15
Les Diables Rouges (Red Devils) Belgian Air Force 13
Les Manchots (Penguins), Belgian Air Force 14
Linton Gin, RAF 53
Lockheed F-80 Shooting Star 113, 114P, 120P
Lockheed T-33A 21P(2), 22, 23, 24P, 33, 87, 88P, 112, 133
Lockheed F-104 Starfighter 14P, 33P
Lockheed C-121J Constellation 129P, 133
Lockheed C-130 Hercules 83, 96, 112, 121, 133P

Macaws, RAF 50
Marine Phantoms, USMC 125
Martin B-57 Canberra 120P, 121
Marksmen, RAAF 9

McDonnell FH-1 Phantom 125
McDonnell F-4 Phantom 108P, 110, 112P, 130, 131P, 133
Meteorites, RAF 38
Meteorites, RAAF 9
Mikoyan MiG-15 135P, 136
Mikoyan MiG-17 136
Mikoyan MiG-19 93P, 136
Mikoyan MiG-21 74, 136
Minute Men, USAF 113
Mitsubishi T-2 84, 85, 86P
Morane 225 28P
Morane 230 28P
Morane Saulnier Paris 18

New Hellenic Flame, Greek Air Force 73
North American P-51 Mustang 77, 120
North American T-6 Texan/Harvard 16P, 17, 18P, 23, 77, 90, 91P(2), 97, 126, 133
North American F-86 Sabre (see also Canadair & Commonwealth) 26P, 42, 76, 84P, 85P, 86P, 92P, 93, 94, 95P, 113P, 114P, 117P, 118P(2), 120, 121P(2), 135, 136P
North American F-100 Super Sabre 105P(2), 106P, 107, 108, 112P, 116P, 117P
North American FJ-3 Fury 133
Northrop T-38A Talon 110P(2), 111P, 112, 119P(2)
Northrop F-5A Freedom Fighter 26, 76, 92P, 95, 98P, 135
Northrop F-5E Tiger II 26, 75P(2), 76P

Pakistan Air Force 93
Paybill, Pakistan Air Force 93
Penguins, Belgian Air Force 14
Phoenix Five, Royal Navy 64
Philippine Air Force 94
Piaggio P-149D 33P
Pilatus PC-7 Turbo-Trainer 135
Pitts Special 135
Peoples' Republic of China Air Force 135
Poachers, RAF 52
Prairie Pacific Team, RCAF 20

RAF SE-5A 34
Red Archers, Indian Air Force 74
Red Arrows, RAF 56
Red Checkers, RNZAF 90
Red Devils, Belgian Air Force 13
Red Devils, Royal Navy 60
Red Devils, Portuguese Air Force 96
Red Devils, USAF 120
Red Diamonds, RAAF 9
Red Diamonds, Royal Netherlands Air Force 87
Red Knight, RCAF 22
Red Pelicans, RAF 48
Red Pitch, Belgian Army 15
Redskins, RAF 44
Republic F-84E/G Thunderjet 26, 29, 71P, 75, 76, 80, 87, 98P, 103P, 109P(2), 112, 114, 115P(2), 116
Republic F-84F Thunderstreak 79P, 81P, 82P, 83P, 86P, 87, 88, 96, 104P(2), 112
Republic F-105B Thunderchief 107P, 108P, 112
Republic of Korea Air Force 135
Roulettes, RAAF 10
Royal Air Force 34
Royal Navy 60
Royal Canadian Air Force 19

Royal Australian Air Force   9
Royal Netherlands Air Force   87
Royal New Zealand Air Force   89
Royal Norwegian Air Force   92
Royal Swedish Air Force   99
Rough Diamonds, Royal Navy   62

SAAB J-29   99, 100P
SAAB J-35 Draken   100, 101P(2)
SAAB 105   11P(3), 99P, 101
Sabre Dancers, USAF   121
Sabre Knights, USAF   121
Sandbag Diamonds, R. Netherlands Air Force   88
Sharks, Royal Navy   65
Scottish Aviation Bulldog   55P
Sidewinders, Philippines Air Force   94
Silver Birds, Austrian Air Force   11P
Silver Eagles, Army Air Corps   70
Silver Eagles, U.S. Army   134
Sherdils, Pakistan Air Force   93
Silver Falcons, South African Air Force   97
Silver Sabres, USAF   120
SIAI-Marchetti SF-260   14, 15P
Simon's Sircus, Royal Navy   64
Sharks, Royal Navy   65
Siskins, RCAF   19
Sky Lancers, RCAF   20
Slivers, Belgian Air Force   14
Skylarks, RAF   49
Skyblazers, USAF   114
Skyblazers, Royal Netherlands Air Force   87
Skyblazers, Greek Air Force   71
Smoke Squadron, Brazilian Air Force   16, 17
Snowbirds, CAF   24, 25
Sopwith Snipe   34
South African Air Force   97
Southern Cross Aerobatic Flight, Argentine Air Force   135
Soviet Air Force   136
SPAD 510   28

Sparrows, RAF   40
Spanish Air Force   136
Sparrow Hawks, Army Air Corps   69
Stampe SV-4   14P 29
Sud-Aviation Alouette II   15
Sud-Aviation Alouette III   88P
Supermarine Scimitar   61, 62, 63P
Supermarine Attacker   93
Swallows, Belgian Air Force   14
Swiss Air Force   102
Swords, RAF   55

Team-60, Royal Swedish Air Force   101
Telstars, RAAF   9, 10
T'Gallant'ls, US Navy   124
Three Flying Fish, US Navy   124
Three Sea Hawks, US Navy   122
Thunderbirds, USAF   103
Thunderbolts, Indian Air Force   74
Thunder Tigers, Chinese National Air Force   26
Tigers, RAF   45
Tigri Bianche (White Tigers), Italian Air Force   80
Tomahawks, RAF   50
Turkish Air Force   136

United States Air Force   103
United States Navy   122
United States Army   134

Vipers, RAF   51

Westland-Bell 47G Sioux   50P, 67P, 69P
Westland Gazelle   55P, 56, 60P, 65P, 66P
Westland Lynx AH.1   70P
Westland Scout AH.1   70P
Whisky-Four, Royal Netherlands Air Force   87
White Swans, Turkish Air Force   136
Wings of Portugal, Portugese Air Force   96

Yellowhammers, RNZAF   89
Yellowjacks, RAF   49